AN INTEGRATED JOURNEY BACK TO HEALTH AND HAPPINESS

with a Focus on Recovery from Lyme Disease, Its Co-infections and Other Mysterious Illnesses

AN INTEGRATED JOURNEY BACK TO HEALTH AND HAPPINESS

with a Focus on Recovery from Lyme Disease, Its Co-infections and Other Mysterious Illnesses

Dr. Kate Wood

DISCLAIMER

This book is not intended as medical advice or substitute advice from a medical or health practitioner, and it is also not intended to prevent, diagnose, treat or cure disease. The book has been compiled to present the informal experiences and opinion of the author and should not be considered as any more important or valid than any other informal information or conversation you may have.

The information, protocols and treatments described in this book may have side effects and create unknown health risks. Please consult with your primary health care practitioner before beginning or implementing any of the information included in this book. Do not change or stop any recommended treatment protocols without the advice of your primary health care provider and/or therapist.

Lyme disease is a controversial topic. At this time, there are some doctors and government officials who claim that Lyme disease does not even exist in Australia. This book has not been evaluated by any such parties, and use of the information is at your own risk.

To my amazing husband, Nick Wood, who has given me the three greatest gifts I could ever ask for—unconditional love, the will to live and our beautiful son, Maxim

Table of Contents

CHAPTER 3 – DETOXIFICATION AND METHYLATION: IMPORTANCE & INFLUENCES

CHAPTER 4 – DIAGNOSIS OF LYME DISEASE

CHAPTER 6 – PHYSICAL TREATMENT

CHAPTER 8 – EMOTIONAL TREATMENT AND STRATEGIES

CHAPTER 9 – SPIRITUAL STRATEGIES

CHAPTER 10 – OTHER HANDY DIAGNOSES AND TREATMENT TIPS & TRICKS

CHAPTER 11 – TRAVEL TIPS

CHAPTER 12 – PETS AND LYME DISEASE

Dedication

My husband, Nick – I married him for a reason, but never did I realise the strength and support I would need from him so soon after being married. You know you have found your soul mate when they give up 18 months of their life for you. He had to stop working for four months just to look after me, he barely saw his friends, rarely rode his beloved bike, and not once did he ever complain or make me feel guilty. He was a source of inspiration when I could no longer help myself. He never gave up on me, even when I told him to. He stayed up with me all through the night when I couldn't breathe or sleep. He held my hand and patted my head when I couldn't stop crying for days on end. He carried me up our hill to take me to the beach when I didn't have the strength to get there myself. He adjusted me chiropractically and did kinesiology work on me every day, and sometimes more than once a day. He took on my jobs within the business, he cooked, he cleaned and at times, he even had to wash and dress me. From the bottom of my heart, I thank you. I couldn't have asked for a better husband, best friend, soulmate, business partner, and now, father to our beautiful baby boy, Maxim. I love you.

My son, Maxim – The thought of never experiencing motherhood and depriving my amazing husband (your 'dadda') of fatherhood was a driving factor in my recovery. I dreamed of you long before you were conceived and visualising being a mum was all that kept me going some days. My true purpose was fulfilled the day you were conceived. Being sick not just taught me life lessons that I hope will make me a better mother but also prepared me for sleepless nights. No fatigue will ever compare to the fatigue I experienced when I was ill and I think that is why I have transitioned to motherhood so easily. You are my world. Never have I understood a love this deep.

You make me happy beyond belief. You have taught me more life lessons in your first 6 months of life than in my previous 34 years. You ground me, help me to live in the moment and I appreciate every second I have with you. I am beyond grateful to have you in my life. I consider you the miracle child, not just because I didn't know if I would ever be granted this amazing gift of motherhood, but because every day in every way you show me the magic of life and love. My health journey has motivated me to share my story and knowledge with the world and in doing so I promise to teach and inspire you to optimal health. Hopefully you will never have to go through what I did and can have the life of your dreams (and mine!).

My Dogs – No matter whether I was happy, sad, sick, at home or out, Megsie and Alfie were always there for me. They are the only ones who saw every step of my journey and, literally, never left my side. Dogs teach you what true, unconditional love is; it's never angry or upset or frustrated. I never ever felt alone due to their presence, and they had this uncanny way of making me smile even through the pain and suffering. Megsie could always make me laugh with her jutting out teeth and weird breathing noises. Alfie is such a sensitive soul and would put his paw on my hand whenever I would cry to let me know he was there protecting me. One of the saddest days of my life was the 12th of March, 2014, when Megsie tragically lost her life in a hit-and-run car accident. It was the day I realised I had more strength than I knew, as not even the pain and trauma of losing my baby and my best friend could set back my health. Although I know Megsie will always be with me and guiding me, it was hard to let go of someone who had been so instrumental in my healing journey. I truly believe someone else needed her love and guidance more than I did, and I hope they realise just how lucky they are. I couldn't imagine my life without my dogs and am so lucky to still have Alfie by my side, loving and protecting me unconditionally.

My Family – My family has always been there for me whenever I needed them, and this time was no different. Although my immediate family doesn't live in Sydney, they were never far from my thoughts. Mum and Dad did many trips to visit, and my sisters called and texted me during every spare moment they had. My parents were a huge emotional support but also provided much needed financial support that allowed us to travel to Germany for treatment without having to sell our beloved waterfront property.

My sister Lauren kept my humour alive with stories and pictures of her gorgeous children who would often call me to tell me, "We love you, Aunty Kate." I know you can't choose your family, but even if I could, I wouldn't change a thing. I love you all.

The Health Space Team – *There is no way Nick and I could have had the amount of time off work and not gone bankrupt without the amazing support from the Health Space team. Not only did they really step up and take on the running of the clinics as if they were their own, but they gave us countless free treatments to help in our healing process. Special mention to the practitioners who helped me with regular treatments - Maggie Godin, John Holmes, Jacqui Johnson, Martyna Fedyk, Jarad Bianchi and Taylor Harrison. Thank you all for your integrity, loyalty and love.*

Dr. Kate Norris– *My doctor, Kate Norris, was an absolute angel (and still is). There is no way I would have even thought to go down the road of investigating Lyme disease without her. She left no stone unturned. It was her passion and thoroughness that helped me get my diagnosis of Lyme disease, and I was finally able to treat the disease that had been plaguing me for 17 years. Never once did she say it was in my head. She was always so loving and supportive and even squeezed me in when I was having bad days and just had to see her. She went above and beyond what I could ever ask for in a doctor. She restored my faith in the medical system. Thank you.*

Jen May– *I don't deal well with being sick. I am also not someone who is very good at asking for help. Jen was there for me in the early stages before I was diagnosed and right through the entire process. Not once did I ever ask for help, but somehow she knew I needed it. Although she was super busy with her gorgeous new baby, Tyler, she still managed to visit me every week without fail and would call and text me on the other days. She never judged me, and she never gave up on me, even when I didn't have the energy to return her calls. She treated me like a normal person and shared the ups and downs in her life, which was so precious, as it took me out of my "poor me" state and gave me the energy to help her and give her advice. This was really healing in itself. She was so positive and always gave me really practical advice. I always felt so happy when Jen was around, and I can honestly say that when I hit rock bottom, it was her, with help from Nick,* *that dragged me up. Jen, I will never forget what you have done for me and am here for you whenever you need me.*

Close Friends – *You really learn who your true friends are when you are sick. Funny enough, it's not always who you expect it to be. My best friend, Lizzie Gale, is always on my doorstep with only a moment's notice. Kate Barbat was always thinking about me, buying me fruit boxes and cooking organic soups for me when I could stomach nothing else. She was just so thoughtful. I met Skye Prendergast and Barbara Zarounas as clients, and they will be lifelong friends because of their regular visits all the way up to Sydney's Northern Beaches and their continuous support. Nadine Webber came and looked after Maxim for a few hours a week while I finished editing this book. Kristin Wakelin, Laura Newall, Maggie Godin, Taylor Harrison and Amy Houlton were always checking in on me and making me feel loved and supported. Thank you to all my friends who were there for me.*

Kuve Bradley, Mark Padd and Kevin Millet – *Thank you Kuve for the weekly Reiki and clearing sessions, Mark for the weekly Rife treatments and Kevin for the daily (sometimes multiple times a day) TBM kinesiology sessions for over a month when you were in Australia. You all gave me hours of your time and were such positive spiritual supports. You must have saved me tens of thousands of dollars by providing me with free treatments. You are all true angels. Kevin, the knowledge you have shared with me over the years has not only helped me but also all the clients I treat, and now it will hopefully help the people who read this book. Thank you.*

Kelly Galvin – *A huge thank you goes to my naturopath, Kelly, who is so much more than a naturopath. She knows more about the body than most doctors and has a unique and intuitive gift to guide and heal from the soul outwards. You spent countless hours going over my millions of blood and other tests and put them into tables that I could understand and make sense of. Your recommendations and functional testing referrals proved invaluable in my healing process. Without your guidance, homeopathy and Bach flower remedies, I honestly don't think I would have made it through the emotional trauma while I was sick and the emotional aftermath that followed during my physical healing post-Germany.*

My Publishing, Editing and Proofreading Team– Firstly, a big thank you to Bryan Rosner of Biomed Publishing who gave me the confidence and opportunity to publish this book. My editor, Kim Junker – although we have never met face-to-face, you have been absolutely amazing at keeping me on track and making sure everything read well and was referenced correctly (which was no mean feat!).The gorgeous people who helped me to proofread – Bonnie Stedman, Kylie DeRouw, Stephanie Brindal, Debbie Miller, Greg Schreeuwer, Lara Coleman, Petra Behuliak and my mum. Thank you for your time and love.

A Health Guide

This book was written as a handbook for you to arm yourself with the latest information, options, ideas and supports. With this knowledge, I hope you're empowered to take healing into your own hands. It is to share with your family, friends and health practitioners so they are able to help you in the very best way they can. Multifactorial health conditions require multifactorial treatment plans that cater for individual variations. For this reason I have tried to add as many options as I can, understanding that, unfortunately, no one treatment program is the magic bullet for us all. I have tried to add as many references and research support as possible, so you don't have to just take my word for it but can explore and understand the information yourself. Some of the information will be familiar to you. I have tried to break down the more complex concepts into usable information, but having said that, some of it is still quite complex, even to me! Take your time with it, and remember that each little gem has the potential to get you one step closer to optimal health.

My Story

I was never sick or injured as a child. From the age of 10, I was the Australian 800m track champion and was undefeated for many years. I left our rural property in the northwest of New South Wales (NSW) and went to boarding school when I was 13. While I continued to train and race, I put running on the back burner while I competed in other team sports at the state and national level.

I can now say that in 1996 my life changed forever. I went on a school camp in northwest NSW for seven days. Eight days after I returned, I realised that the itchy lump on my back was neither a mole nor a pimple; it was a tick. The school nurse removed it, and I thought nothing more of it. I'm pretty sure I didn't get the characteristic erythema migrans (EM) rash that looks like a bullseye and indicates with 100% certainty that you have contracted Lyme disease, but not long after I had my first proper flu. My glands became sore and swollen and I became extremely fatigued. Tests showed that I had glandular fever and very low iron stores. I was prescribed an iron supplement and rest was ordered until I recovered.

I had qualified for an international athletic tour of the US later that year and didn't want to stop training, as I was really looking forward to traveling and competing again. I had a few weeks off and did the best I could with my training leading up to the trip. I ran well considering my lack of preparation and picked up a few medals but came back exhausted. At least I had the rest of the year off to recover.

I will never know if it was that tick in NSW that gave me Lyme disease or even if I picked up something while competing in the US. Either way, my health issues began with that tick bite. If only my doctors or I had known to test for Lyme disease back then, how different my life might have been. Having said that, I have no regrets. I have learned many valuable life lessons and have had many wonderful things come out of my Lyme disease journey.

I continued to train and compete but never at the same level as I had before the glandular fever diagnosis. The right gland in my neck never went down, and I often had a sore throat, dry cough and lost my voice. I would become easily fatigued, had headaches for the first time in my life and developed this weird rash on my hands and feet, that I was told was a fungal infection. Doctors said it was because I had gone through puberty and my body was different. As a teenager, it sounded logical to me.

At the end of 1997, I convinced my parents to let me leave boarding school and return home to train with my coach, Mr. Manning, while completing my year 11 and 12 studies at the local high school and via correspondence. I was so excited to have the opportunity to train like I used to and regain my national title, but it didn't go to plan. Even though I put hours of extra training and stretching in, fine-tuned my diet, started visualising and did more than I had ever done to get my health and fitness back, something just wasn't quite right. It wasn't coming as easily as it had before. I was getting niggling injuries and often felt rundown and fluey. I blamed it on hormones and puberty, because now I was carrying a little more weight than I used to as a young girl.

I was picked for the 1998 Australia Oceania under-21 team and traveled to Tonga to compete. Although I came home with three silver medals, I was quietly disappointed, as the times I was running were equivalent to times I ran when I was 13 (and I was 17 at the time). After that trip my health declined and I started getting really bad cramping and stabbing pains in my calves. The more I ran, the worse the pain and cramping became. One day I was racing school cross country and my legs gave way on me; I couldn't stand up or feel my feet. I had a stack of tests done which indicated that my iron levels were dangerously low and that I was extremely deficient in magnesium and potassium. I started supplementing with both iron and magnesium, and also ate three or four bananas a day as the doctor had instructed, but the pain persisted. I had been taking iron on-and-off for a couple of years, so some questions were raised as to why my iron stores were still so low. I missed winning the national 800m final that year by one-hundredth of a second and realised it had to be more than just a nutritional deficiency.

My mum and I traveled to Sydney during the school holidays to see all the top sports doctors, and it was then that I was diagnosed with compartment syndrome (where the fascia doesn't expand as the muscle does during exercise, limiting blood flow in and waste products out). The options were either surgery to slit the fascia or six months with no running and limited walking to see if the fascia would recover naturally. I chose the latter, throwing myself into weekly physiotherapy and acupuncture, and daily deep tissue massage and stretching to try to stretch the fascia. This meant driving to Dubbo (3 hour round trip), once or twice a week for treatment, which my taxi driver mum did without the blink of an eye.

In April 1999 I did my first walk / jog session and slowly began to train again. My calves felt fine, but I just couldn't get fit. I could barely run the 2 km warm-up (even as a 10-year-old, I used to run 8-10 km with my eyes closed, and here I was nearly 18 barely able to jog 2km), and the more I trained, the more unfit I felt. I kept telling myself it was because I hadn't exercised for six months and my body was just really unfit. Then I started getting headaches, heart palpitations and severe chest pain. My short-term memory was affected, which really impacted my study for my Higher School Certificate (HSC), because by that time I was in my final year of school.

I felt sick, my glands were swollen and inflamed, I had a dry cough that wouldn't shift, and I'd often have a sore throat and lose my voice. I could barely get out of bed some days, let alone run. My mum took me to the local doctor who did an ECG. The result? The strongest, healthiest heart he had ever seen. My mum then took me to a cardiologist who gave me every test under the sun including an exercise ECG, angiogram and ultrasound. Everything was normal.

After multiple exams and tests by a plethora of doctors around the state, including a SPECT scan of my brain (by this stage, I was having excruciating headaches daily), many of the doctors I had seen decided that it was all in my head, and I should be prescribed antidepressants. My parents and I were exhausted and were still none the wiser as to what was wrong with me. Even I began to wonder if it was all in my head. My poor parents were beside themselves and thought that maybe I should try to take the antidepressants to see if that helped. I had rarely even taken basic over-the-counter pain medications except for Panadol®, so I wasn't about to start taking some psychotropic drug; deep down I knew it wasn't in my head.

Besides my parents, I was lucky that at least one other person truly believed I wasn't faking it or creating it in my head, and that was my coach, Mr. Manning. He found a biochemist and suggested that my mum take me to see him. By this stage I was sleeping up to 18 hours a day and was starting to get seriously depressed. I wondered if I would ever be well again. I felt helpless and hopeless and would often cry myself to sleep with my head under my pillow so as not to worry anyone.

The biochemist in Rutherford believed that I had picked up a parasite in Tonga because I had been much sicker after returning from there. He said my liver had a fatty buildup (possibly affected by the glandular fever) and that my ATP levels were affecting my energy levels (ATP stands for adenosine triphosphate, the biochemical way the body stores and uses energy for every cell in the body including your muscles). As a biochemist, he made all of his own supplements and medications, so to this day I still don't know what he prescribed, but it worked! Initially, I became really sick and had a huge rash all over my body. He said it was my liver detoxing and that I needed to have lots of water and veggie juices to support the detox pathway. Within eight days, the rash died down and my head cleared a little. Over the next few months, I went from strength to strength and had enough energy to return to school for the entire day and do some social activities. My right gland never went down and to this day, if it gets sore, it is a warning for me to slow down. My short-term memory has also never been the same, but I learned ways around it by writing things down and getting good at using diaries and reminders.

Note: The biochemist who helped me is now in jail for fraud because he claimed that he could cure cancer and one of his patients died. Although I'm sure his claims were not communicated well at his trial, I know his intentions were sound, and I truly believe that he saved my life at the time.

In 1998 I finished my final exams and slowly started back into my athletic training. I received a scholarship from the Australian College of Physical Education at Homebush Bay to study Sports Science and moved to Sydney in early 2000 to pursue my beloved athletic career while also getting an education. Over the next few years, I worked my way back and was ranked #3 in Australia in the 800m event, but my body was never the same. I had many injuries that kept setting me back. I would often get sick in my easy training week and I would always struggle to run well if I had to travel. I had blood tests every 4 to 6 weeks to monitor my low iron levels, and I also had many other tests, such as stool tests, gastroscopes, a colonoscopy and other blood tests, to determine why my body was either losing iron or not absorbing it. Once again, many doctors were involved and no one could work it out, so they decided low iron was "normal" for me!

In 2006 I broke the navicular bone in my foot in a race after a stress fracture was misdiagnosed. I was absolutely devastated, as I was in contention to earn a spot on the Melbourne Commonwealth Games' Team. I was told I would never run again if I didn't have an operation to put a screw in the bone. Whether I had the operation or not, I wasn't going to recover in time for the Commonwealth Games, so once again I opted for the natural route. That meant having my foot in a cast and then a boot for three months, followed by another three months of daily rehabilitation.

By this time I had graduated from Sports Science from ACPE and was studying chiropractic part-time. I decided to study chiropractic full-time so I could rehab my foot properly and also earn my Master's of Chiropractic, so I could always pursue an exciting career of helping others once I had finished competing. After finishing my Master's of Chiropractic, getting a job, meeting the man of my dreams and starting Health Space with my now husband, I never did go back to racing.

Fast forward to 2012... Both my husband and I were bitten by a tick in February. Once again, we didn't think anything of it after removing it. In April we did a whirlwind trip to Las Vegas and Los Angeles, and I returned feeling a little tired. Because we were planning to start a family at the end of that year, I researched and found a good holistic doctor. I thought I should get some blood tests, have my iron levels checked and make sure I was ovulating, all while doing a six-month preconception detox. I hadn't been to a doctor since I had retired from athletics in 2006, so it was time!

After what I thought would be some routine blood tests to give me the green light, my second visit to the doctor was both surprising and scary. My white cell count was dangerously low, my liver enzymes were through the roof and there was likely something seriously wrong with me. Differential diagnoses that needed to be ruled out included cancer, leukaemia, Lyme disease and HIV, to name a few. From the start, my doctor, Dr. Kate Norris, thought that I had Lyme disease, and it was really only because she was so thorough and dedicated that I was diagnosed with Lyme five months later.

At first I was in denial. I had researched medical sites but the symptoms and diagnosis didn't exactly fit. As more tests came back positive, such as Mycoplasma pneumonia (which explained all the sore throat and dry cough symptoms I had had over the years), EBV (Epstein-Barr virus, which causes glandular fever), HSV1 (herpes simplex virus), a strong case was building up. All the Australian testing came back negative for Lyme disease, so I thought I was in the clear and went on a holiday to Europe for the month of July. While I was traveling, I realised something was really wrong. I was so fatigued that I had to have a sleep every day, my hair was falling out, any scratch or sore I had would take ages to stop bleeding and heal, I became extremely constipated and I had all these sores on my skin that just wouldn't heal. Once I arrived back home, I met with Dr. Norris. She convinced me to get a western blot test for Borrelia, which was sent to IgeneX Labs in California to test for Lyme disease. Five weeks later the results came back. They were positive for Lyme disease.

I struggled to come to terms with the treatment recommended: three different types of antibiotics at very high doses, indefinitely. I reached out to many doctors, friends and health professionals for advice and came to the conclusion that if I didn't do the antibiotic regime along with all the natural options, I wouldn't get better. Once I made my decision I never looked back, and I have no regrets. I was committed to everything I put my mind to and had in my head that I would be better in 3 to 6 months maximum. I convinced myself that in the scheme of things, it wasn't such a long time, especially because I had been sick on-and-off since I was 16!

I cut all dairy, gluten, caffeine, processed foods and sugar from my diet, bought all certified organic produce, made sure all my home products (cleaning, cosmetics, etc.) were all certified organic and stopped aerobic exercise so I could give my adrenals a rest and allow my white cells a chance to recover. I took all the supplements that were recommended, started meditating every day and committed to treatments such as Rife, acupuncture, Reiki, kinesiology, lymphatic massage and, of course, chiropractic. Sometimes I would drive hours each day just to get these treatments. I was blessed to have so many colleagues, friends and clients to help me, and it was rare that I paid for a treatment, for which I was extremely grateful.

Six months later I was so much worse. I was blacking out, extremely fatigued, had severe headaches and jaw pain, my eyesight had diminished to a blur, my hearing was super sensitive (to the point that even the hum of a dryer could drive me crazy), I had a rash all over my fingers and toes that would burn like my hands were being held in a fire, and my short-term memory and brain fog were so bad that I couldn't remember a simple word like *honey* or even my close friends' last names. I was stressed and depressed and began to give up hope of ever getting better.

I had a consultation with Dr. Nicola McFadzean who recommended that I focus on the treatment for Babesia, as she believed that I had 90%+ of the symptoms. I also started looking into other treatment options and came across a clinic in Bali, which I had decided I wanted to go to. Then a friend of a friend suggested Germany, as there was a well-established clinic in Bad Aibling that was getting great results with Lyme disease patients. I spoke to both clinics and realised that I needed to detox before I could do either program. The next day I woke up and decided that I had given antibiotics a good go and was done. That was it—no more antibiotics as of March 2013! The other thing that made a huge difference was getting a root canal tooth removed, as I believed it was harbouring infection.

I chose to go to the St. Georg Klinik (SGK) in Bad Aibling, Germany. In hindsight, I wished I had gone as soon as I was diagnosed. I truly believe that this is what helped me turn the corner to full health again. There is more information about this clinic later in this book and on our Health Space website: www.healthspaceclinics.com.au/service/lyme-disease-consulting.

While writing the end section of this book, I received the all-clear from my doctor that not only was I physically better, but all my blood tests and functional tests were in the normal range. This was an 11-month journey post-Germany. After I left the German clinic, I worked very closely with Dr. Kate Norris and my naturopath, Kelly Galvin, doing in-depth functional and gene testing, and using nutritional changes and supplements to ensure every system of my body was functioning optimally.

The most exciting news came in May 2014. My husband and I decided to start trying for the family we had longed for, and I fell pregnant on the very first try! Not only that, but the pregnancy was a breeze—no nausea, no sickness and not even a hint of tiredness. All I can say is that my healthy pregnancy was a great sign that my body was functioning optimally.

On February 17th at 7:19am, my life changed forever with the birth of our son, Maxim Cruz McMaster Wood. It was not the serene home water birth we had planned, but the end result was the same—a beautiful, healthy baby boy. All the heartache and suffering from Lyme disease (and labour!) were worth it to have this beautiful little miracle in my arms. The baby I had longed for and at many times in my life thought may never happen was finally here. He is such a miracle, and every single day I am grateful to have him ground me and make me fully understand the beauty of life. I am so thankful that I didn't give up on life when it would have been so easy to.

I tell you my story not because it is so different from many other Lyme disease sufferers, but because I want to inspire you to listen to your heart and know that there is life after Lyme disease. It is my hope that I can be the one person who makes a difference for you by providing up-to-date and specific information about Lyme disease and its treatment options, so you can get back to being the best version of yourself, just like I am. Take it one step at a time, and remember that you are never alone.

All the different treatments I did are outlined in detail in this book, including details about the SGK in Germany.

Chapter 1 –
Introduction

WELCOME TO THE CRAZY WORLD OF LYME DISEASE

Anyone who has Lyme disease or knows someone who has Lyme disease (Borreliosis) will probably already understand, or at least they will have heard about the complexity of this disease.

The main bacterium responsible for Lyme disease is Borrelia burgdorferi (Bb, as I will refer to it from now on), and it is transmitted mostly by ticks. There is now emerging research that transmission may also occur via other vectors, such as mosquitoes, lice, fleas and mites, through sexual intercourse and via the placenta to unborn babies. Blood transfusions are also another likely transmission route, especially because Lyme disease is believed to be under-diagnosed, especially in Australia.

Borrelia is a type of bacteria that can affect the whole body. It is initially in the blood but can move to the muscles and joints, and even cross the blood-brain barrier and the placenta. With Bb comes a host of co-infections, such as Bartonella, Babesia, Rickettsia and Ehrlichia, and opportunistic infections such as mycoplasmas, Chlamydia pneumoniae, Epstein-Barr virus, human herpes virus 6 (HHV-6) and human cytomegalovirus (HCMV). These are just a few microbes that might complicate the picture.

1

Bb can escape most antibiotic treatments and can morph into various forms, including the spirochete and cell wall-deficient (L-form) forms, and a cyst form that can hibernate for many years at a time. The various stages of Lyme disease depend on how long you have had it and include acute, early and late disseminated, and chronic.

Whether this sounds familiar or not, it still sounds depressing, right? You hear stories of people who are debilitated, dying or have died.

My book is not written as a commercial venture. When I recovered, I wanted to document what I had experienced and what I found helpful to hopefully make it easier for people who are suffering and want to learn about the possible causes and treatments available. It is to help you, your family and your health support team with information about treatments and tools available to help you on your healing journey. With this book, I hope to inspire you to look beyond the disease and trust in your body's power to heal itself. If you honour your body and understand that illness is not bad luck or even bad genes, you will feel empowered to get back your most cherished possession...... optimal health.

There are many great books and websites that explain what Lyme disease is, how it's contracted, all the stages and the various treatment options (find these in Appendix A: Recommended Reading List). I highly recommend that you research the literature of all the professionals so that you have a really good understanding of Lyme disease, the theories about it, how it spreads, the co-infections and the various treatment options. Be careful to distinguish between textbook diagnoses and treatment options, and Lyme-literate recommendations.

This book will not only help you become Lyme-savvy so that you know the difference between Lyme disease, its co-infections and other ailments, but it will also provide you with the tools and resources to hopefully beat it. At the end of the day, it doesn't really matter how, when or why you contracted it. What matters is that you have it, and you can heal your body if you want to. You have the control, so don't forget that like I did when I started on my Lyme journey. I was so caught up in thinking and talking about Lyme disease that I lost track of the task at hand: to strengthen my body so the Bb bacteria and its co-infections could no longer survive there.

You can get your body healthy again physically, biochemically, emotionally and spiritually, so there is no way any disease (Lyme or anything else bad) can possibly reside in your body long-term or even short-term. It is my belief that the experiences I share in this book can put the pieces of the puzzle together for you so that you can do what you were born to do in this life—shine, thrive and share your gifts with the world. Sometimes we just need a bit of help to get there!

"Even muddy water, let stand, becomes clear."

Lao Tzu

LYME DISEASE IN AUSTRALIA AND BEYOND

At the time of writing this book, the Australian government still does not recognise Lyme disease in Australia, despite its prediction as the biggest epidemic of the 21st Century.

The Karl McManus Foundation, the Lyme Disease Association of Australia (LDAA), Lyme-literate practitioners led by Dr. Peter Mayne (who started the group ACIDS [Australian Chronic Infectious Disease Society]), and many other passionate people are working hard to change this. ACIDS is a group of savvy doctors and other health professionals whose aim is to develop Lyme disease treatment guidelines, educate the public and mentor other health professionals to help as many people as possible who have or may have Lyme disease.

Lyme disease is complex to diagnose and treat, in part I believe, due to ignorance. My colleagues and I have worked with many patients who have never left Australia yet have confirmed lab results and clinical diagnoses for Lyme disease and its co-infections. Anyone who has been afflicted by Lyme disease in any way knows it exists in Australia.

A 2011 study by Peter Mayne (Mayne 2011) strongly supports the contention that Lyme disease is a neurological disease transmitted in Australia, despite the government's claims that it is not transmitted in Australia. There are certain places in Australia known as tick hotspots, particularly in the coastal areas of NSW, including Mid North Coast (from Forster up to Coffs Harbour), the South Coast and Sydney's Northern Beaches. The Lyme Disease Association of Australia (LDAA) is working to identify areas where known tick bites have led to Lyme disease in order to record epidemic areas relative to Australians.

Ticks have been found on every continent except Antarctica (though they have been found on birds in Antarctica!). The first official case of Lyme was recorded in 1975 in Old Lyme, Connecticut (a town in the US), although there are many other reports and evidence that it existed long before that in many regions of the world. Today, South America (especially in Brazil), much of Europe (especially Russia), Germany, Bali, and almost every part of the United States and Asia are affected. Although it's yet to be recognised in Australia, diagnosed cases are popping up all over Australia. The treatment is costly, as is the effect it has on your health and your life.

Chapter 2 –
Getting Savvy
With Lyme Disease

WHAT IS LYME DISEASE?

Lyme disease is caused by a spiral-shaped spirochete bacterium called Borrelia burgdorferi (Bb), typically from an infected tick bite. There are varying opinions about how long the tick must be attached before it can transmit the bacteria, ranging from 4 to 36 or more hours. Tick saliva, which contains substances that disrupt the immune response at the site of the bite, accompanies the spirochete into the skin during the feeding process. This allows an often unnoticeable protective environment to be set up, enabling the spirochete to establish the infection in a stealth-like mode.

Here, the spirochetes multiply and migrate outward within the dermis (outer layer) of the skin, which is often what creates the characteristic erythema migrans (EM, or bullseye) rash. For some reason, neutrophils (a type of white blood cell that is essential for innate immune system healing) fail to appear in the developing EM rash. Neutrophils are essential in eliminating the bacterial invasion. In their absence, the Bb are able to survive and spread throughout the body, often undetected.

Days or weeks after Bb transmission, the spirochetes spread via the bloodstream to the joints, heart, nervous system and distant skin sites, which may give rise to the symptoms of the disseminated stages of the disease. If left untreated, the bacteria may persist in the body for months and even years, despite the production of antibodies by the immune system. The spirochetes may avoid detection and/or elimination by the immune response in many ways, including decreasing their expression of surface proteins that are targeted by antibodies, deactivating key immune components, or changing their form to either the L-shaped or cyst form that can either resemble normal bodily tissues or hide in the extracellular matrix.

It is also believed that if under threat from an antibiotic, antimicrobial or immune response, the cyst form can clump together and form clusters protected by a biofilm that is very hard to break down or penetrate. Diagnosis of late stage, chronic Lyme disease is often complicated by multifactorial, non-specific symptoms, which is why it is known as "the great imitator." Lyme disease is often misdiagnosed as MS (multiple sclerosis), Parkinson's disease, rheumatoid arthritis, chronic fatigue syndrome, lupus, fibromyalgia, Motor Neurone Disease, Crohn's disease, Alzheimer's or other autoimmune and neurodegenerative diseases.

WHAT ARE TICKS AND HOW DO THEY INFECT US?

Ticks are ectoparasites (external parasites) that live on the blood of mammals, birds and sometimes reptiles and amphibians. They are the vectors of several diseases including Lyme disease. They tend to live and hibernate in wooded, forested and long-grassed areas throughout the world. Ticks feed and then hibernate, which is why they may seem more abundant at certain times of the year. They feed using their cutting mandibles, which cut the skin in order to insert a feeding tube into your bloodstream. They also insert a small amount of anesthetic in the process, which is why most people don't know that it's happening. Unlike a mosquito bite, even after the tick has had its fill and dropped off its host, you often won't feel a thing! So, unless you actually see it or happen to get the classic bullseye EM rash, you will be none the wiser to its visit! Remember that ticks need direct contact with your skin to latch on.

Generally, ticks carry diseases in their gut. There is debate as to how long a tick needs to be attached before it can infect you, but information on the Lyme Disease Association of Australia website suggests that most ticks infect people in the nymphal, or immature stage of development, when they are the size of a poppy seed. This is another reason why many people don't see or remember being bitten; ticks at this stage of growth are so small that they are easy to miss.

For further information on the prevention of tick bites and removal techniques, skip forward to the start of the Prevention Is the Best Treatment section in Chapter 5.

"Turn your wounds into wisdom."

Oprah Winfrey

TRANSMISSION OF LYME DISEASE

The most common mode of transmission for Lyme disease is via a tick. While there is much debate as to other transmission modes, there is no doubt that ticks can and do carry bacteria that have the potential to cause Lyme disease as well as countless other co-infections.

Other possible modes of transmission include:

❖   Other vectors such as mosquitoes, lice, fleas and mites

❖   Sexual intercourse (in the bodily fluids)

❖   In utero via the placenta to unborn babies

❖   Blood transfusions (if blood is taken from an infected person)

Up to a point, I agree with the theory that many doctors have, including Dr. Horowitz, that if it were sexually transmitted, it would be a much bigger problem than it already is. It will be interesting to see what research emerges, because we know that Bb can make its way into seminal and vaginal fluids, as these fluids can and have tested positive for Bb in many people.

However, the question is, how much sexual exposure would someone need to have to contract it? It seems reasonable that a couple who have regular, unprotected sex have a greater chance of sexually transmitting the disease, not just due to sexual transmission, but due to an increased load being transmitted over time.

Once again there are many things to take into consideration, such as the immune capabilities of the partner, how much Bb is contained in any one fluid sample and how often they have sexual intercourse. Only time will tell, but my opinion is that if you have a partner diagnosed with Lyme disease, then safe sex is best and treating both partners is essential!

COMMON LYME MYTHS

Myth: Lyme-infected ticks don't live in Australia.

Truth: There is a growing body of evidence that disproves this theory (although at the time of writing this book, the government still does not recognise Lyme disease in Australia). Ticks have now been found on every continent in the world. There are many cases of people who have been diagnosed with Lyme disease in Australia who have never left the country. The truth is, we know it exists here, so it's time to get proactive and educate our fellow Aussies as well as the world. I have personally removed a tick (and I had not travelled for more than two years, so I was definitely bitten in Australia) and had both the tick and bite site biopsied and found positive for Borrelia.

Myth: You can't contract Lyme disease from a tick bite in winter.

Truth: Ticks can live for up to two years, depending on the breed, and can survive very cold climates. Although it's much less likely to get bitten by a tick during the winter while you're inside and sheltered from the cold, it is still possible.

Myth: You only have to worry about contracting Lyme disease if you get an EM (bullseye) rash after a tick bite.

Truth: Only 15-50% of people (depending on what research you read) will develop the EM rash. Also, many people who don't get a rash have been diagnosed with Lyme disease (including me), so using the EM rash alone as a diagnostic tool is not recommended.

Myth: There is no point treating chronic Lyme disease, as people don't get much better anyway.

Truth: The sooner you treat Lyme disease, the quicker the recovery will usually be. Having said that, many people recover fully from chronic Lyme disease; it just takes longer and you may have to address more aspects of your health to get there. The better your genetics and lifestyle are, the better your chances of a full recovery. Unfortunately, in Australia, I don't believe we always have the tools and the treatments required to beat chronic Lyme disease. Hopefully that will change soon.

Myth: If you test negative for Lyme disease on labs, then you don't have Lyme disease.

Truth: Not necessarily. At this stage there is no lab test that can provide 100% accurate results. The testing still has false negatives and positives. Diagnosis via labs is only one part of the diagnosis; the history and the clinical symptoms will give the full picture. Labs are handy to give people more certainty, but the existence of positive co-infections with a Lyme-like clinical picture and history of a tick bite is enough for a diagnosis.

Myth: If the person with Lyme disease doesn't look sick, then it's possible that they don't have Lyme disease

Truth: This couldn't be further from the truth. Everyone with Lyme is affected differently and goes through different symptoms at different times. One of the most ignorant things that people say to chronic Lyme sufferers is, "You look fine to me." Many of the symptoms, such as fatigue and neurological deficits, may not change the outward appearance of the Lyme sufferer. Remember, too, that when the person is at their sickest and in bed, people don't tend to see them. Some people who are severely affected may lose or gain significant amounts of weight or even become wheelchair-bound, and in these cases, people tend to be taken more seriously.

Myth: There is a gold standard for testing for Lyme disease.

Truth: At this stage, there is no universally accepted method for testing accurately for Lyme disease. There is still debate as to which labs are the best, and this changes constantly. Borrelia is known for its antigenic shifting, so antibody testing isn't always accurate. PCR tests are available for certain tissues and fluids. While PCR testing is very accurate, a negative PCR doesn't mean you don't have Lyme disease; it just means that there was no evidence of Borrelia in that specific sample. There is more information about the different testing modalities in the Diagnosis chapter.

STAGES OF LYME DISEASE

From a Lyme-literate viewpoint, there are various stages to Lyme disease. Some experts use three categories and some use four (I have included four). When you are reading the literature, you need to be aware what each stage represents, as the symptoms, treatment options, and healing time will all be affected depending on the duration of the infection and how many complicating factors are present.

Early Localised: begins the days to weeks after transmission of Bb, before the infection has become widespread in the body. This is the time that symptoms, such as the EM rash, will be seen. Only 15–50% of people get this rash depending on who you talk to and what research you read. Flu-like symptoms, fever, muscle soreness, general malaise and headaches may set in. Please note that some people may be totally asymptomatic.

Early Disseminated: occurs weeks to months, but less than one year after the transmission of Bb bacteria, as the infection begins to spread throughout the body. This stage is usually marked with a change in symptoms and severity of symptoms as the infection invades and becomes more systemic. Symptoms may include the expansion of skin rashes; joint problems, such as swelling, redness and/or pain; early nervous system issues such as pain and weakness, especially in the arms and/or legs and face; muscle pain, especially in the large joints such as the knees; and occasionally heart issues, usually palpitations, arrhythmia, or slowing of the heartbeat that can cause dizziness. Pain and symptoms are often migratory.

Late Disseminated: symptoms present more than one year after the initial transmission of the Bb infection (if known), which has had time to spread throughout the body. These patients are usually quite ill and often immune suppressed. Joint problems can resemble or even become arthritic. Late nervous system issues include pain, weakness, numbness, headaches, migraines, memory loss, brain fog, loss of short-term memory and stiff neck. Patients can experience emotional instability such as anxiety and depression; heart issues, including tachycardia, arrhythmia, palpitations and heart pain; and speech and movement that may be impaired if severe.

Chronic (Persistent / Recurrent): an active, persistent infection of prolonged duration in which the person is significantly co-infected. Initially, they often get misdiagnosed or not diagnosed at all, so the infections have had a long time to permeate the body and weaken the immune system. They are often severely ill, chronically immune suppressed, have higher spirochete loads, issues with detoxing and methylating, and have significant amounts of opportunistic, concurrent and collateral infections. All of the symptoms outlined earlier are also likely. Plus others, such as loss of libido, hypotension, persistent fatigue, blackouts / fainting, vertigo and paresis, if severe, can be present as well.

On page 3 of Joseph Burrascano's clinical data (Burrascano 2008), he indicates that the following criteria must be present to diagnose someone with chronic Lyme disease:

1. *"Illness present for at least one year (this is approximately when immune breakdown attains clinically significant levels).*

2. *Have persistent major neurologic involvement (such as encephalitis/ encephalopathy and meningitis), or active arthritic manifestations (active synovitis).*

3. *Still have active infection with B. burgdorferi (Bb) regardless of prior antibiotic therapy, if any."*

CO-INFECTIONS

A co-infection is broadly defined as the simultaneous infection of a host by multiple pathogen species. In the case of Lyme disease, Bb is considered the primary infection, and the co-infection is any pathogen that is transmitted at the same time of Bb transmission via a single vector, namely a tick. Co-infections are often present in humans affected by Lyme disease. Over 20 different co-infections have been identified to-date, and more continue to be found. Studies compiled by Joseph Burrascano have shown that co-infections result in a more severe clinical presentation with more organ damage, and the pathogens become more difficult to eradicate. In addition, it is known that Babesia infections, like Lyme Borreliosis, increase the chance of immunosuppression.

The most common co-infections are:

Babesiosis *caused by Babesia*

Babesia is a microscopic protozoan parasite that causes a hemolytic disease, or Babesiosis, by infecting the red blood cells of the host. Once the protozoan is inside the red blood cell, it splits in half to form two new protozoa. This splitting continues until they can't fit inside the cell which causes it to burst and release them into the bloodstream to continue the process.

There are more than 100 species of Babesia, a malaria-like parasite that is also known as a piroplasm. The most common transmission in humans is via the tick bite via the species B. microti and B. divergens, although it can be contracted via blood transfusion and in utero. A study done by Dr. J Schaller in 2008 showed that 60% of Lyme sufferers also have Babesiosis. (Schaller 2008)

Bartonellosis *caused by Bartonella*

Bartonella is a genus of Gram-negative bacteria that live inside the cell of the host. Bartonella are said to be the most common co-infection of Lyme disease. Bartonella bacteria are carried by fleas, lice, ticks, and some dust mites and sand flies in certain countries. It can be passed on in utero. It can also be carried by other mammals, including cats, and can cause cat scratch disease, endocarditis and several other diseases in humans. There are also Bartonella-like organisms referred to as BLOs.

Rickettsias *caused by Rickettsia*

Rickettsia is a genus of non-motile, Gram-negative, non spore-forming, highly pleomorphic bacteria that are intracellular parasites typically invading the epithelial cells (a type of membranous tissue that line the cavities and surfaces of structures throughout the body and also form part of glands). Rickettsia, unlike most bacteria but similar to viruses, requires a living host, or living cell, to survive. There are various categories of Rickettsia that cause a variety of different diseases in different parts of the world, including conorii, rickettsii, helvetica, slovaca, and prowazekii, which all have varying symptoms. Most rickettsial pathogens are transmitted by vectors such as ticks, lice, mites and fleas, during feeding. Rodents, dogs and humans are also carriers. It is possible to contract it by being exposed to the faeces from an infected vector via open skin wounds or by inhaling dust contaminated with infected vector faeces.

Ehrlichiosis and Anaplasmosis *caused by Ehrlichia and Anaplasma phagocytophilum (rickettsial parasites)*

Ehrlichiosis is the general name used to describe several bacterial diseases that affect both humans and animals. Ehrlichia are tick-borne rickettsial parasites that infect different parts of the white blood cells of the host causing two types of Ehrlichiosis:

4. *Human Monocytic Ehrlichiosis (HME)* where the monocytes (a type of white blood cell important in the innate immune response) are infected.

5. *Human Granulocytic Ehrlichiosis (HGE)* where the granulocytes (a type of white blood cell that has secretory granules in its cytoplasm) are infected. HGE is now known as Anaplasmosis or HGA (Human Granulocytic Anaplasmosis).

There are at least three recognised species of Ehrlichia that can be transmitted via the vector of a tick to humans.

Mycoplasmas

The Mycoplasma species are smaller than usual bacteria and lack a cell wall, and therefore, can invade human cells more easily, causing disruption to the immune system. There are at least 200 known species of *mycoplasma.* Most are innocuous and do no harm and only four or five are pathogenic. The two mycoplasmas most commonly linked to Lyme disease are Mycoplasma fermentans and Mycoplasma pneumoniae. Mycoplasma fermentans is universally accepted as a tick-borne disease. There is some argument as to whether M. pneumoniae should be classified as a co-infection or an opportunistic infection, as the accepted mode of transmission is infected respiratory droplets (i.e., from coughing and sneezing the bacteria is passed through the air into the lungs). The debate continues, but I have added M. pneumoniae as an opportunistic infection at this time. The other species of Mycoplasma that are associated with Lyme disease are Mycoplasma hominis, M. genitalium and M. penetrans, which are not included in this book.

Mycoplasma Fermentans

Mycoplasma fermentans (incognitus strain) is believed to come from the nucleus of the Brucella bacterium. Therefore, it is not a bacteria or a virus. Rather, it is a mutated form of the Brucella bacterium combined with a visna virus from which the mycoplasma is extracted. Mycoplasma fermentans is not recognised as a disease or illness in itself, but the bacteria are believed to be linked to various ailments (including Gulf War Syndrome, which is very similar to chronic fatigue syndrome, fibromyalgia and rheumatoid arthritis) and has been found in necrotising lesions of organs in AIDS patients. Some species of ticks are known to carry and transmit Mycoplasma fermentans.

OPPORTUNISTIC INFECTIONS

An opportunistic infection is an infection by a microorganism that normally does not cause infection or disease but can when the body's immune system is impaired and unable to fight off infection. In the case of Lyme disease, the Bb and co-infections weaken the body's immune function, allowing a host of other infections the opportunity to invade or reactivate within the body. Essentially, any infection can become an opportunistic infection when the immune system is compromised. The following infections are opportunistic infections commonly found in Lyme disease patients. Some are contracted as the "environment" within the sick person's body makes conditions more ideal for the bacterium to infect and replicate, and other infections are reactivated from past latent, or dormant, infections.

Respiratory Infections

Mycoplasma Pneumonia Caused by Mycoplasma Pneumoniae

M. pneumoniae is a respiratory tract, Gram-positive, spindle – shaped, pleomorphic bacterium in the class Mollicutes and is pathogenic in humans. It causes atypical pneumonia and respiratory symptoms, although it is possible to have no pneumonia-like symptoms. It is principally transmitted by coming in very close contact with respiratory secretions (e.g., phlegm or large droplets from sneezing, coughing, laughing or talking) from the respiratory passage of an infected person. The infection is often mild and self–limiting unless the immune system is compromised as seen in Lyme disease patients. When the immune system is unable to suppress the Mycoplasma pneumoniae, the bacteria are able to contribute to ongoing or recurrent low-grade symptoms, and sometimes serious respiratory complications.

One of the first diagnoses I had was M. pneumoniae. I had experienced sore, scratchy throats, loss of voice and an irritating dry cough that was always attributed to exercise-induced asthma since I was 16. All these symptoms went away once M. pneumoniae was treated! The elimination of those symptoms alone made a huge difference to my health, as the dry cough would often prevent me from sleeping well.

Chlamydia Pneumonia [CPN]aka Chlamydophila Pneumoniae

C. pneumoniae, a species of chlamydia, are small Gram-negative bacteria that are airborne but not sexually transmitted. These bacteria have a complex life cycle and need to infect another cell to be able to reproduce. As its name suggests, it is one of the bacteria that can cause pneumonia. However, it usually causes a relatively mild form called walking pneumonia with mild flu-like symptoms. Just like Mycoplasma pneumonia, this respiratory illness is often mild and self-limiting unless the immune system is compromised.

Viral Infections

Herpes Viruses

There are nine herpes viruses known to have humans as their primary host. The word herpes comes from the Greek word *herpein* which means "to creep." This aptly describes what herpes viruses do—they creep in and either infect or sit patiently and often latently. Once the infection is inside the host, it may become active or inactive at any time depending on the surrounding conditions. Common symptoms include fatigue that is worse after exercise and swollen glands (especially in the neck) often accompanied by a sore throat. Blood tests may show a decreased white blood cell (WBC) count and elevated liver enzymes.

HUMAN SIMPLEX VIRUS 1 AND 2 – HSV-1 & HSV-2

HSV-1 (which produces mostly cold sores on the lips) and HSV-2 (which produces mostly genital herpes) are also part of the herpes virus family called Herpesviruses, which use humans as their host. Symptoms include blisters on the skin or mucous membranes of the lips, mouth and genitals. These can be painful, burn, tingle or itch. The virus is transmitted via contact with infected sores whilst the virus is active, although evidence suggests that a latent virus can be passed on in certain circumstances. HSV is also passed on via saliva, intercourse or oral sex. It is possible for HSV to be passed from mother to child during childbirth. However, it's highly unlikely unless she has a primary infection late in her pregnancy or a reactivation that is still active during labour. Although HSV-1 typically causes cold sores around the mouth and lips, it is becoming increasingly common for it to express as genital herpes, especially if the immune system is compromised as it often is in Lyme disease. Some people are totally asymptomatic, even during the primary infection, leading people to theorise that some people may be carriers. The virus can be reactivated by illness, eczema, emotional and physical stress, gastric upset, fatigue and menstruation. When the immune system is compromised by Lyme disease and its co-infections, it is common for reactivation of HSV to occur.

I have HSV-1 and still to this day have never had a cold sore. However, I was one of the unlucky people who had the virus activate on my genitals. Whenever I was rundown or had even the slightest emotional upset, it would flare up and sometimes be so uncomfortable that I would scream while I urinated. Often just walking would be out of the question. I used drugs like Valtrex when the pain was unbearable but found that as my immune system recovered post-Lyme disease, the outbreaks became less frequent and less severe. I later found homeopathics that were enough to control the symptoms if I felt tingles (particularly Nat Mur). I can happily say that since the severe reaction during my hyperthermia treatment in Germany, I have not had any more reactivations. It's another great sign that my immune system is working well!

EPSTEIN-BARR VIRUS (EBV) – HHV-4

The Epstein-Bar Virus is a complex virus of the herpes family (also known as human herpes virus 4 [HHV-4]) and is one of the most common viruses in humans. It is best known as the cause of the infectious mononucleosis (glandular fever) and is also implicated in Burkitt's lymphoma, Hodgkin's lymphoma, nasopharyngeal carcinoma and multiple sclerosis (MS). There is evidence suggesting that EBV is associated with a higher risk of certain autoimmune diseases such as lupus, rheumatoid arthritis, Sjogren's syndrome and MS. Transmission is via saliva (which is why it is often called the kissing disease) and genital secretions. EBV infects B cells of the immune system and epithelial cells. Once the virus's initial lytic infection is brought under control, EBV exists latently in the B cell forever. The virus will not reproduce when in a latent phase but can reactivate to lytically reproduce when the B cells are responding to other infections, as seen in Lyme and other chronic diseases.

HUMAN CYTOMEGALOVIRUS (HCMV) – HHV-5

CMV is also a part of the herpes viruses family, with the species that affects humans commonly known as HCMV (human CMV) or human herpes virus 5 (HHV-5). Although the virus may be found throughout the body, HCMV infections are synonymous with the salivary glands. HCMV typically goes under the radar in healthy people but can be life-threatening for the immunocompromised (such as chronic Lyme disease patients) and may cause complications if contracted during pregnancy by endangering the developing foetus. Transmission can be via bodily fluids such as saliva, blood, semen, vaginal secretions, breast milk and urine. Close bodily contact from coughing and sneezing are also possible routes of transmission.

Like all herpes viruses, HCMV has the ability to remain latent for long periods of time. In the vast majority of cases, HCMV will be asymptomatic, but signs and symptoms that may occur in an acute primary infection (especially in immunocompromised patients) include prolonged fever, night sweats, sore throat, swollen glands, joint pain, lack of appetite, weight loss, malaise and a general feeling of uneasiness. Signs and symptoms of a reactivated infection include fever, gastrointestinal tract (GIT) issues (especially diarrhoea), ulcerations and bleeding, shortness of breath, pneumonia with hypoxemia or low blood oxygen, mouth ulcers, problems with vision (such as blurry, floaters or blind spots), hepatitis and encephalitis which may cause behavioural changes, seizures and even coma. Sound like Lyme disease and other chronic illnesses? As you can see, these are very similar sets of symptoms. If you are not responding to treatment for Lyme disease and these are your main symptoms, I highly suggest having a blood test for CMV. A blood test can detect antibodies that form when there is an immune response to the presence of CMV, and a PCR can detect an active virus.

HUMAN HERPES VIRUS 6 (HHV-6)

HHV-6 is a collective name for HHV-6A (the more neurovirulent infection that is associated particularly with neuroinflammatory and autoimmune diseases) and HHV-6B (a common cause of the childhood disease roseola infantum). Transmission is most frequently via saliva containing the viral particles and can be reactivated in transplant patients and those who are severely immune compromised.

Once the infection is inside the cell, it may become active if the conditions are favourable, or it may become inactive. It is believed that 100% of humans have been exposed to HHV-6 by three years of age with the virus sitting in the salivary glands. Some people get the rash and high fever associated with an acute active infection and then acquire primary immunity, whilst others have no symptoms as the virus becomes inactive, hiding away in the salivary glands waiting until it is favourable to reactivate and replicate. Primary infection in adults is very rare, but when it does happen, the symptoms are much more severe. Reactivation in HHV-6 is not well understood, but is believed to be influenced by stressors such as serious physical injuries, emotional stress and hormonal imbalances. HHV-6 has been implicated in MS and as a co-factor in chronic fatigue syndrome, fibromyalgia, cancer, optic neuritis, temporal lobe epilepsy and now, Lyme disease.

Fungal Infections

Candidiasis Infections (yeast overgrowth)

Most people suffering from a chronic illness, such as Lyme disease, are immunocompromised and have often taken multiple types of antibiotics and drugs over prolonged periods. The combination of the antibiotics wiping out all the favourable bacteria in the GIT and the weakened immune defences within the body often contributes to an overgrowth of yeast, most notably Candida albicans, also known as Candidiasis. Candida albicans' growth is usually limited by optimal immune system function and competition with other bacteria, and in the case of the skin, its dryness, as Candida requires moisture to thrive. It is important to note this, as everyone has some yeast in their body (mainly in the colon) along with millions of other types of "good" and "bad" bacteria in the digestive tract. When in balance, the "good" and "bad" bacteria create an ecosystem that allows optimal digestion and protection from infection. If certain bacteria, such as Candida (which is a yeast-like fungus), get out of balance and create an overgrowth, then the body's balance is thrown off. This can cause problems in the bowel and gut, and subsequently the immune system, as it's believed that 70+% of our immune system resides in our digestive tract.

Candidiasis can be categorised as mucosal (including thrush and vaginitis), cutaneous, onychomycosis (nail infections) and invasive. Invasive Candidiasis occurs in severely immunocompromised patients and is either systemic with one organ involved or disseminated with multi-system involvement. Symptoms of yeast overgrowth may manifest physically and behaviourly with various signs and symptoms:

Signs	Symptoms
Thrush in the mouth including a white coating on the tongue	Headaches
Thrush on the genitals	Emotional instability from an unknown origin
Skin rash or eczema	Stomach pain
Red ring and itchiness around the anus	Sleep disturbance
Rash or cracking between toes or joints	Lack of sphincter control (wet pants)
Nail infections	Fatigue
Itchy genitals	Sugar cravings
	Constipation
	Bloating / gas / digestive issues
	Confusion / fogginess

Causes of yeast overgrowth include anything that affects the delicate balance of our digestive tract and/or immune function allowing yeast to proliferate, such as poor diet / nutrition (especially excess sugar), dehydration, physical, chemical or emotional stress, medications, lack of or poor quality sleep, poor detoxifying capacity, hormonal imbalances (such as from the pill and hormone therapy) and allergies, to name a few. In relation to chronic illness, Candida is not a new topic, but allopathic medicine is slow to agree that yeast can cause chronic conditions and also be caused by chronic conditions that have left the immune system weakened. See the Biochemical Treatment chapter for treatment protocols.

BIOFILM CONSIDERATIONS

What Is a Biofilm and How Is It Created?

Biofilms are created by bacteria aggregating together to weave a protective web or polymeric matrix around themselves. This matrix is a sticky, gooey, mucous layer that contains fibrin to give it more structure. It is believed that minerals as well as heavy metals, especially those that are positively charged, can be leached from the body to assist the biofilm structure. Once this protection has been established, the bacteria shed their outer membrane, which consists of proteins, to serve as antigens and trick the immune system. This mechanism allows the bacteria to hide, survive and multiply away from the detection of the immune system as well as antibiotics and other herbal treatments.

How Does the Biofilm Negatively Affect Healing and Health?

The protective matrix that the bacteria create allows them to hide and live. Not only that, but the bacteria are still multiplying, fermenting, metabolising and leaching toxins into the bloodstream. The biofilm gives bacteria protection from anti-infectious agents, treatments and even the immune system! The biofilm can often affect testing by blocking evidence of the infection in fecal matter when stool cultures are performed. It allows the bacteria to stay alive and hide until the body is compromised so the bacteria can attack again when the immune system is at its weakest. The biofilm can also contain other nasties within its structure, such as heavy metals, so it's important to be aware of this if treatment is targeted to break down the biofilm. A chelator is needed to bind and safely release these neurotoxins and metals from the bloodstream.

Is It Important to Address the Biofilm in the Treatment of Lyme Disease and Any Other Chronic Bacterial Disease?

I believe that biofilms could be one of the missing links in Lyme treatment (and indeed any autoimmune-type chronic infection). For the immune system to remain in a state of dysfunction for so long, there has to be something going on. Either the immune system has been corrupted or the organism has transformed itself in such a way that the immune system can no longer recognise it or find it.

Is There a Test for Biofilm?

The answer, which may surprise most people, is yes! Fry Labs has an Advanced Stain for Biofilm which involves a staining technique that gives an idea of the degree of biofilm involvement. This test can be particularly helpful in patients who are making slow or no progress in order to see whether the biofilm might be a major player affecting healing.

"If you are distressed by anything external,
the pain is not due to the thing itself, but to your estimate of it;
and this you have the power to revoke at any moment."

Marcus Aurelius

COLLATERAL CONDITIONS

Collateral conditions (also called concurrent conditions) are terms I use for either a condition you:

1. Had prior to contracting Lyme disease, or

2. Now have as an indirect or direct result of disruptions to the body caused by Lyme disease and its co-infections.

Either way, these imbalances and conditions need to be addressed in order to get better, feel better and ideally, stay that way. No single treatment is likely to heal the patient. The more complex the co-infection/ opportunistic infection / concurrent conditions, the more complex the treatment and healing process will be. Even with a full and specific diagnosis, the patient's compliance is paramount to the healing process. Sometimes it is the concurrent / collateral conditions that run parallel to chronic illnesses like Lyme disease and its co-infections that create the most havoc, as they can change the symptom picture by exacerbating or masking symptoms and even preventing a solid diagnosis in the first place. Damage to any bodily system is possible. Once other bodily functions are affected, such as sleep, hormones, adrenals and thyroid, then the concurrent condition can end up making you feel worse than the chronic disease itself, and it can certainly slow down the healing process. These conditions are often found in people who have been sick for a long time, as the body keeps trying to adapt and compensate. Sometimes it is a diagnosis in this category that prevents people from establishing the true cause of all their symptoms. This is why Lyme disease is often called "The Great Imitator."

Some collateral conditions to look for:

Nutritional Deficiencies

Iron, magnesium, manganese, potassium, sodium, copper and vitamins B, C, D, and K are particularly important to monitor. Speak to your doctor about testing these nutrients so you can monitor your treatment and outcomes. IV therapy may be necessary to correct deficiencies.

Endocrine System Dysfunctions

Endocrine glands (such as the pineal, pituitary, pancreas, ovaries, testes, thyroid, thymus and adrenals, and the neuroendocrine organ the hypothalamus) secrete hormones directly into the blood rather than via a duct. If disrupted, they can affect or contribute to hormonal imbalances, adrenal fatigue, thyroid dysfunction and issues with the hypothalamic-pituitary axis.

ADRENALS

The adrenal glands produce cortisol, one of our stress hormones. Stress can result from: physical causes such as excessive exercise or a chronic infection; biochemical stress such as drinking too much caffeine or eating too much sugar; or from any emotional stress, real or perceived. In a healthy body, the release of cortisol to boost energy in times of stress is an important mechanism controlled by the autonomic nervous system and, more specifically, the sympathetic nervous system. If the adrenals continually have to secrete stress hormones because the body has been in a "fright, fight or flight" state for too long, then they become depleted and exhausted. Adrenals are implicated in most chronic health issues, and if not resolved, can affect energy levels (and Lymies need every ounce of energy they can get!) as well as the amount of inflammation in the body, as cortisol is inflammatory. Symptoms of adrenal stress include fatigue, weight loss or gain (especially around the midsection), lightheadedness, darker skin or freckles, nausea or anorexia.

A saliva test over 12 hours can give you a good indication of your adrenal health. Samples are usually taken 4x a day at 6am–8am, 12pm, 6pm and 10pm. Some tests do slightly vary with collection times. Levels should be high in the morning (which is one part of the mechanism that wakes you up) and naturally slump at night to allow the body to rest and heal. You can also do a base hormone panel that measures all your fertility hormones at the same time. See the section Other Testing to Consider in Chapter 10 for further information.

THYROID

Thyroid dysfunction can often go hand-in-hand with adrenal fatigue. Some reasons why Lyme sufferers and people with chronic illnesses may have thyroid dysfunction include:

❖ During chronic bacterial infections, such as Lyme disease, increased enzymatic activity can deplete the amino acid tyrosine. Tyrosine is a precursor for thyroid hormone production.

❖ Lyme and its co-infections can disrupt the hypothalamic-pituitary axis which has the ability to affect all hormone balance in the body, including thyroid hormones.

❖ The thyroid is already quite susceptible to autoimmune disease, and as we know for many people, Lyme can trigger autoimmune or autoimmune-like diseases that can create hyper (increased) or hypo (decreased) thyroid function.

❖ Testing iodine levels is also important when addressing thyroid issues.

Reproductive Hormone Imbalance

It's not just the endocrine organs that can be impacted by dysfunction of the hypothalamic-pituitary axis, but also the reproductive hormones. If you have not had children or wish to have more, this especially concerns you. Even if that is not the case, if these hormones are out-of-whack, they can create a variety of other unwanted symptoms. A test for base hormones that includes adrenal and reproductive hormones exists because they are interlinked. The adrenal glands are required to produce at least one-third of the reproductive hormones, such as estrogen, progesterone and testosterone, in women AND men! When reproductive hormones are out of balance, symptoms you might experience include: PMS, decreased libido, fatigue, menstrual irregularities, weakness, insomnia and early onset menopause (not to be confused with the night sweats from Babesia).

Inflammation

Inflammation has been linked to many health issues which may be acute or chronic, local and/or systemic and may also contribute to other collateral conditions. When the methylation cycle is impaired, it decreases the body's ability to detox and repair itself on a cellular level. At the same time, it allows an influx of uncontrolled inflammatory substances that not only cause inflammation, but disrupt the natural healing process. Lifestyle factors, such as stress and excessive exercise, and nutritional factors, such as consuming processed sugar, caffeine and alcohol may exacerbate this inflammation. Inflammation can be from tissues in the body creating pain (such as in ligaments, muscles and tendons), internal inflammation of the vessels and heart, neurological inflammation or inflammation that contributes to autoimmune processes such as rheumatoid arthritis or allergies.

WHAT IS ACUTE INFLAMMATION?

Inflammation is a natural and necessary healing mechanism in our body that allows immune activity to respond rapidly to infection, injury, allergens, toxins or temporary stress. When inflammation is temporary, it is known as acute inflammation, and the healthier we are, the more effective and efficient this process is. When people shrug off the body's amazing self-healing abilities, do you think they have pondered how the body heals a wound? It's not like we say to our body, "Right body, I want you to increase blood flow to the wound please! Can you please shoot over some specific hormones, proteins and other inflammatory mediators to dilate the surrounding blood vessels? Once that's done, send me some cytokines, eosinophils, prostoglandins, leukotrienes and interleukins to flush out the tissues. And while you are at it, you might as well start making specific antibodies to fight the infection and crank the white cells over here to clean up the mess, please!" This all happens quickly without any conscious thought! That's pretty amazing!

Symptoms of acute inflammation may include pain, heat, redness, swelling or immobility as the body goes about healing itself.

<u>HOW DOES INFLAMMATION BECOME CHRONIC?</u>

Once inflammation becomes chronic and prolonged due to unresolved acute inflammation or a multitude of factors, such as stress, poor diet and other lifestyle factors, it is then linked to a whole host of chronic illnesses. The weakened immune system believes it is still under attack and continues its attempt to clear away inflammation and heal the body. In some cases of Lyme and other chronic diseases, the body IS still under attack, so the key is to get the inflammation under control; otherwise, the body starts to attack itself. This is known as an autoimmune dysfunction. I believe the key to this is optimal nutrition and lifestyle. If we go back some two and a half thousand years, there was a man called Hippocrates who said, "Let food be your medicine, and let medicine be your food." Why did we wait this long to actually realise he was right all along?!

GIT Disturbance

An imbalance of microbes directly contribute to GIT disturbances, such as Leaky Gut Syndrome (intestinal permeability) and Irritable Bowel Syndrome (IBS), which indirectly increase inflammation and suppress the immune system. This can then exacerbate allergies, intolerances and sensitivities. So getting the gut right is paramount, not just so you can digest your food, get the nutrients you need and feel good, but for optimal immune system function. Depending who you talk to, people say that 70–90% of your immune system is located in the GIT, so it's kind of an important thing to get right!

If you have any GIT symptoms, such as bloating, diarrhoea, constipation, food intolerances or gas, to name a few, then before you do anything, you will need to consult with your primary health care practitioner to work out a treatment program to heal, seal and support the GIT. You can test for food intolerances and do a stool test (I use the company Bioscreen) to have a look at your natural gut flora. This takes out the guess work. You will need a doctor's referral to do these tests. Your doctor may also suggest testing for microbes, including parasites. My doctor uses a company called Histopath to do this testing. Both the Bioscreen and Histopath tests involve stool testing, so get ready to play with poo!

Detoxification and Methylation Issues

If your detoxification is not optimal, no matter what the reason (genetic defects, lifestyle, environment or disease) it will not only slow the healing process overall, but also impact methylation and create other collateral conditions, as the detoxification organs affect many other bodily functions. I consider detoxification and methylation so important that I have dedicated a whole chapter to it called Detoxification and Methylation.

Mould Toxicity

Moulds are everywhere and mould spores are commonly found in dust. Toxic mould refers to the moulds that excrete mycotoxins, which are secondary metabolites produced by fungi under certain and favourable environmental conditions. Temperature, pH and water activity are the main factors influencing the production of these mycotoxins, and most people are aware that mould mycotoxins are most commonly found in damp locations. Some people are more susceptible due to genetic predisposition (they can't effectively eliminate mould when exposed and can't make antibodies to fight mould and the toxins it produces) and others, like in Lyme disease, are more susceptible because they are immunosuppressed. The longer you are exposed, the worse the symptoms often are and the slower your healing progress may be. I know many people who have moved out of their mouldy homes and had almost immediate improvements in their health and healing. The more immunosuppressed a person is, the more they will struggle to eliminate mould, and the more mould a person has, the more susceptible they are to the symptoms from tick-borne diseases, so it's a double-edged sword that must be addressed.

SYMPTOMS OF MOULD TOXICITY

Acute mould exposure usually causes hay fever-like symptoms such as sneezing, itchy eyes, headaches and skin irritation. If the body is able to detoxify the mould mycotoxins, then the symptoms will only last for as long as the exposure or for a short period after as the body detoxifies.

Chronic mould exposure occurs when the exposure to the mould is potent and/or prolonged causing a buildup of mould in the system that the body can't get on top of naturally. As mentioned earlier, genetic susceptibility and immunosuppression play a big part in this process. Symptoms are very similar to those of Lyme disease, so certain symptoms may be exacerbated, or as the Lyme symptoms decrease, you may not notice due to the concurrent exposure and effects of mould. Symptoms include:

Brain-related symptoms – fog, confusion, concentration issues, memory problems, mood issues

Neurological disturbances – numbness, tingling, weakness, muscle tremors, headaches

Musculoskeletal symptoms – stiff joints, pain, aching, cramps

Respiratory symptoms – coughing, sneezing, dry or sore throat, sinus problems, shortness of breath

Other symptoms – excessive thirst, visual disturbance, red / itchy eyes, night sweats

Sound familiar? There are many cross-over symptoms, especially with Lyme disease and Babesiosis. See Addressing and Treating Mould Toxicity in the Biochemical Treatment chapter for treatment tips and advice to eliminate mould.

Metal Toxicity

Some people get confused between the term *heavy metals* and *metals*. To clarify, a heavy metal must weigh at least five times more than water. Not all metals are bad. In fact, the body requires some trace metals, such as zinc and copper, to function optimally. Some heavy metals, including mercury, lead, arsenic, cadmium, tin, thallium and nickel, are dangerous for humans, and some, such as copper, are toxic but only at high levels. The most common heavy metals that cause toxicity in the body are lead and mercury. (Aluminium is a toxic metal but is not classified as a heavy metal). Metal toxicity can come from environmental exposure such as soil, building supplies, pollution, coal burning and incinerator smoke; absorption from beauty care products such as cosmetics, skin care and deodorants; absorption from cleaning products, medications, some vaccines; and even food.

If your body is clogged up with heavy metal toxicity, not only can it put a great strain on the immune, digestive, respiratory and detoxification systems, but it can slow or even stall the body's natural self-healing ability. Because heavy metals can bind to proteins, they can end up in the major organs such as the liver, brain, kidneys and heart. They can also insert themselves into the matrix of biofilms. Mercury and lead may contribute to liver problems, and cadmium and lead can build up in the bones. Many of the symptoms of heavy metal toxicity are similar to that of Lyme disease such as dysfunction in neurological, musculoskeletal and cognitive functioning. It's hard to know if the Lyme sufferer had the heavy metal toxicity all along and it was only identified due to the already decreased detoxification and healing capacity of the body, or if their compromised detoxification systems did not allow the body to excrete the heavy metals as usual and so they accumulated. Either way, heavy metals need to be addressed.

TESTING FOR HEAVY METALS

If you suspect heavy metal toxicity or show no improvement with treatment, then I highly recommend that you see your doctor or a doctor who specialises in the detection and safe removal of heavy metals from the system. If this is not done properly, it can be extremely dangerous.

❖ **Blood Test:** You can test for heavy metals in the blood but remember that most metals end up in your tissues, so a negative blood test for metals does not mean you don't have any in your system; they just aren't in your blood.

❖ **Urine Tests:** You can do an unprovoked urine test first, but like blood tests for heavy metals, it won't give you insight as to what's in the tissues, and it will usually only be positive if there has been recent exposure to heavy metals. In a provoked urine test, a dose of heavy metal chelator is given to release the metals from the tissues into the bloodstream so the kidneys can filter it. Urine samples are then taken over a six hour period. This test highlights which metals are in the tissues but not specifically how much is stored there. Comparing an unprovoked and provoked test can give you an idea about the amount of the metals. Over time you should see each provocation release fewer and fewer metals if the treatment is working. Usually DMSA is used as the provoking agent.

❖ **Hair Analysis:** This type of testing is controversial, because it's hard to say whether excess heavy metals show up in the hair due to the body's ability to effectively excrete them or because they are at toxic levels and it's the body's way of trying to dump the excess. Add to that the factor that anything you put in your hair, such as shampoo, conditioner, styling products and dyes, can affect results. It's an option to use for those who are super sick and don't feel they can tolerate provocation urine testing, or as information for retesting purposes.

Heavy metals have to be moved from the tissues to the blood to be removed, but correct binding agents need to be prescribed to ensure safe excretion. If you are someone who is quite sensitive to treatment, then go easy. If you are a bit more robust, you may be able to tolerate more aggressive treatments. See the Biochemical Treatment chapter for heavy metal treatment options.

Sleep Issues / Insomnia

Many Lymies will find it hard to sleep. Some find it hard to fall asleep (even though they are tired), some wake up often and have broken sleep, and some may have poor sleep routines or be in pain. Please be aware that sleep needs to be addressed, as it is essential to the healing process. If you aren't sleeping, then it will be very difficult to heal. See the Physical Treatment chapter for information about the stages and importance of sleep as well as tips on how to get a better night's sleep and heal quicker.

Neurally mediated hypotension (NMH)

NMH can occur in Lyme disease, often concurrently, due to dysautonomia (dysfunction of the autonomic system) which affects the sympathetic nervous system function. Symptoms according to Dr. Burrascano include "palpitations, lightheadedness / shakiness especially after prolonged standing or exertion, heat intolerances, dizziness, fainting (or near fainting), *and an unavoidable need to sit or lie down*." (Burrascano 2008) Often just simply increasing mineral salts (NOT iodised salt) and water intake will be enough to control it, and many of the symptoms will disappear once Lyme is treated and other autonomic dysfunctions are addressed. If NMH is really bad, you will need to consult a cardiologist to have testing done, and at extreme measures you may be put on a beta blocker. Keep hydrated, ensure your minerals are balanced (especially sodium, potassium and magnesium) and get up slowly if you have been sitting or lying for long periods.

Neurological Complications

Lyme disease affects multiple systems in the body. Neurological symptoms include numbness, pain, weakness, visual disturbances, nerve damage in the arms and legs, meningitis symptoms (fever, stiff neck and a severe headache) and Bell's palsy (paralysis of the facial nerve causing one-sided facial paralysis). If the brain is affected, you could experience symptoms like brain fog, irritability, memory loss (especially short-term memory), decreased concentration, mood swings and sleep disorders.

Cognitive Impairments

Laboratory tests, such as SPECT scans, MRIs, PET scans, and psychological testing have demonstrated physiological and anatomical findings associated with the dysfunction of the cerebral cortex in patients with Lyme and tick-borne diseases. The examination of human and animal brains has further supported these findings.

Robert Bransfield, M.D, says that Lyme disease predominantly affects the white matter in the brain (as seen in SPECT, PET and MRI scans), which particularly affects memory association, recall, and associations. (Bransfield 2013) Many Lymies have attention impairments that were not apparent before they contracted Lyme disease, such as difficulty sustaining attention, increased distractibility when frustrated and a greater difficulty prioritising which perceptions are deserving of a higher allocation of attention. It's not only cognitive function that is affected, but also other cortexes of the brain including visual, auditory (hearing), olfactory (smell), gustatory (taste), vestibular (balance) and somatosensory (touch).

Auditory hyperacusis (hyperacusis is an oversensitivity, so in this case, it's an oversensitivity to sound), where sounds seem louder and more annoying, is the most common impairment. Sometimes there is selective auditory hyperacusis to specific types of sounds. Visual hyperacusis may be in response to bright lights or certain types of artificial lighting. Tactile hyperacusis, which can be painful, may be in response to tight-fitting or scratchy clothing, vibrations, temperature and touch. Some patients prefer to wear loose-fitting clothes and are frustrated that being touched can be painful. Olfactory hyperacusis may result in excessive reactivity to certain smells such as perfumes, soaps, and petroleum products. The slightest scent may cause dizziness, nausea and even vomiting.

I had very sensitive hearing. Certain sounds, like the beeping one hears when they don't buckle their seat belt, would drive me crazy. I couldn't have background noise like music or run the washing machine, or I couldn't concentrate. I was extremely jumpy, and even something as innocent as someone talking to me would often scare me if I wasn't ready for them. Bright lights would exacerbate or create headaches and lightheadedness.

Memory

Memory is the storage and retrieval of information for later use. There are often several different memory deficits associated with chronic disease that can affect how your memories are coded, stored and retrieved. Short-term memory seems to be affected first, although in my experience, recall of names, places, words and even faces can be affected.

My short-term memory was severely affected right from the start of my illness; however, I wasn't diagnosed with Lyme disease until 17 years after the initial symptoms began. By then, my memory had became so bad that I could not remember whole conversations that I had had the day before, I couldn't recall friends' names, and I would write appointments in my diary but not remember doing it or even what they were for. I lost the ability to put sentences together for many months, and even though, for example, I knew what a knife was, I couldn't remember or even say the word. I had always been a good speller, but no matter how many times I looked at certain words, sometimes I could not work out if it was spelt correctly. I felt like I had the symptoms of Alzheimer's disease, and at one stage, I remember being so scared that I would forget who my family and friends were. After extreme heat hyperthermia treatment, most of these memory functions returned; however, I still don't have the memory I used to have pre-Lyme disease. I am always very careful to write everything in my calendar and diary so I don't miss anything.

Processing

Processing allows you to break down complex information in order to understand it better and communicate it more effectively. This can include information you have read or heard, or from information received through your other senses such as smell and touch. Processing is required for things like spatial awareness, knowing your left and right, speaking and writing fluently, calculating numbers in your head and imagery (real or perceived).

I was unable to read properly for many years, not just because I was so tired and had constant headaches, but because I felt like my eyes were playing tricks on me; words didn't make sense anymore. I had to really concentrate when watching TV or when others spoke to me, and often I just couldn't keep up, which left me unable to understand what was going on around me. My spatial awareness was severely affected, and I would often bump into things or reach for a door handle and completely miss it. My speech was very broken, as it took me awhile to put words together and make sense of what I was trying to communicate. I was unable to write due to pain in my hands and the inability to put words together quickly enough for my brain and hand to coordinate. My ability to understand a map was gone (not that I was awesome at it before!). I had very vivid and scary dreams, and often found it hard to tell the difference between what was real and imagined. These are all deficits caused by poor processing.

ORGANISING AND PLANNING

Organising and planning are dependant upon processing and having a proper working memory. The ability to concentrate, multitask, show initiative and problem solve are all affected when your brain can't organise or plan efficiently and is often described as "brain fog."

Read Robert Bransfield's article "Lyme Disease and Cognitive Impairments" for more in-depth information on how Lyme and other chronic illnesses can affect your cognitive ability.

MORE ON BRAIN FOG

In Lyme disease, a frequent complaint is brain fog, or cognitive dysfunction, which interferes with concentration, memory, word recall and performance. Often the insomnia and constant fatigue that sufferers of Lyme disease have contribute to their decreased cognitive ability as well. As we know, Bb can cross the blood–brain barrier, and research studies suggest that Borrelia affects the circuits in the brain that are responsible for executive processing. In addition, our immune system decides that higher brain functions are not a priority during chronic illness and essentially diverts blood and nutrients from the brain to the immune system so it can do its job more effectively. That's why when we get sick, we often don't feel hungry, don't have much energy and definitely do not feel like having sex. Our immune system is demanding more power supply to help heal us! Children are much more affected and often mood, behaviour and learning are severely affected.

My concentration was severely affected and my once amazing ability to multitask was completely gone. Not only that, but I would often start a sentence or walk into a room to do something and completely forget what I was saying or doing. My creativity was non-existent, and there was no way I could have done puzzles or any type of problem solving activities. My brain fog was debilitating, my head felt heavy and cloudy, and that coupled with my blurry eyesight made it impossible to drive or watch TV (before I went to Germany).

Another aspect of brain fog is believed to be caused by inflammation of the brain due to all kinds of toxins in your system. These toxins can come from ingestion (food, drinks, medications, toothpaste, parasites), inhalation (mould spores, dust mites, microbes, allergens), skin absorption (cosmetics, soaps, body products, sunscreen), injections (vaccinations, party drugs, blood transfusions), radiation (flying, x-rays) and system(ic) disturbances (infections, microbes). If the body is toxic, chances are that detoxification is also affected and elimination of these toxins is diminished as well (through expiration, sweat, urine and faeces primarily).

Inflammation and toxins can also affect the limbic brain (emotional brain) and may prevent you from getting well because you are unable to think clearly and rationally or without unnecessary emotion attached. Some examples of things that people may feel, say or do are:

❖ Let false fear control them, always in reaction without thinking it through.

❖ Jump from one treatment to another imagining that what they are doing isn't working.

❖ Be so confused that they are unable to follow a treatment plan.

❖ Mix herbs, drugs and support products together without considering their interactions.

❖ Imagine (just like it is real) that someone or something is trying to harm them, such as the doctor, a loved one, the air, the electricity, the electronic waves, the dwelling, the food, the medication, the vitamins, the minerals, etc.

❖ Decide it is more comfortable to stay in their comfort zone rather than do the work necessary to heal.

❖ Buy and do everything that they have heard helps with their illness, which in the case of Lyme disease includes sauna, frequency devices, pills, herbs, exotic treatments, dozens of books on Lyme and an endless array of what others have claimed to be helpful in the eradication of Lyme disease. Always hoping to find a short cut. Often implementing too many things at once gets you no closer to eradicating the infections.

❖ Drag themselves from doctor to doctor to doctor trying to force those with little knowledge of Lyme and zoonotic diseases to diagnose or treat them—not understanding how their expectations are unrealistic.

❖ Jump from one thing to another, always thinking that this will be the magic pill that eradicates the infections with no Herxheimer reaction!

❖ Feel like they are going crazy (just like everyone said!!)

Most of the previous information was taken from the article "Lyme Disease and Cognitive Impairments" by Robert Bransfield. (Bransfield 2013)

Please check out the Treating Cognitive Dysfunction section in Chapter 5 for tips on treating brain fog and cognitive impairment.

Insulin Resistance / Diabetes

Insulin resistance is a physiological condition in which cells fail to respond to the normal actions of the hormone insulin and become resistant and unable to use insulin optimally, leading to hypoglycaemia. The beta cells in the pancreas go into overdrive to compensate, which causes a further cascade that can lead to hyperinsulinaemia and, if untreated, type 2 diabetes. This can occur as a collateral condition of Lyme disease and other co-infections (due to your body not working optimally already) or as a concurrent condition that you may have had beforehand. It will often exacerbate your symptoms and slow the healing process if not addressed.

Fatigue – Chronic Fatigue versus Fibromyalgia

It's often difficult to distinguish between fibromyalgia (FM) and chronic fatigue syndrome (CFS), and researchers and specialists are still trying to determine whether they are two completely separate illnesses, two distinct disorders with many similar symptoms or different facets of the same disorder. In the Lyme-literate world, there is another theory: FM and CFS are manifestations of Lyme disease and its co-infections. Many Lyme-literate doctors are now treating people diagnosed with FM and CFS as Lyme patients and having remarkable results! Both FM and CFS are diagnoses of exclusion. In other words, because no one knows exactly what causes them or how to treat them, if you have had the symptoms for a specific amount of time and everything else is ruled out, then that's the label you get!

FM AND CFS SIMILARITIES

Some similarities are muscle and/or joint pain, debilitating fatigue, headaches, memory loss, difficulty with concentration, forgetfulness, depression, numbness and generalised weakness. Other clinical similarities include:

❖ Reduced blood flow in the cerebral cortex and midbrain

❖ Suppression of the hypothalamic pituitary axis

❖ Disturbed Stage 4 sleep

❖ Reduced levels of growth hormone

❖ Lower than normal serotonin levels

❖ Evidence of a genetic component

FM AND CFS DIFFERENCES

The simplest explanation of the difference between FM and CFS is that with FM, pain is the most predominant symptom, while with CFS, extreme fatigue is most predominant.

Additional distinct differences include:

❖ Substance P (a neurotransmitter that transmits pain signals) is elevated in FM but not in CFS.

❖ RNaseL (a cellular antiviral enzyme) is frequently elevated in CFS but not in FM.

❖ Often CFS will be triggered by a flu-like or infectious illness, while FM is more often triggered by some kind of trauma to the body (e.g., accident, injury, surgery). (Klippel n.d.)

DIAGNOSING CFS

❖ The patient must have severe chronic fatigue for six months or longer with other known medical conditions excluded by clinical diagnosis.

❖ The patient must concurrently have four or more of the following symptoms:

> ➢ Substantial impairment in short-term memory or concentration

> ➢ Sore throat

> ➢ Tender lymph nodes

> ➢ Muscle pain

> ➢ Multi-joint pain without swelling or redness

> ➢ Headaches of a new type, pattern or severity

> ➢ Un-refreshing sleep

> ➢ Post-exertion malaise (deep fatigue and exhaustion following physical exertion) lasting more than 24 hours. (Klippel n.d.)

Note: The symptoms must have persisted or recurred during six or more consecutive months of illness and must not have predated the fatigue.

2010 FIBROMYALGIA DIAGNOSTIC CRITERIA

The new criteria have more flexibility, take into account more symptoms and provide a method for monitoring symptom severity. The researchers behind this method say the new criteria are about 88% accurate. As with the old criteria, other possible conditions must be ruled out and symptoms must have been present for at least three months. They also include two new methods of assessment: the widespread pain index (WPI) and the symptom severity (SS) scale score.

The WPI – lists 19 areas of the body, and the patient indicates where they've had pain in the last week. Score 1 point for each area, so the score is 0–19.

SS Scale Score – the patient ranks specific symptoms on a scale of 0–3, and the numbers assigned to each are added up for a total of 0–12. These symptoms include:

❖ Fatigue

❖ Waking un-refreshed

❖ Cognitive symptoms

❖ Somatic (physical) symptoms in general (such as headache, weakness, bowel problems, nausea, dizziness, numbness / tingling, hair loss)

For a FM diagnosis you need EITHER:

WPI of at least 7 and an SS scale score of at least 5, OR

WPI of 3–6 and an SS scale score of at least 9
(FM Criteria Work Sheet. PDF 2015)

"Face towards the perfect image of every organ, and the shadows of disease will never touch you."

Robert Collier

ENDOTOXINS AND HERXHEIMER REACTIONS

The full name is Jarisch-Herxheimer Reaction (after the founder), but the more commonly used term is a Herx. There are many theories and ideas about what a Herx reaction really is, what causes it and what it means clinically. Essentially in Lyme disease, a Herx reaction is an immune system reaction to the endotoxins that are released when large amounts of Bb are dying off due to effective treatment. There are a couple of reasons why Herx reactions vary from person to person. Firstly, each person has a different pathogen load. The more pathogens one has, the more endotoxins are released when the pathogens die. Secondly, a Herx reaction is affected by how well your body is detoxing, so if the body can't eliminate the endotoxins quickly enough (either through poor detoxification pathways or pure overload), then a Herx reaction will occur. The severity and duration of the Herx is, once again, affected by the aforementioned factors.

To distinguish between a Herx reaction and a drug / supplement / food or any other reaction, the general rule of thumb is that a Herx reaction will usually be *delayed* (it takes at least 48–72 hours for a treatment to cause a die-off and, subsequently, an endotoxin release), will *worsen* your current symptoms, often be worse at the 4-week mark of treatment and may cause you to experience detox symptoms such as headaches, joint and muscle aches and pains, sore throat, general malaise, fever, nausea, hives or flu-like symptoms. A reaction to drugs or something else will usually occur *quickly* after the drug / food / treatment is administered and bring a new symptom or set of symptoms that you might not have had before. Those symptoms will often flare quickly and then go away just as quickly (e.g., as in food poisoning or an allergic reaction to something).

For example, a drug reaction to an antibiotic treatment will usually occur quite quickly (i.e., headache or nausea within 10 minutes), whereas a Herx reaction may cause the same symptoms (headache and nausea), but the symptoms will be delayed 3–4 days or 3–4 weeks. A drug reaction will cause the same reaction unless the dose is changed, the drug is changed or the body gets used to it. It's often hard to know if treatments are working due to the delayed nature of the Herx reaction, especially if you add or change too many things at once.

Herx "Healing" Reaction	Drug or Other Allergy Reaction
Delayed reaction	Immediate or quick reaction
Worsening of current symptoms	New symptom(s)
Accompanied by detoxification symptoms such as headache, muscle / joint aches & pains, sore throat, malaise, fever, nausea, hives or flu-like symptoms	
Symptoms will calm down slowly as the body gets on top of the detoxification process	Symptoms often resolve quickly
Symptoms are cyclic and usually flare up every four weeks (and often in conjunction with menses, for females) with the worst of the Herx often occurring around the fourth week of treatment.	Symptoms will go away if the treatment or allergy-producing item is removed or the dose, as in the case of medications (e.g., antibiotics), is decreased / changed.

Our bodies are already loaded with many biotoxins that we are exposed to in our daily environment, such as preservatives, additives, mould, yeast, parasites, aspergillus (a common mould), heavy metals, PCBs and phthalates from plastics, to name a few. These biotoxins build up in our systems over time, and if our body is not detoxing efficiently, they can wreak havoc with many of our bodily functions and systems, including the immune system. This becomes an even more important consideration for those who have Lyme disease, because the greater the biotoxin load, the less effective the detoxification pathways will be to deal with endotoxin die-off, the more stress there will be on the immune system that is already struggling, the greater the Herx reaction will be and the slower your recovery will be.

Some practitioners believe that Herx reactions are dangerous and unnecessary, whilst others believe that not only are they part and parcel of healing, but they are a great indication that the treatments you have chosen are working. Although the jury is still out, I can say from personal experience that I felt so much better after a Herx, so I firmly believe it is a healing reaction. However, if you are having severe reactions, you need to reduce, change or stop the treatment that is causing the reactions. Herx reactions can also set you back and be very dangerous if the body can't detox the endotoxins quickly enough, for whatever reason. There is a whole chapter on the importance of detoxification and methylation as well as tips about how to detox your body inside and out (see the Biochemical Treatment chapter)

Useful Tips to Ease Severe Herx Reactions (or Prevent Them in the First Place!)

❖ If the reaction is severe, you may want to reduce or stop your treatment, because chances are, whatever you changed or increased in your regime has caused the reaction.

❖ Go back to basics and make sure your body is detoxing properly. Start with lemon juice in water and body brushing (cheap, easy and effective).

❖ Ensure your diet is as close to nature as possible. Include lots of organic seasonal vegetables and fruits (not too much fruit, as it's still fructose) and lean organic meats. Avoid alcohol, sugar, packaged foods, fast foods and especially caffeine.

❖ Ensure you are getting your water requirements – 43ml of water per kg per day (ideally filtered and room temperature).

❖ Use the supplements parsley and burbur (as used in TCP [The Cowden Protocol] – see Chapter 7 for more information about this protocol).

❖ Supercharge the drawing out of toxins via the skin by applying Bentonite clay to the body first thing in the morning and allowing it to harden before washing off in the shower.

❖ Sit in the Infrared sauna for 30 minutes to help open the pores, increase circulation and give the liver and other detoxification organs a rest by removing toxins and heavy metals via the skin (ensure you drink enough water so you don't get dehydrated and replace essential trace minerals).

❖ Soak your feet in a foot bath. You can buy special detoxing foot baths or just make your own. Fill a bucket or bath with warm water and add a teaspoon each of mustard, garlic and cayenne powders to assist in drawing toxins out through the feet.

❖ Visualise your body detoxing and healing. Although it may be difficult when you are really sick, it can really help. Give it a go, or use a meditation CD or app to guide you. You will get better the more you practice.

❖ Dilute 2 drops of Ylang Ylang in a few ml of olive oil and smear on the soles of the feet morning and night.

Now that you understand what a Herx reaction is and how the microbial die-off creates endotoxins, you will start to appreciate how important the detoxification and methylation pathways are to eliminate these toxins and microbes from the body. There are many reasons why detoxification and methylation are important but the main ones are:

1. To minimise Herx reactions that weaken the body further

2. To continue to clear the body in case any microbes manage to survive. If some of the microbes survive and the body is not able to eliminate them, they can regenerate and continue the assault

on the body. Not only that, but they are often stronger and harder to overcome second time around due to the toxins that they were exposed to during their regrowth. They become "super" bugs which makes them much harder to eliminate.

The importance of detoxification and methylation pathways is covered in-depth in its own chapter, and there are helpful tips and tricks to apply in the Biochemical Treatment chapter.

Chapter 3 –
Detoxification And Methylation: Importance & Influences

As we technologically advance, it's interesting to note that we are still no closer to solving or curing many of the diseases and health issues that have plagued society for so long now. In fact, the occurrences of diseases that are predominantly lifestyle based are increasing! Nearly all diseases have multiple contributing factors, so it is ridiculous to think that we are going to cure them with one treatment or a "magic bullet." There are so many factors that need to be considered when trying to heal from disease or, more importantly, when striving for optimal health (which sadly seems to be a thing of the past for many people!) Detoxification, I believe, is one big part of that puzzle.

Our bodies can only take so much, and the threshold is different for each individual depending on a variety of factors including genetic make-up, environment, lifestyle, exposure to toxins (in food, drinks, air pollution, plastics, cosmetics, skin and cleaning products, etc.), EMF and heavy metal levels. Knowing how the body detoxes is one thing but knowing your body's genetic make-up, susceptibility and genomics is just as important (if not more so) in creating health and treatment protocols specific for detoxification for YOUR body at any one time. If you want to create an efficient and effective detox program, you have to individualise the assessment and treatment by looking at:

❖ Body biochemistry

❖ Levels and locations of toxins as different toxins are stored in various places – especially "fat-loving" organs (such as brain, adrenal glands and thyroid), and fat itself (especially the stomach, bottom and breasts)

❖ Vitamin and mineral status

❖ Hydration

❖ Lifestyle – including the possibility of further toxic exposure.

There's no point detoxing if you are just going to "re-tox" it as soon as you step back into your old lifestyle and environment.

The best advice is to pay attention to your body and what it is telling you. Each and every sign and symptom is a message to you that you are not on track, and often those symptoms are measurable. A severe symptom often tells you that you are way off track and vice versa.

DETOXIFICATION

Detoxification is the metabolic process by which the toxic qualities of a poison or toxin are reduced by the body (predominantly the liver) and removed. It is not a simple process and involves many systems, hundreds of enzymes and multiple genes. When you think of detoxification, which organ do you think of? The liver, right? Whilst the liver is very important in detoxification, there are many other organs that also have roles to play. The liver breaks down and converts toxic material into less harmful substances that are then eliminated through the lungs via respiration, the kidneys via urine, the bowels via faeces and/or the skin. The lymphatic system has a big role to play, too. So pooing, weeing, sweating and breathing are essential functions! Unfortunately, the combination of a poor Western diet, increased toxic chemicals and a more sedentary lifestyle has increased the work the liver and other detox organs have to do to rid the body of toxins. It has also put a huge strain on our overall health, making us much more susceptible to disease.

"TOXIFICATION"

Whilst toxification is not a technical word, it is important to note that, for every route of detoxification, there is the ability for "toxification," or toxins to reenter the system and circulate. For example, we can breathe in toxins from the air (such as air pollution or chemicals from perfumes), and the skin (which is our largest organ and an effective way of detoxification especially via sweat) can also reabsorb these same chemicals into the system from things like cosmetics, deodorants, skin products and toxic cleaning products. The creation and overuse of toxic chemicals is a big contributor to the toxification of our systems, so the body is constantly working overtime just to rid itself of toxic substances (i.e., detox organs can't do their normal jobs as they are so busy ridding the body of excess toxicity). So although addressing detoxification is paramount, addressing the reduction (or elimination, where possible) of toxins in whatever form, and the possibility of reabsorption is just as important. For more information, see the Decreasing the Toxic Load section in the Biochemical Treatment chapter.

THREE PHASES OF DETOXIFICATION

Phase I: fat-soluble toxins such as bacteria, endotoxins, medications and hormones are broken down into water-soluble toxins

Phase II: free radicals from Phase I are neutralised and toxins missed in Phase I are deactivated

Phase III: broken down toxins are eliminated (usually by the bowel or bladder in faeces and/or urine).

Charles Poliquin uses a great analogy to explain the three phases of detoxification. He says that Phase I is like emptying all the smaller bins in the house into the big bin outside in your yard. Phase II is like moving the big bin from your yard to the curb. Phase III is like the garbage truck coming to remove the rubbish out of your bin for good. It's so important that each part of the process occurs; otherwise, there is a buildup of waste that has to go somewhere! If waste is not efficiently eliminated, then not only can it build up, but the body can reabsorb and store it. In addition, the methylation cycle should be optimal so that toxic substances can be broken down into safe levels that won't harm the body before they are eliminated.

I once heard at a seminar that it takes more than 50 enzymes under the direction of at least 35 genes for Phase I detoxification to be carried out! Not only does that make me marvel at how amazing our body is, but it shows the importance of having an optimal genetic make-up (or knowing and understanding our genetic profile so we can up-regulate mutated genes, if necessary).

Both phases of liver detoxification require the right balance and amount of nutrients, including vitamins, minerals, fatty acids and amino acids, to detox efficiently and effectively. The more deficient you are in these nutrients, the slower and harder your body has to work to detox. The higher your toxic burden, the more of these nutrients will be needed. So don't underestimate the importance of nutrition and supplements in optimal detoxification!

SIGNS AND SYMPTOMS OF IMPAIRED DETOXIFICATION

Healthy detoxification underpins many of the body's systems and processes that are essential for homeostasis, so any effect to the detoxification process has widespread signs and symptoms. The key is to look at the symptoms and, instead of treating the symptom, try to correct the underlying cause. For many people, one of the underlying issues for their health problems is poor detoxification capacity, which can result in the following:

❖   Constipation

❖   Skin rashes / disorders

❖   Lung infections / coughs

❖   Fatigue or energy problems

❖   Brain fog or cognitive issues

❖   Hormonal imbalances

❖   Kidney or bladder dysfunction

IMPORTANCE OF THE LYMPHATIC SYSTEM IN DETOXIFICATION

It is essential to consider and support the lymphatic system, as it is an important filter for catching and redirecting toxic debris and microbes (such as bacteria and viruses) back to the liver and immune system to be detoxified and eliminated. It essentially works to filter and keep our blood clean. The lymphatic system does not have a pump like the circulatory system does with the heart, so it relies predominantly on movement and hydration to function optimally. Exercise, infrared saunas, deep breathing, hydration and skin brushing are all great ways to stimulate lymphatic function. See Chapter 6 for in-depth information about these supportive treatments.

METHYLATION

The methylation cycle is a key biochemical cellular pathway that not only helps the body to detox efficiently and effectively, but is involved in hundreds of chemical reactions in our bodies. You need to look at this as a whole picture including the liver, kidneys, gallbladder, pancreas, stomach, intestines, thyroid, adrenals, other hormones and homocysteine levels. Having genetic testing done can help show where you are strong and where you are weak, and what lifestyle, nutrition or supplementation may be able to up-regulate your genetics to assist you to methylate more efficiently. Some of the important processes the methylation cycle is involved in include:

❖ Synthesis and regulation of important hormones which are important for hormone balance (such as the adrenals, thyroid, liver, and pancreas) and can cause anything from menstrual cycle irregularity and infertility to adrenal fatigue and thyroid issues.

❖ Neurotransmitter synthesis and regulation – e.g., serotonin, which regulates appetite and emotions, increases the chance of anxiety and depression if methylation is not optimal

❖ Formation of enzymes and proteins for growth and repair of tissues (including muscle mass)

❖ Up and down-regulation of genes

❖ Mental clarity (causing brain fog and decreased cognitive function if affected)

❖ Folate metabolism

❖ Reduction of inflammation

❖ Manufacture of CoQ10 for energy production and heart health

❖ Building and repair of DNA and RNA

❖   Heavy metal detoxification

❖   Myelination

❖   Immune Function – contributes to the production of T-Cells

❖   Digestion

❖   Elimination of microbes

❖   Balancing

Optimal methylation requires adequate levels of B12 and folate as well as other key nutrients (such as B6 and betaine).

Homocysteine: Homocysteine is a non-protein amino acid that is biosynthesised by another amino acid called methionine. When the body is functioning optimally, homocysteine in the blood is converted into SAM-e (S-adenosyl methionine) and glutathione. Folate, B12, B2, zinc and magnesium are required for conversion to SAM-e, and B2, B6 and zinc for conversion to glutathione. High levels of homocysteine in the blood means there is an inefficient conversion of homocysteine to glutathione. Decreased glutathione levels in the body mean decreased antioxidant activity and increased free radical activity (speeding up the ageing process, decreasing immune system capacity and increasing pain and inflammation).

SAM-e: An optimal methylation cycle not only creates SAM-e but recycles it. SAM-e is the most active methyl donor in your body. It donates methyl groups to important chemical processes and is essential in acting upon neurotransmitters to convert them to other compounds such as:

❖   serotonin to melatonin (supports sleep)

❖   noradrenalin to adrenalin (regulates the stress response)

❖   glutathione synthesis (supports detoxification)

❖ mitochondrial support via the creation of CoQ10, creatine and carnitine (helps energy)

❖ protein production

Vitamin B12: Without getting too technical, B12 is required in the methylation cycle to convert homocysteine into methionine as well as support the Kreb's energy cycle. Liver function is important in this process as it converts the inactive B12 to the active B12, which is the more usable form for detoxification and methylation.

Folate: It's very rare that folate deficiency is caused by an inadequate dietary intake. More likely, the cause is a defect in one or more of your MTHFR genes. MTHFR has received a lot of press lately, and some doctors think it's the new fad to test for this gene defect. However, there is no denying that its role in methylation is crucial. Statistics indicate that more than 30% of people are likely to have an MTHFR defect in some form and that it will decrease the function of one of the key regulatory enzymes for homocysteine metabolism in the body by 7–70%, in which case, it's definitely something we should take notice of. More on this later.

MAIN CAUSES OF IMPAIRED DETOXIFICATION

Underlying Genetic Susceptibility

Genetics is the study of genes, what they are and how they work (includes gene molecular structure and function, distribution, variation in populations and behaviour in the context of a cell or specific organism, e.g., dominance, nutrigenomics and epigenetics). Genes are units inside a cell that control how living organisms inherit features from their ancestors. For example, children usually look like their parents because they have inherited their parents' genes. Genetics tries to identify which features are inherited and explain how these features pass from generation to generation.

In genetics, a feature of a living thing is called a trait. Some traits, such as eye colour, height or weight, are part of an organism's physical appearance. Other traits are not easily seen and include blood types or resistance to diseases. The way our genes and environment interact to produce a trait can be complicated. For example, the chance of somebody dying of cancer or heart disease seems to depend on both their genes and their lifestyle.

Genes are made from a long molecule called DNA that is copied and inherited across generations. DNA is made of simple units that line up in a particular order within this long molecule. The order of these units carries genetic information, similar to how the order of letters on a page carries information. The language used by DNA is called the genetic code. It allows the genetic machinery to read the information in the genes in triplet sets of codons. This information is the instructions for constructing and operating a living organism.

The information within a particular gene is not always exactly the same from one organism to another, so different copies of a gene do not always give exactly the same instructions. Each unique form of a single gene is called an allele. As an example, one allele for the gene for hair colour could instruct the body to produce a lot of pigment, producing black hair, while a different allele of the same gene might give garbled instructions that fail to produce any pigment, giving white hair. Mutations are random changes in genes, and can create new alleles. Mutations can also produce new traits, such as when mutations to an allele for black hair produce a new allele for white hair. This appearance of new traits is important in evolution. Find out more in this YouTube video: https://www.youtube.com/watch?v=R4lJrBo4eX8

In 2000 scientists finished mapping of the genome. We now know that there are 25,000 genes in a human organism. The problem is that the character of each gene is relatively unknown, and there are only minimal genes to which health care professionals can apply their understanding in order to make a difference in day-to-day practice.

Whilst genes can't be changed, they can be influenced both positively and negatively. The good news is that there are tests to determine which of your genes are more "susceptible" to disease. And by "susceptible," I don't mean that if you have the breast cancer gene, you will get breast cancer, or if you have a defective methylation set of genes, you can't methylate. I mean that we test and take charge of our health and choose lifestyle factors that are going to enhance and up-regulate our genetics, not down-regulate them. This includes the study of nutritional genomics, and using nutrition and supplements to bypass certain genetic mutations and increase the body's resilience in its environment. There is some information about genetic defects that affect methylation (and, hence, detoxification) in the Methylation Defects section and more information on genetic testing and gene defects in the Biochemical Treatment chapter.

Environmental influences (or Epigenetics)

Epigenetics refers to the ability our environment has to affect our genetic predisposition due to exposure to toxins, stress and infectious agents. As you well know, environmental toxins and stress are more abundant now than when our ancestors were living. Much of our soils are depleted of nutrients, our foods are full of chemicals, people eat more and more toxic substances like unfermented soy, unprepared whole grains and vegetable oils, our environments are often polluted, we don't move as much as we used to, our posture is compromised and we are exposed to all sorts of stress! No wonder our bodies don't work so well! Our livers were not designed to be exposed to the amount and diversity of toxins we are exposed to today, which is often why the increased toxic burden often exceeds the body's ability to safely and easily detoxify and eliminate toxins.

Epigenetics literally means "above" or "on top of" genetics. It refers to external modifications or environmental influences on DNA that turn genes "on" or "off." These switches can actually control the way our genes behave! Everything from our emotional well-being to how much we eat and even the diseases we are susceptible to! Not only that, research now suggests that what our ancestors' lifestyle and environment was like (that influenced their genetic potential) can also be passed on! The modifications to DNA do not change the actual sequence of the DNA as once thought but instead change the expression of the physical structure of DNA. So epigenetics effectively influences how cells "read" genes. One of the main examples of an epigenetic change is DNA methylation in which there is an addition of a methyl group, or a "chemical cap," to part of the DNA molecule. This prevents certain genes from being expressed. But more about this later!

Another key point to mention with our modern lifestyle is the effect that chronic depletion of glutathione has on our bodies. In one of his podcasts, Chris Kresser (Chris Kresser, M.S., L.Ac is a globally recognised leader in the fields of ancestral health, Paleo nutrition, and functional and integrative medicine) described glutathione, a mega antioxidant, as a bulletproof vest; if you have enough glutathione, then you are well protected against oxidation (free radical damage). All disease processes, including ageing, are in part caused by oxidation. Our bodies can naturally produce glutathione, which works much like a Pac man against free radicals; it has an unlimited capacity to neutralise those free radicals that race around your body causing cellular damage and affecting your detoxification capacity. Unfortunately, natural glutathione production is greatly impacted by toxins (e.g., environmental, endotoxins, medications), stress (physical, chemical and emotional), exposure to infectious agents and nutrient deficiencies. You can supplement with glutathione, but depending on who you talk to, it is believed that the body does not absorb it well, and anything that is absorbed only works on a one-to-one basis (i.e., one glutathione for one free radical), so the detoxification capacity is greatly reduced. The best way is to ingest nutrients or supplements that boost natural glutathione production. There is more on this at the end of Chapter 7 in the Detoxing and Decreasing the Toxic Load section.

So the key message here is that our lifestyle and our environment (and the lifestyle and environment of our predecessors) affect the way we express our genetic makeup! Way to make us accountable for our lives! No longer can we solely blame the genetics we were born with! Dr. Bruce Lipton, who is one of the world leaders in stem cell research, realised early on that although genes can affect our genetic expression, our environment can too. Bruce is a biologist who uses his scientific background in combination with new age ideas about spirituality and health. He has some great podcasts and three books—*The Biology of Belief, Spontaneous Evolution* and *The Honeymoon Effect*—that are great if you want to learn more about this. His most recent book, *The Honeymoon Effect,* explains his belief that one's perception of the environment is even more powerful than the environment itself!

Infectious Agents and Toxic Load

People who come in contact with toxins and infectious agents will manifest different symptoms depending on the "toxic load" that already exists in their body. So if two people come in contact with the same toxin, it makes sense that the person who has the least toxic load and is detoxing the best will respond better than the person who is quite toxic, not detoxing well or fighting an infection already. Detoxification becomes even more important in someone with a chronic disease like Lyme disease, and even more so when there are opportunistic and co-infections present. Think of the toxic load like your car. When there is clean fuel and not much in the car, it runs smoothly and uses less energy (fuel), depending on how you drive it of course! However, the more load you put on the car, the harder the engine has to work and the more fuel that is used. If the fuel is low to start with, if the car is not serviced and well maintained or if the fuel that was put in it was dirty or not premium fuel, then the car isn't going to get very far, is it? Our bodies are no different: The cleaner you eat, the more you look after and service your body (with treatments like massage, acupuncture and chiropractic, to name a few), the better balanced your exercise regime is and the better your body is detoxing, the healthier you are.

The immune system is supposed to detect and work with the other bodily systems to eliminate toxins such as heavy metals and microbes (bacteria, viruses, fungi and parasites), but when the toxic load is already too great and/or the methylation cycle is compromised, then the immune system becomes suppressed and these toxins and microbes set up shop in our bodies, replicate and basically take over!

Methylation Defects

Optimal methylation allows the body to break down substances to safer levels and detoxify the body with less effort. If there are mutations to methylation genes, then detoxification of toxins and infectious agents are affected. Defects in methylation decrease the body's resilience to environmental toxins and infectious agents, such as Bb in Lyme and the various other microbes involved in the co-infections of Lyme disease. Our bodies are equipped with systems to naturally detox the toxins that accumulate, but if someone has methylation defects, then more toxins are accumulated than excreted, and this is where the problems can begin! The medical term for someone who under-methylates is histadelia.

One gene that you may have heard of about recently is the MTHFR gene. Anyone with significant health problems or who sees an Integrated GP (trained through ACNEM) will often have genetic testing done to identify specific mutations called SNPs (single nucleotide polymorphisms). This is useful because it can identify individual genetic risk factors to more specifically target treatments and preventative health strategies. This is especially helpful with the treatment of Lyme disease, because anything that you can improve in terms of the healing process will better your chances of getting on top of the disease and moving towards optimal health. See the Biochemical Treatment chapter: Genetic and Genomic Testing for more information on genetic testing.

I suggest reading some of Amy Yasko's work if you want to learn more.

Overview of Histadelia – Under-methylation

Histadelia is an inherited condition characterised by elevated blood levels of histamine. Individuals with high histamine levels may have a metabolic imbalance as a result of under-methylation. As a consequence, these individuals overproduce and retain excessive levels of histamine, a substance in the body that has wide-ranging effects. There are receptors for histamine in the brain, stomach, skin, lungs, mucus membranes, blood vessels, etc. High histamine levels are caused by a metabolic imbalance (under-methylation) which is a biochemical process responsible for the elimination of histamine as well as other functions, such as the production of certain neurotransmitters. When this process is disrupted and excess histamine accumulates, it can cause a deficiency in serotonin, dopamine and norepinephrine, which is why sufferers often exhibit psychological, behavioural, and cognitive symptoms. 15–20% of schizophrenics and many sufferers of depression may have undiagnosed histadelia. Sufferers may be suicidally depressed and fall prey to obsessions, compulsions, and addictions.

Signs and symptoms of histadelia

- ❖ Histamine excess can manifest as asthma, vasomotor rhinitis, allergic skin disorders with pruritus (itching), excess stomach acid production, saliva, tears, thin nasal and bronchial secretions, and certain types of vascular headaches.

- ❖ Histamine speeds up the metabolism, which produces a tendency towards hyperactivity, OCD, frequent colds / flu, phobias, a highly motivated and hard-driving personality, good creativity / imagination, high libido, joint pain / swelling / stiffness, excess perspiration, warm skin, chronic depression and strong suicidal tendencies.

- ❖ Other symptoms include: poor tolerance of heat, unexplained nausea, poor pain tolerance, and excess / abundant saliva in the mouth.

- ❖ Excessive histamine results from the inadequate methylation in liver detoxification.

- ❖ Histamine opposes adrenalin (stress hormone), so fatigue as debilitating as that of adrenal exhaustion may occur.

- ❖ Physical signs can include: low tolerance for pain, rapid metabolism, lean build, profuse sweating, seasonal allergies, and frequent colds.

In severe cases involving psychosis, the dominant symptom is usually delusional thinking rather than hallucinations. Those afflicted tend to speak very little and may sit motionless for extended periods. They may appear outwardly calm, but suffer from extreme internal anxiety.

Diagnosis of histadelia

A blood test with a basophil count greater than 50 cells / cu mm and histamine levels greater than 70 ng/ml (0.629umol/L) is considered diagnostic for histadelia. It is common for sufferers to also have low copper levels, as copper is part of the enzyme histaminase which is involved in the metabolism of histamine. Copper should also be tested by either 24-hour urine copper or serum ceruloplasmin.

Other clues to histadelia may be low calcium, magnesium, methionine, vitamin B6 and excessive levels of folic acid.

People suffering with Lyme disease have enough to deal with without having something like histadelia affecting their methylation and detoxification capacity.

Genes Important in Methylation and the effect of SNPs (mutations) in these genes

MTHFR (aka Methylenetetrahydrofolate Reductase) is a common genetic variant that causes one of the key regulatory enzymes for homocysteine metabolism in the body to function at a lower than normal rate (this is hugely important to detoxification and methylation in the body). When homocysteine is affected, it can lead to a variety of medical problems, especially when a person is exposed to more toxins than their body can handle, as seen with people with chronic diseases such as Lyme disease. There are over 50 known MTHFR variants, but the two main variants that are consistently studied and tested are called C677T and A1298C. The numbers refer to their location on the gene. The 677 variant is associated with early heart disease and stroke and the 1298 variant with a variety of chronic illnesses. The MTHFR gene is reported as heterozygous or homozygous. If you are heterozygous , you have one affected gene and one normal gene. Basically, the MTHFR enzyme will run at about 55% to 70% efficiency as compared to a normal MTHFR enzyme. If you are homozygous for the MTHFR gene, then you have two defective genes (thanks mum and dad!) and enzyme efficiency drops down to 7% to 10% of normal, which of course makes a huge difference to anyone, especially if your body is already struggling with Bb and other co-infections. The worst combination is when you are heterozygous to both 677/1298 genes (i.e., you have four defective genes).

MTHFR can increase your susceptibility to illness because this pathway is the primary source of glutathione production in the body. Glutathione is the body's primary antioxidant and detoxifier. People with MTHFR anomalies usually have low glutathione, which makes them more susceptible to stress and less tolerant to toxins. This is, once again, a huge issue for people with Lyme disease, as their toxin load is already high and their detoxification and methylation pathways often compromised.

MTHFR problems get much worse the older we get due to the accumulation of toxins and the cumulative effect of oxidative stress over our lifetime. So, generally, the older you are, the worse you are affected, which is why it may not come into play symptomatically until later in life (especially if you have a healthy lifestyle).

Non-mutated MTHFR is one of the leading regulatory enzymes of homocysteine metabolism, an extremely important factor in our metabolic systems. This process touches many aspects of our general health and is, therefore, very important. The MTHFR mutation is a defective enzyme that hinders this process.

This is a huge topic and quite confusing even for me, and I have a health and medical background and training. The website http://www.stopthethyroidmadness.com/mthfr/ has a great summary based on a 2003 genetic study called the Human Genome Project if you want further information.

What a healthy MTHFR gene does for you

When it's working correctly, the MTHFR gene begins a multi-step chemical breakdown process, (aka methylation), which in simplified terms is like this:

❖ The MTHFR gene produces the MTHFR enzyme.

❖ The MTHFR enzyme assists the breakdown of folate vitamins (B9, folic acid) into a more useable form (*5-methyltetrahydrofolate*). 5-methyltetrahydrofolate helps convert the amino acid homocysteine into another essential amino acid, methionine, which is used by your body to make proteins, utilise antioxidants, and assist your liver to process fats. Methionine helps with depression and even inflammation. It also helps convert estradiol (E2) into estriol (E3), which are important hormones, especially for fertility!

❖ Methionine, which is converted in your liver into SAM-e (*s-adenosyl-methionine*), has many jobs. It acts as an anti-inflammatory, supports your immune system, helps to produce and breakdown chemicals important for your brain, sleep and mood (such as serotonin, dopamine and melatonin), and is involved in the growth, repair and maintenance of your cells.

So a proper methylation pathway ensures you will have a better chance of eliminating toxins, heavy metals and, of course, endotoxins from the die-off of Bb and other co-infections.

What a defective (mutated) MTHFR gene does to you

A defective MTHFR gene produces different varieties of the *defective MTHFR enzyme* (i.e., it functions less than optimally, 7–70% less, depending on the defective gene it produces, so your ability to break down and eliminate toxins is compromised).

The defective enzyme doesn't break down folate (B9) or B12 properly, which can affect *homocysteine*, increasing your risk of coronary heart disease (arteriosclerotic vascular disease or venous thrombosis) and related heart and BP conditions as well as your risk for dementia.

Homocysteine is poorly converted to *glutathione*, which is your body's chief antioxidant and detoxifier. You are then more susceptible to stress and toxin buildup (which is already exacerbated for Lymies due to their high toxin load).

Homocysteine is poorly converted to *methionine*, and less *methionine* can raise your risk of arteriosclerosis, fatty liver degenerative disease, anaemia (which Lymies are already susceptible to due to Bb's affinity for iron), increased inflammation, and increased free radical damage.

Less SAM-e can increase mood-related disorders, such as depression, which many Lymies are already prone to due to the accumulated stress of the illness itself.

Testing for MTHFR

It's fairly easy to test for MTHFR by checking homocysteine levels in the blood (mutations will cause high homocysteine levels) or having genetic testing done. In Australia, you can do functional testing (I use Health Scope or Nutripath) to do a blood test for MTHFR defects, and it costs about $50. Other companion or follow up tests might include vitamin B12 levels, red cell folate, a salivary hormone profile and/or a functional liver detoxification profile.

CBS (cystathionine-beta-synthase) The CBS gene, when working optimally, will convert homocysteine into cystathionine, and it regulates the enzymes that assist conversion of homocysteine to glutathione. CBS mutations cause an "up-regulation" that makes the gene work too fast. This can cause low homocysteine levels, an excess of urinary sulfates, ammonia and taurine, and a decreased breakdown of glutathione.

So, in short, speak to your doctor about getting tested. Remember, it is genetic; so if you test positive for any mutations, it's important to have the rest of your family tested, too.

NUTRITIONAL GENOMICS

Nutritional genomics is the science that looks at the relationship between the human genome, nutrition and overall health. It can be divided into two groups: nutrigenetics and nutrigenomics. These may sound similar, but they are actually very different.

Nutrigenetics studies the effect of genetic variations (individual differences in genes) that influence the body's individual response to diet and nutrition and, therefore, someone's susceptibility to diet-related diseases. Basically, it's the study of genetic differences to explain why people who live a similar lifestyle may have different health outcomes. The ultimate goal of nutrigenetics is to provide specific nutritional recommendations—known as *personalised* or *individualised nutrition*—for individuals to get the most out of what they are eating.

Nutrigenomics is the study of how food and nutrition affects gene expression (i.e., the way the information in our genes are translated by the body). By altering the genome, proteome and metabolome, one can investigate the resulting physiological changes. Nutrigenomics is a discovery science which aims to understand how nutrition influences metabolic pathways and homeostatic control, and how this regulation is disturbed in the early phase of a diet-related disease. Testing is available to examine a person's genetic uniqueness in order to customise protocols, such as nutritional supplements, in order to bypass genetic mutations and up-regulate healing and health.

GENETICS VERSUS EPIGENETICS AND ITS IMPORTANCE TO METHYLATION

Susceptibility to disease is believed by Dr. Manual Estseller to be 50% genetics and 50% epigenetics. If you apply this theory to the methylation cycle, then 50% of methylation is based on pure genetic susceptibility and 50% upon the environment, but because methylation is also part of the modification of DNA, they are directly linked. The good news is that these mutations can be bypassed by understanding the results from your genetic testing and applying nutritional genomics. In her e-book, *Autism: Pathways to Recovery* (Yasko 2008) Amy Yasko uses a computer analogy to explain the difference between genetics and epigenetics: If your computer keyboard had a broken M key, then all words needing an M would always be spelled incorrectly; that would not magically fix itself or change overtime. She says these words are like mutations, as they will also not change over time. However, if you ran spell check on the document, then substitute words would pop up that you could click on to override your mistake. Epigenetics is like spell check. It can create change by compensating for what is missing. But spell checker also relies on an optimally functioning computer and power source to work, just as your body requires optimal methylation and nutrition to work. This analogy helps you to see what mutations are present and what changes to your personal environment and nutritional support may help to override these mutations.

GENETICS VERSUS GENOMICS

Whilst genetic research focuses on individual genes, genomics studies the entire genome (a complete sequence of DNA that essentially determines who we are). Genomics can be used to evaluate specific mutations in genes or SNPs (single nucleotide polymorphisms) which can give valuable information, such as predisposition to certain diseases, potential drug reactions / responses, identification of people with chemical sensitivities and individual detoxification capacity. Genomic testing can tell you exactly what treatments, lifestyle changes, nutritional support and supplementation would be best for your specific genetic make-up or to up or down-regulate certain genetic mutations that you have inherited (depending whether up or down-regulation is needed). Pretty exciting stuff! (Nutrigenetics 2014) (Nutrigenomics 2015)

Chapter 4 –
Diagnosis Of Lyme Disease

"This world, after all our science and sciences, is still a miracle; wonderful, inscrutable, magical, and more to whoever will think of it."

Thomas Carlyle

TEXTBOOK VERSUS A LYME-LITERATE DIAGNOSIS

The entire clinical picture must be taken into account when diagnosing a chronic illness. In the case of Lyme disease, the diagnostic process may involve ruling out other illnesses and diseases before Lyme can be ruled in. Ideally the diagnosis should then be supported with laboratory evidence, but this is not essential.

Please note that the Centres for Disease Control and Protection (CDC) have surveillance criteria for Lyme disease on their website. As stated on their website, the criteria were not devised to DIAGNOSE Lyme disease and only represent a very narrow band of cases for epidemiological purposes. Some doctors and health practitioners use the criteria to diagnose Lyme disease or discourage patients from having testing done for Lyme disease.

I recommend using ILADS treatment guidelines, Dr. Nicola McFadzean's books and Burrascano's *Advanced Topics in Lyme Disease: Diagnostic Hints* and Treatment Guidelines for Lyme and other Tick-borne Illnesses for extra guidance.

Dr. Peter Mayne recommends using the words "unlikely,""possible" and "highly likely" to diagnose Lyme disease and to consider any case with an EM rash and positive serology or PCR as an "absolute" (i.e., one definitely has it!)

"Keep your mind as much as you can from dwelling on your ailment. Think of strength and power and you will draw it to you. Think of health and you will get it. "

Prentice Mulford

CLINICAL DIAGNOSIS OF LYME DISEASE

Using a Patient's History in Diagnosis

❖ Have you had a known tick bite?

❖ Where were you when the tick was found on you?

❖ How long was the tick on you?

❖ How was the tick removed, if it was found?

❖ Have you had a bulls-eye looking rash (EM rash)?

❖ Have you had any other rash in relation to this illness?

❖ Were there any flu-like symptoms within two weeks of the bite that possibly never ceased?

❖ Did you have general malaise (tiredness) that may have persisted?

❖ Have you ever travelled outside of Australia?

❖ Summarise your health history prior to being symptomatic or bitten by a tick.

❖ Are the symptoms cyclic, and if so, can you establish a pattern over days, weeks or months as to when symptoms are worse and then better? (Classically, symptoms of Lyme disease cycle every four weeks, especially with females, as it often coincides with their menstrual cycle).

Using Signs and Symptoms of Lyme Disease and Its Co-infections in Diagnosis

Because Lyme disease can essentially migrate to any part of the body, the symptoms are widespread and numerous. Depending on how long the bacteria has been in your body, factors such as co-infections and the state of your health before you contracted the bacteria will all affect the signs and symptoms, and the diagnosis. The symptoms you have can be useful in diagnosis, but even more importantly, they are signals or information to your body that you are out of balance and can sometimes indicate what part of your health is most affected and which area you need to address first. Our bodies are smart and they communicate to us with symptoms. If you ignore these messages for too long or override the signals (e.g., with medication), then the body will be overloaded, which allows disease to afflict other areas of your body and health. The more symptoms you have, the more areas that need your attention. This symptomatic information can then be used with other diagnostic techniques, such as pulse and tongue diagnostics, live blood analysis, kinesiology testing and biofeedback (more on these later), to create a strong clinical or working diagnosis. Laboratory testing can strengthen and support this diagnosis but is not definitive. So start listening: what is your body telling you?

I recommend using a symptom checklist to monitor your symptoms over time, as it's sometimes difficult to keep track or even remember. I have included copies of a few different ones in Appendix E.

I've included a brief list of the signs and symptoms of Lyme disease and its co-infections (see AppendixE:1 for a full list of symptoms for Lyme disease and its co-infections and how they affect each bodily system). A good way to see patterns is to highlight the symptoms you currently have and underline the symptoms you have had in the past. Please remember that there is a lot of crossover with symptoms, and these summaries of each infection only consider scenarios where the patient has ONE infection. Once a patient has more than one infection (including co-infections and opportunistic infections), the clinical picture can change and the onset of symptoms may be more rapid and often more severe.

Lyme disease caused by Borrelia burgdorferi (Bb)

(the life cycle of a spirochete is about 28–32 days)*

In the normal 28 to 32 day life-cycle of a spirochete, as adult bacteria reproduce and die, a person experiences a Herxheimer usually during this same period.

ACUTE / EARLY / LOCALISED

EM rash, flu-like symptoms, general malaise, headaches, fever, sweats, muscle soreness

CHRONIC / LATE

Please see signs and symptoms listed in the Stages of Lyme Disease section and in more detail in Appendix E.

Overall general well-being is affected with symptoms such as loss of libido, extreme fatigue, migrating and cycling symptoms, increased allergies and sensitivities, continual infections and illness, unexplained weight loss / gain or fluctuating weight, the feeling of being hung over all the time, insomnia and emotional instability.

Babesiosis

(incubation period 5 days to 9 weeks)*

Problems with temperature regulation

Drenching sweats (often at night)

Ringing in the ears

Visual issues including blurry vision or floaters

Nausea

Nightmares (vivid and/or violent dreams)

Breathing issues including shortness of breath, wheezing or air hunger

Skin issues including capillary angiomas and white blotches

Anxiety

Head / neck and/or jaw pain

Loss of appetite

Left undiagnosed and/or untreated, Babesia can cause severe immuno-suppression which can cause further complications such as hormonal imbalances, haemolytic anaemia, liver dysfunction, thrombocytopenia, leucocytopenia, hemoglobinuria and low blood pressure.

Bartonellosis (aka cat scratch disease or trench fever)

(incubation period 3–38 days)*

Severe stabbing headaches (often described as an ice pick headache)

Pain or burning in the soles of the feet (and sometimes hands) especially in the morning

Lymph node enlargement, especially in the extremities

Severe joint pain and/or swelling

Muscle twitches / tremors / cramps / shivers

Severe anxiety / depression

Insomnia

Arthralgia / myalgia / neuralgia

Rib pain

GIT issues – including bowel disturbance, lower abdominal pain, gastritis

Malaise

Skin issues such as scratches, nodules, striae (streaked rash that may resemble or be misdiagnosed as stretch marks) and other rashes

Cognitive deficits – confusion, personality changes or exacerbations in habits such as obsessive compulsive behaviour (OCD)

Rickettsias

(incubation period 5–7 days)*

Fevers

Nausea / vomiting

Abdominal pain – especially the right upper quadrant

Headaches knife-like and/or behind the eyes

Severe muscle pain

Low WBC

Neurological symptoms (seizures, shooting pains)

Tendon pain

Encephalitis

Hypotension

Acute renal failure

Respiratory distress

Ehrlichiosis and Anaplasmosis

(incubation period up to 4 weeks)*

Because these two diseases are caused by rickettsial bacteria, they have similar symptoms to each other and Rickettsia (see the previous sections). However, the symptoms often have a rapid onset and respond quickly to treatment. Flu-like symptoms and diffuse erythema (reddening of the skin), including the palms of the hands or the soles of the feet, might help discriminate between them. On blood tests, it can cause a decreased WBC count and elevated liver enzymes.

*Incubation dates come from research at Infectolab in Germany (Infectolab Australia 2014)

Mycoplasmas

Some general mycoplasma symptoms include fatigue, fever, joint pain, swollen joints, headaches, insomnia, anxiety, emotional instability, confusion, lack of concentration / alertness / memory.

MYCOPLASMA PNEUMONIA

Cough (usually dry)

Recurrent sore throats

Hoarseness or loss of voice

Excessive sweating

Fevers

Chest pain

Headaches

Problems with breathing, wheezing, asthma

Fatigue

Possible complications include ear infections, haemolytic anaemia, severe pneumonia and skin rashes.

MYCOPLASMA FERMENTANS

Flu-like symptoms

Intermittent fevers and night sweats

Muscle cramps and spasms

Irritability, nervousness, anxiety and even depression

Memory loss

GIT issues including abdominal pain, nausea, bloating, diarrhoea

Headaches

Light sensitivity and visual disturbances

Chlamydia Pneumonia

Gradual onset of cough which can include hoarseness of voice

Common cold symptoms including sore throat

Pharyngitis or laryngitis or sinusitis

Pneumonia / bronchitis / bronchiolitis / myocarditis

In the absence of any positive lab tests or EM rash, your symptoms in conjunction with your history may help with the clinical diagnosis of Lyme disease and its co-infections. And remember, a negative lab test does NOT rule out Lyme disease.

USING LABORATORY TESTING TO ASSIST IN THE DIAGNOSIS OF LYME DISEASE IN AUSTRALIA

Diagnosing Lyme disease is very tricky using laboratory testing alone. Unfortunately, there are no tests that definitively rule in or out Lyme disease 100%, as it is very difficult to culture Borrelia bacteria in the laboratory. Lyme disease can be diagnosed clinically, but there are many different factors that need to be considered such as co-infections, opportunistic infections, collateral / concurrent conditions, health history and travel history. There is also a lot of crossover with other illnesses and diseases due to Lyme's widespread symptoms. There are tests available, however, that can shed some light or strengthen a diagnosis in a clinically suspected case, but none are diagnostic in their own right. Remember, the type of test ordered and the interpretation of the results by the laboratory and your health care practitioner may vary, so be sure they are Lyme-literate, or become Lyme-literate yourself! (Golightly and Thomas 2002)

Recommended Laboratories for the Testing of Lyme Disease and Its Co-infections

Currently Australian patients are being tested through three main labs. Please note that both international labs IgeneX and Infectolab are accredited by the government as "specialty" Lyme disease testing laboratories. At this stage, Australian Biologics is not.

IgeneX in California – www.igenex.com.au

Infectolab in Germany – www.infectolab.com.au

Australian Biologics in Sydney – www.australianbiologics.com.au

I agree with the LDAA that current testing for Lyme disease in Australia is controversial. I also agree that it is best to do initial testing with Australian Biologics using a PCR, or with Igenex or Infectolab using a western blot, rather than doing the two-tiered "screening" test using ELISA. ELISA is covered under Medicare, but its sensitivity and reliability is not high enough to be used as a screening tool. (Diagnosis 2015).

Laboratories for Lyme Disease Testing in Australia and What They Test

Australian Biologics is located in Pitt St, Sydney NSW. The chief Scientist, Jenny Bourke, is very knowledgeable and helpful. *Lyme tests include*

PCR *(blood, urine, serum), Elispot®-LLT, immunoblot, IgG and IgM of key bands of the western blot, and the Lyme lymphocyte transformation test (LLTT).* They also do PCR testing on blood for mycoplasma and chlamydia. Dr. Peter Mayne believes that the Australian Biologics PCR for Borrelia is more sensitive than IgeneX, perhaps due to its ability to identify Australian genotypes. Australian Biologics one of the few labs in the world that can perform a blood culture for Borrelia (Advanced Labs in America also does this test), and their IgG and IgM kit detection of key bands on the western blot are believed to have great sensitivity and are based on testing done in Germany.

Palms Laboratory is associated with North Shore Hospital in Sydney NSW – tests ELISA, IgG, IgM

The Australian Rickettsia Reference Laboratory (located in Geelong VIC) is a NATA-accredited (National Association of Testing Authorities) laboratory that tests for Rickettsia via serology culture and PCR. They also offer serology and PCR for both species of Ehrlichiosis (HGE and HGM). Australian residents may be bulk-billed through Medicare for testing (so there are no out of pocket expenses).

Sullivan Nicolaides Pathology is located in Brisbane QLD and conducts PCR for Bartonella (skin, blood), serology and PCR tests.

IMPORTANT DEFINITIONS TO UNDERSTAND

Laboratory tests are rarely definitive, especially in the case of Lyme disease, and all tests have a proportion of results which are **false positive** (test indicates disease in someone without the disease) and **false negative** (test indicates that there is no disease in someone with the disease). It's important to understand the reliability and sensitivity of the testing; if it is not close to 100%, then don't rely on the test as much as the clinical picture. Remember, a negative test does not rule out Lyme disease in those with a positive clinical picture. It's nice to have a piece of paper that confirms your diagnosis with positive lab results (for your own sanity and also some of the practitioners), but it isn't the be-all or end-all.

Early Stage Lyme Disease Testing and Diagnosis

After Bb is transmitted, it will take about six weeks to six months before Bb serologic testing will become positive. Even though only 5-50% of people will get the classic bullseye EM rash, if the rash is present, then treatment must start IMMEDIATELY, as there is only a short window of time to eliminate or weaken the infection in its early stages. In my opinion, if you have been bitten by a tick and have either the EM rash, flu-like symptoms, sore and inflamed glands or fever within a few weeks, it is best to get treated with antibiotics immediately, as during this time, the success rate for treating with antibiotics is the highest. This is one of the very few times I would recommend having antibiotics without a confirmed diagnosis. In my experience, rebuilding your immune system after a course of antibiotics would be safer than contracting Lyme disease. Of course natural follow up treatments would be required, such as high doses of probiotics and lifestyle changes, to restore gut flora and optimal immune function. You would need to see a Lyme-literate doctor immediately. In the case of a suspected acute Lyme disease diagnosis, many Lyme-literate doctors wouldn't even bother ordering expensive lab testing; they would treat you straight away with antibiotics. Please read further about the EliSpot® iSpot testing, as at the moment, it is the most accurate test for detecting Borreliosis.

Late Stage Lyme Disease Lab Testing

Blood Tests

When I chatted with Dr. Peter Mayne, he suggested the following tests to help determine the severity of Lyme disease and detect if co-infections are present. Your doctor will know these tests, but I have explained some of the tests I know about and think are important:

❖ FBC, LFT, ESR, CRP, MBA-20, CK

❖ IRON STUDIES, VIT B12, Plasma zinc, copper and red cell folate

❖ ANA, ENA, ANCA, Rheumatoid factor, CCP antibody

❖ TSH, T4, Reverse T3, Anti-thyroid antibodies, TRab, insulin

❖ ASOT, Anti-DNase, ACE, Coeliac Disease, Anti-gliadin antibodies, IgG, IgA, Tissue Transglutamase and Coeliac Disease genetic test, CD57, IgG Subset and IgA

❖ Rickettsia, Q Fever, Borrelia, Bartonella, Mycoplasma and Chlamydia Pneumoniae antibodies

❖ Ross River Fever, Barmah Forest Virus, Flavavirus, EBV, CMV, HHV6 and Toxoplasmosis

❖ 25OH Vit D, 125DiOH Vit D

The FBC, ESR, LFT and TSH are four of the most commonly ordered pathology tests. Often you will look at a blood test request form and have no idea what these abbreviations mean, I am sure! So here is a quick summary for you.

FULL BLOOD COUNT (FBC)

Doing a full blood count is a good start to see what is happening in the body. Monitoring your biochemistry and haematology is advisable monthly to track your progress.

RED BLOOD CELLS (RBCS) AKA ERYTHROCYTES

Hb is haemoglobin, the main substance in the red cells which carries oxygen.

RCC is red cell count which is measured by how many red cells are in a cubic millimetre of blood as well as characteristics of the RBC (such as size and shape). MCHC stands for mean corpuscular haemoglobin content, and MCV stands for the mean corpuscular volume.

WCC is the white cell count, again measured in one cubic millimetre of blood. There are many different types of white cells, and these subgroups are also counted and reported. These include neutrophils, lymphocytes (with many types), monocytes, eosinophils and basophils. All of these have special functions. Platelets are another type of small white cell involved with the clotting process.

ESR – ERYTHROCYTE SEDIMENTATION RATE

This is where a column of blood is left to stand for an hour. There should be very little settling of the RBCs, as they should be suspended in the blood. Anything that does settle is referred to as the ESR and, if elevated, may indicate a disease state. It is not diagnostic on its own.

LFT – LIVER FUNCTION TESTS

Bilirubin is a breakdown product from haemoglobin and is excreted by the liver. Its level in the blood gives an accurate measure of the liver's ability to excrete.

Total protein, albumin and globulin levels in the blood reflect the liver's manufacturing ability.

Liver enzymes The liver has special functions and the liver cells contain unique enzymes. When a liver cell dies, the enzymes in it are liberated and can be measured in the blood. When the level of enzymes in the blood increases, it indicates the increase / death / turnover of liver cells, which can occur in certain disease processes.

The following enzymes are measured in LFTs:

ALP – Alkaline Phosphatase (normal range 25–110 U/L)

GGT – Gamma Glutamic Transpeptidase (normal range 10–49 U/L)

ALT – Alanine Transaminase (normal range 5–40 U/L)

AST – Aspartate Transaminase (normal range 5–40 U/L)

LDH – Lactate Dehydrogenase (normal range 100–310 U/L).

TSH THYROID STIMULATING HORMONE

TSH is produced by the pituitary gland and travels via the blood stream to the thyroid gland where it stimulates the thyroid gland to produce and secrete thyroid hormone, which controls the metabolic activity of the body.

VITAMIN D

Vitamin D is a pro-hormone with several active metabolites that act as hormones. There is no agreed upon optimal level of Vitamin D; however, most people agree that low vitamin D levels are linked to and could potentially be a factor in many diseases. Vitamin D status is assessed by blood-testing serum 25-hydroxyvitamin D (25(OH)D) concentration. Due to many factors that cause a lack of direct sun exposure, people across the world (especially in Australia) are lacking in vitamin D. Vitamin D has many essential functions, hence, why it is routinely tested. According to the Health Scope Pathology website, optimal levels should be between 60-80nmol/L (Vitamin D Insufficiency n.d.), but people I have spoken to recently believe it should be a lot higher than that to be "optimal."

C-REACTIVE PROTEIN (CRP)

CRP, which rises in response to inflammation, is a protein found in the blood and is an acute-phase protein. Measuring CRP levels is a screen for infectious and inflammatory diseases. CRP is synthesised by the liver in response to factors released by macrophages (white blood cells in the tissue that are often found at the site of infection) and adipocytes (fat cells). The acute phase response develops in a wide range of acute and chronic inflammatory conditions (e.g., bacterial, viral, or fungal infections; rheumatic and other inflammatory diseases; malignancy; tissue injury or necrosis) and is often quite high in people diagnosed with Lyme disease. During the acute phase response, levels of CRP rapidly increase within two hours of acute insult, reaching a peak at 48 hours. With resolution of the acute phase response, CRP declines with a relatively short half-life of 18 hours. Rapid, marked increases in CRP occur with inflammation, infection, trauma, tissue necrosis, malignancies, and autoimmune disorders. Because there are a large number of disparate conditions that can increase CRP production, an elevated CRP level does not diagnose a specific disease. An elevated CRP level can, however, provide support for the presence of an inflammatory disease and be another clue to support Lyme disease diagnosis.

CD-57+

CD-57+ testing was discovered and used for a long time as a screening tool in Lyme diagnosis and to monitor the immune status of a patient, but at the time of writing, this has been debated heavily and also taken off the PBS (Pharmaceutical Benefit Scheme) register (i.e., it could no longer be tested in Australia using Medicare benefits) and then put back on again! I believe it may be useful as a screening tool for Lyme disease and to track your immune systems markers, but it is not 100% predictable and should not be relied upon fully for a diagnosis either way. Dr. Peter Mayne believes that if your CD-57 is not suppressed, then you are likely suffering from something other than Lyme disease; a high CD-57 count could indicate Babesia.

Let me give you a quick review. Some of our white blood cells contain lymphocytes. The main types of lymphocytes are T cells, B cells and natural killer (NK) cells. B cells produce antibodies in response to infection or vaccination, whereas T cells and NK cells are the "destroyers" and target foreign or infected cells. Each of these cells has specific markers on it. Just like doctors use T cells as a marker of how active an HIV infection is, there are those who believe that CD-57NK cells can be a marker to indicate how active a Borrelia infection is. CD-57NK markers can also be used to predict the likelihood of relapse after a patient has undergone treatment and is asymptomatic. So, if your CD-57 marker returns to "normal" after treatment and your symptoms are gone, then you are less likely to relapse and vice versa.

Many Lyme-literate professionals at Infectolab in Germany have tracked chronic progression of a Lyme infection, which is seen symptomatically and on labs as a weakening of the immune system. This suppressed immune system is often reflected by the decrease of the CD-57+ NK cells (Infectolab in Germany also uses CD3) where, in contrast, other clinically similar diseases, such as MS, SLE and ALS, do not reflect a decreased CD-57+. It is believed that the CD-57+ cells reflect the activity of chronic Lyme disease but unfortunately don't show the progression. So, as long as your body is suppressed or affected, your CD-57+ levels will be, too. For this reason, it should NOT be used as a progressional marker.

There are very few diseases associated with a LOW CD-57NK count. Drs. Stricker and Winger (Stricker and Winger 2001) discovered that CD-57 levels were low in most of their Lyme disease patients, and subsequently, the levels improved as the patient clinically improved. They found that those whose CD-57 count returned to normal range during and after treatment often had long-lasting results, whereas those whose CD-57 levels didn't recover relapsed more often than not. There is an overseas test for CD-57 often referred to as "Stricker CD-57," or the "Stricker Panel," that can be done at Labcorp. In a CD-57 panel, Dr. Burrascano believes that a high CD-57 count in a patient who is sick is more likely to be caused by a co-infection or another disease rather than Lyme disease. This can be especially helpful when clinical symptoms are not clear enough to point to one particular infection. Once again, clinical status of the patient is paramount, and no one test or marker should be used in isolation in the diagnosis of Lyme disease.

Interpreting CD-57 Values

Experts who use the CD-57 testing as a screening test or indication for treatment success believe a healthy person will usually have a "normal" CD57 NK cell count of >180. 0–20 is considered severe illness (mine was as low 4 at one stage), 20–60 is the most common reading in chronic Lyme patients, 60–120 indicates minimal Lyme activity and 120+ indicates a relapse is unlikely after discontinuing treatment. (Stricker and Winger 2001),

Serologic tests – Elisa, PCR, IFA, Western Blot, EliSpot®

Please note that most serologic tests, when reactive, only indicate EXPOSURE to the infection, not whether it's a CURRENT infection. Bb serologies are often unreliable, so it is very important to test at reputable labs.

ELISA (ENZYME-LINKED IMMUNOSORBENT ASSAY)

There are a large number of commercial tests available that use antibodies and colour to identify a substance (for Lyme disease, the substance is Bb). Many mainstream doctors still use the ELISA as a screening tool for Lyme disease because it is simple and inexpensive. Unfortunately, it's also unreliable and not very sensitive. In order for a test to be used as a screening tool, it must have at least 95% sensitivity; ELISA for Lyme disease only has a sensitivity of 65%. If the test results are negative, Lyme-literate doctors, who rarely use this type of test, will recommend other labs such as the western blot. In some cases, they will bypass this test completely for a more reliable test. If money is a consideration, then other, more cost-effective testing may be done first. Be aware that if your doctor orders an ELISA and the results are negative, you must insist that other testing be done.

PCR (POLYMERASE CHAIN REACTION)

The PCR name is derived from an actual lab technique used to detect the presence or amount of DNA or RNA of a specific organism. The PCR test is often the only marker that is positive in all stages of Lyme disease. PCR testing is very specific, but contrary to what many people will tell you, it's not terribly sensitive when testing for Bb. Because Bb may become dormant in cyst form and "hide" in the body, the PCR can often be negative even with an active infection.

Burrascano (Burrascano 2008) believes that the PCR has a sensitivity of just 30%. Per his guidelines, Bb causes a deep tissue infection, so a negative result doesn't rule out Lyme disease, but a positive result is extremely significant. Most accurate results are likely to be achieved by running PCRs on whole blood, serum and urine simultaneously when the patient is most symptomatic. It is also a good option to test after a round of treatment if the patient is asymptomatic to see if the bacteria are still active. Burrascano recommends waiting at least six weeks post-antibiotic therapy to get the most accurate results. Australian Biologics currently runs the most recognised PCR testing in Australia. PCR testing can be performed on many fluids / tissues including semen and breast milk.

LYME IFA (IMMUNOFLUORESCENT ASSAY)

This test detects IgG, IgM and IgA antibodies specific for Bb. Specific titers of IgM often persist in the presence of Lyme disease while antibody levels tend to rise 2–3 weeks after infection and can remain elevated in chronic Lyme disease. Many Lyme-literate practitioners say this is even less specific than an ELISA test, but it is still used.

WESTERN BLOTS

The western blot tests for the exact antibodies (IgM and IgG) you are making **in response to Bb.** When tested, not all patients have antibodies at all times. Antibodies are more commonly detected between 6–12 months after infection and after a reinfection on a western blot. A positive IgM is generally interpreted as an antibody response to a current infection, whereas a positive IgG is generally regarded as the body's immune response over time, indicating a more chronic infection. The more immunocompromised the patient, the greater chance there is that these results can be skewed. Research also shows that patients with acute culture-proven Lyme disease will still show up seronegative on serial western blot sampling. www.ilads.org

ELISPOT® – ISPOT LYME (ENZYME-LINKED IMMUNOSORBENT SPOT)

This is believed to be a more effective method for assessing the T cell immunity by measuring the frequency of antigen-specific T cells that are specific for Lyme antigens (which is indicative of exposure to Lyme disease). The EliSpot® method is used in a new test (at the time of writing) called iSpot Lyme. This test detects a cellular immune response against the Bb-specific T cell response in people who have been exposed to the Bb spirochete. Anyone who has been infected with Bb will harbor the Bb-specific immune T cells in their bloodstream. Generally a T cell response will only be positive two weeks after a tick bite and generally last 2–3 months past the acute infection. However, Bb-specific memory T cells develop and last for years! This test accurately detects, measures and performs a functional analysis of these immune cells. iSpot Lyme is a highly reliable and accurate test with 84% sensitivity and 94% specificity. It can even detect antigen-specific T cell responses in seronegative patients. For more information, go to: https://neurorelief.com/index. php?p=cms&cid=486&pid=149 (Chenggang Jin 2013)

Urine Tests – LDA (Lyme Dot Blot Assay)

This test looks for the presence of Lyme bacteria in the urine with a specificity of 90%+.

CSF tests: Spinal Tap – PCR and LDA

There are also spinal taps available in order to study CSF (cerebral spinal fluid), which is essentially the blood of the brain. If patients have negative blood and urine tests and have neurological symptoms, they often have positive results with CSF. A PCR and LDA can be performed on CSF.

The diagnosis of Lyme disease is controversial at the best of times, especially in Australia, even as confirmed cases rapidly increase. Hopefully the high sensitivity and specificity of the cellular-based iSpot Lyme test in combination with the western blot testing will improve the accuracy of a Lyme disease diagnosis. Then, people who are affected can get treated quicker and more effectively.

INTERPRETING THE WESTERN BLOT RESULTS FROM A LYME-LITERATE VIEW

It is critically important that you or your practitioner is experienced in reading western blots. When interpreting the results, don't look at the NEGATIVE or POSITIVE summary that comes with the results. These criteria are based on the CDC guidelines that many Lyme-literate practitioners argue are not appropriate for the diagnosis of Lyme disease. For example, certain bands that are specific to Lyme disease (bands 31 and 34) were excluded from the criteria by the CDC because they were used to create the Lyme vaccine that's no longer available.

The results of a western blot look similar to a bar code. The reports show which bands are reactive (i.e., the strength of the immune response specific to the bacteria being tested) by using the symbols +, ++, +++ and IND. The stronger the immune response, the more pluses (+) there will be. ++ and +++ are considered strong immune responses to the bacteria. If a patient is immunocompromised (this is particularly evident with patients that are severely co-infected, have neurological involvement and/or have been infected for a long time), it is believed that a + and an IND should be treated as a positive result, as even a small immune response from these patients is significant.

Currently there are nine bands specific to Lyme disease—18, 23–25, 34, 37, 39, 83, and 93. ANY response to two or more of these bands should be considered a positive result. It is also believed that bands 31 and 34 (as mentioned earlier) as well as 22, 28, 30, 41, 45, 58, 66, and 73 should be considered significant, though at this stage not specific for Lyme disease. (Diagnosis 2015)

LABORATORY TESTING AVAILABLE TO ASSIST IN THE DIAGNOSIS OF OPPORTUNISTIC AND CO-INFECTIONS

There are many different strains of each organism that can cause Lyme disease and related co-infections, but remember that lab testing only tests for a few of the identified strains. You can refer to the **IgeneX** website (http://www.igenex.com/) for their recommendations, but you will need a doctor's referral to test for any tick-borne diseases. IFA and PCR tests that detect parasites / bacteria directly on air-dried blood smears are available as well as FISH tests for Babesia and Bartonella. (What Tests to Order n.d.) **Infectolab** (refer to their English website http://www.infectolab.com.au for further information and forms) recommends the following tests for co-infections:

❖ **Babesia:** Direct detection – PCR in blood (EDTA blood), Blood smear. Indirect detection – Antibodies of Babesia-IgM and Babesia-IgG

❖ **Bartonella:** Direct detection – PCR on Bartonella in blood (EDTA blood). Indirect detection – Antibodies on Bartonella henselae-IgM and Bartonella henselae-IgG, Histology (hemangiome / lymphadenitis)

❖ **Rickettsia:** Direct detection – PCR on Rickettsia in blood (EDTA blood). Indirect detection – Antibodies on Rickettsia IgM and IgG

❖ **Ehrlichia / Anaplasma:** Direct detection – Ehrlichia PCR in blood (EDTA blood). Indirect detection – Antibodies for Ehrlichia-IgM and Ehrlichia-IgG.

(Infectolab Australia 2014)

SO WHICH LAB TEST IS BEST FOR LYME DISEASE TESTING?

IGeneX is a well-respected reference laboratory specialising in state-of-the-art clinical and research testing for Lyme disease and other tick-borne infections. According to their website, their recommendations for first-line testing are either an IFA or a western blot. If these come back negative, they recommend PCR on serum and whole blood or the LDA/Multiplex PCR panel on urine, which they believe may be more sensitive at the start of menses. There are also antibiotic protocols developed by physicians to enhance the sensitivity of the LDA.

Infectolab has great testing available and also some indirect testing that is useful for monitoring the progression of disease. (Infectolab Australia 2014)

Fry Labs Advanced Stain for Biofilm (Fry Laboratories, L.L.C.) is an independent clinical diagnostic and research laboratory located in Scottsdale, Arizona. Although I don't have much knowledge or experience with their testing, many people in the Lyme community believe their testing, especially for co-infections, is excellent. Their Advanced Stains test for biofilm is of particular interest. This test was originally used in the assessment of Bartonella and other protozoa in the blood of chronically ill patients. However, over time biofilm involvement was seen in all sorts of blood samples. Fry Labs' staining techniques have been further developed and can provide a picture as to the degree of biofilm involvement.

Their website http://frylabs.com/services-list/biofilm/ has some great information on Lyme, co-infections and biofilm. (Biofilm: Background n.d.)

Australian Biologics works hard all the time, and it is my hope that as Australians, we will have access to state-of-the-art testing in our own country sooner rather than later. The testing gets better and better every day, so as we move forward, there will be less wait times for laboratory diagnoses and, therefore, quicker treatment response times!

WHY IS IT SO HARD TO DIAGNOSE LYME DISEASE?

The Lyme Disease Association of Australia (LDAA) has great information on their website. Included are some of the reasons why it is so hard to diagnose Lyme disease, especially in Australia and countries that don't specifically recognise Lyme. It is important that you understand this so that you can explain to your friends and family when they ask why it's not recognised or easy to diagnose or treat! Here is a summary to help you.

1. Lyme disease symptoms are so similar to other diseases that misdiagnosis is common.

2. There are so many Lyme disease symptoms that can be migratory and intermittent, so it's not uncommon for patients to be told the illness is "in their head," especially when test results come back negative.

3. Many doctors in Australia are unfamiliar with Lyme disease (or follow current government recommendations and believe it doesn't exist in Australia), so they don't test for it or they order less specific and less sensitive tests.

4. Bacteria Bb doesn't necessarily reside in the blood but can morph and move into tissues, organs, nervous system, joints, muscles, etc., which makes it very hard to isolate the bacteria in a blood serology test.

5. Most blood tests conducted for Lyme disease test for the immune system's response to the bacteria rather than its presence. The longer the patient has been infected and the sicker they are, the less likely they are to return a positive test, as their immune defenses are often weakened or inhibited.

6. There are currently 14 known strains of Bb with more being discovered all the time. The western blot only tests for two of these strains, so it is possible that the strain specific to Australia hasn't even been isolated yet, making it difficult to accurately test.

7. Due to medical politics in the USA, which directly affects patients in Australia, the ISDA (Infectious Lyme Disease Testing Association) still recommends that Lyme disease testing follow a two-tier procedure that uses ELISA (which is not known for its sensitivity) as a screening test. Unfortunately, many patients who have a negative ELISA result often aren't referred for a western blot.

8. A western blot test still has its downfalls if you use the CDC criteria for test reporting, as the CDC has stipulated that certain bands in the western blot must be positive in order for Lyme disease to be diagnosed "positive." The problem is that those bands were chosen for statistical rather than diagnostic purposes. It is important to be familiar with interpreting western blot results or work with a Lyme-literate practitioner who is. For example, the most specific bands for Lyme disease are bands 31 and 34 which were excluded from the CDC criteria because they were used to make the Lyme disease vaccine that is no longer available. These bands are believed to be highly specific for Lyme disease, yet are not included in the results; therefore, their absence affects valuable diagnostic criteria. So, chances are, if you test positive (+) or indeterminate (IND) to bands 31 and 34, you have Lyme disease (assuming you did not have the Lyme disease vaccine when it was available for a short period before being pulled off the market, as this may affect how your markers react). The CDC also includes a number of bands that are not necessarily specific for Lyme disease. This also increases the chance of a false negative test result. (Diagnosis 2015)

FUTURE TESTING AND RESEARCH

At the time of writing, there is a Lyme disease research project underway at the University of Sydney. Dr. Ann Mitrovic is using volunteers with diagnosed Lyme disease and a control group to develop standardised testing procedures for ELISA, western blot and PCR that can be used to reliably diagnose Lyme disease and its co-infections in Australia.

Chapter 5 –
Treatment Of Lyme Disease

INTRODUCTION

Just as diagnosing Lyme disease is tricky, so too is treating the disease. There is no one way guaranteed to treat or cure Lyme disease, not yet anyway! There are many different treatments, supports and supplements (and the list goes on), so how do you know which one to do first, second or at all? The answer is… you don't! This chapter is broken up into physical, chemical, emotional and spiritual components. I believe to truly heal from Lyme disease, and indeed any disease, you need to address all these facets of healing. Too often I see people in my clinic who say, "I went to the naturopath and that didn't work, and then I went to the acupuncturist and that didn't work, and then I had one life coaching session and I noticed a huge difference straight away." Or, "I changed my whole diet and that helped a little bit. Then I gave up coffee and alcohol and that didn't make much difference. And then I started taking this supplement and I felt better straight away!!" Usually the latter treatments are the ones which finish the jigsaw puzzle and, hence, get the biggest rap for healing and helping even though all parts of the puzzle were essential (regardless in what order they were done!). Had you not done all those other things, it may not have worked out that way or seemed that miraculous.

As a chiropractor and a kinesiologist, I often get to be that person who gets the "miracle" results. Often people have tried other therapists, treatments or health changes before they see me, so I just get to put it all together for them. So please know that no matter what you do for treatment, it is never a waste of time. Each change or treatment is a building block on your journey back to health.

The Four "Must-Dos" for a Successful Treatment Program

I believe that there are four essential elements in any healing program for chronic illness. No matter what treatment protocols you choose, it is absolutely essential to get these four elements right in order to give yourself the best possible chance of healing. If you are not compliant, don't get enough quality sleep, are stressed and/or drink alcohol (or indeed use any illicit drugs), then there is no doubt your healing will be slower or stalled indefinitely.

Compliance – Complying with the treatment you choose is essential. Choosing a primary practitioner and having a good support network will be imperative for helping your compliance as well as really understanding why you are doing certain treatments; if you enjoy and/or believe in the treatment and have faith in your practitioner, you are more likely to be compliant and, hence, get great results.

Sleep – If you can't or don't sleep enough, you won't get well. Some people with Lyme disease really struggle with sleep, so if this is you, your primary focus should be to get your sleep right before doing anything else. If your body is tired or you're not sleeping, it makes it very hard to heal.

Stress – It can be physical (e.g., poor posture and repetitive movements), biochemical (e.g., dehydration, nutrient deficiency, toxicity, hormonal imbalance etc.), or emotional (e.g., family, work, finances, death). Mainly, I'm referring to stress that causes an increase in adrenaline and cortisol hormones, which can start a cascade of issues that slow down healing even in healthy people.

Alcohol – Alcohol suppresses the immune system, increases inflammation, decreases your detoxification and methylation capacity and has a myriad of other side effects. My advice: Don't drink alcohol if you ever want to get better. If you really must have a drink, then choose wisely. You may be able to get away with a glass of preservative-free organic, red wine here and there if you are not symptomatic or immunocompromised. If you need to drink or have a night out, be gentle with yourself and know that it will set you back. The important thing is to jump back on the horse as soon as you can. Who knows? Maybe a hangover will be all the reminder you need to stop drinking again!

Factors to Consider When Choosing or Combining Treatment Protocols

Lyme Disease and Modern Chinese Medicine: An Alternate Treatment Strategy Developed by Zhang's Clinic written by Dr. Qingcai Zhang and Yale Zhang (Zhang and Zhang 2006) highlights some factors that can affect the outcome of your treatment:

1. **The sensitivity and resistance of different strains of bacteria to different antibiotics:** In short, different strains of bacteria will react differently to different types of antibiotics, and every person has different genetics and resistance depending on their past exposure to bacteria and antibiotics. So an antibiotic treatment that works for one person may not work for another.

2. **How long you have had Lyme disease:** The longer you have had Bb and its co-infections in your system, the more ingrained they are and the longer they have had to adapt and dissemble your immune system. Also expect that the longer you have had the disease, the longer your treatment will take. If there is cyst form, it is even harder to eradicate because it can lie dormant when the immune system fights or the treatment is effective, only to reactivate when the body is sick or stressed later on.

3. **The virulence and load of the Borrelia bacteria:** Every tick carries different strains and microbial loads, so the type of microbe(s) present, how long the tick is attached, the location of the tick bite

and the person's immune response at the time can affect the transmission and subsequent severity of the disease.

4. ***The presence of autoimmune complications:*** Direct cell and tissue damage can induce the production of excessive cytotoxic and inflammatory factors that can contribute to autoimmune complications. All aspects of the disease must be addressed, and stand-alone treatments rarely work in these instances.

5. ***Multiple pathogenic factors:*** There are multiple pathogenic factors (including co-infections) of Lyme disease that not only cause the disease in the first place, but affect everyone very differently. Because it is unlikely that just one protocol is going to address all these factors, treatment protocols are often cycled, changed or tiered accordingly.

Choosing a Primary Practitioner

When choosing a practitioner, I recommend someone you can connect with, someone who has a good understanding of your disease or illness (or is willing to work it out if you are undiagnosed) and someone who is a healer, of course. This person can communicate with your other practitioners to ensure your program is coordinated, you are compliant and that you remain focussed and positive. I used a kinesiologist as my primary practitioner and highly recommend using one. Acupuncturists, integrated doctors and naturopaths also make great primary practitioners.

Keeping a Lyme Log

It is important that people keep a carefully detailed daily (if possible) diary of their symptoms to help their doctor and/or primary health care practitioner to track patterns (such as the presence of the classic four-week cycle), assess whether treatment is effective and determine their treatment endpoint. Important things to track are: diet, prescribed medications or supplements, exercise, stress levels, energy levels, sleep quality and quantity, temperature readings in late afternoon, notes from health care practitioners and blood or other testing results. Create a folder on your desktop and/or in your filing cabinet so all your information is together. You will be surprised how quickly time will fly. Plus, the better you track everything, the better you will know how you are doing over time. Remember the beautiful quote, "If it's to be, it's up to me."

Creating Schedules for Yourself

The best way to stay on track is to create tables or schedules. If you are anything like me, your memory is not so great, and if you don't write everything down and put an action plan together, it's not going to happen! You will be surprised how fun it is and how good you feel when you create schedules for yourself. It puts you in control of your healing.

To-Do Lists and Reminders

If you are anything like me when I was sick, you are lucky if you remember what you ate for breakfast that morning or your best friend's last name some days. To-do lists and reminders are great for this. The key with to-do lists is to ensure that you are taking stress OUT of your life, not adding more because your list is so long it has become totally overwhelming! There are two things I use religiously.

1. *Calendar in my iPhone:* Even if you don't have an iPhone, most phones these days have calendars and to-do lists. As soon as you organise a meeting or appointment, put it in your calendar with a reminder. If you are visual and OCD like me, then you can colour code things into treatment, meeting, social, exercise, to-do, birthdays, etc.! I always set a reminder for the day before and two hours before. If you are still a good old-fashioned tangible diary person, that's okay, too. You just need to get into the habit of opening your diary at least 2–3 times a day, because it's not going to beep to remind you when something is on (although you can still use your phone to set reminders to

check your diary)! For ease of access, keep the diary small enough so that it can fit in whichever bag you carry.

2. **Wunderlist App:** This is a free app for those who are computer or phone savvy. To be honest I am not blessed when it comes to anything technical and IT, but this app is too easy to use, even for people like me! It's a FREE app (yes, you heard it...free!!) that lets you make lists of things to do. You can enter reminders as well as due dates. It's great for keeping track of RSVPs, to-do lists and shopping lists. The really novel thing about this app is that you can invite people to your lists. So if you have a work list of things to do, you can give access to your work group and you (or they) can tick off each item as it is completed. Just like Facebook, an email and phone message will pop up letting the rest of the group know that someone has added or ticked something off (e.g., Kate has just completed "Finish marketing flyer" from Wunderlist or Kylie has added "Buy tissues" to Wunderlist)! It's great if you run a business or have delegated jobs to family or friends. You don't have to follow up to see if they have done their jobs; Wunderlist will tell you! When you are sick, it is so important to learn to delegate no matter how hard it is to let go, because let's face it, you just can't do everything! Not even if you are a super hero! Wunderlist will make you feel a little more wonderful and super hero-ish. That's something I can promise!

Tracking your Symptoms

As I mentioned earlier, the best way to track your symptoms is to use the Burrascano symptom checklist. It may seem insignificant, but it's a good way to objectively track your symptoms over time. Often there are so many symptoms (and they can change), so keeping track will help you work out what treatments may or may not be working. It will help keep you organised at appointments with doctors and practitioners if you can say, for example, "I had 40 symptoms at the start and now I have 5." Ideally, I have my clients complete the checklist before each monthly appointment, and I do progress evaluations every six months minimum. Try not to get attached to the symptoms. Just track them and then let it go. Easier said than done, I know!!

*"A hundred times every day I remind myself that my inner
and outer life depends on the labors of other men, living and dead,
and that I must exert myself in order to give in the same measure
as I have received and am still receiving."*

Albert Einstein

PREVENTION IS THE BEST TREATMENT

Education and Awareness

It's all well and good to know AFTER you get bitten how to remove a tick properly or AFTER you go for a bush walk that you were walking through tick central, isn't it? Hindsight is a wonderful tool! At this stage, we know the government does not recognise Lyme disease in Australia (many other countries are the same), so it's silly to think that they are going to educate the public on where the tick "hot spots" are, how to prevent tick bites or how to remove them safely! It's up to us! Unfortunately most people learn this information AFTER being exposed to a tick bite. However, if each and every one of us tells our network of family, friends and work colleagues, then at least we can get the ball rolling. The power of one is very effective. It only takes the power of one person to create an educated nation, but someone has to start! Make it your mission to educate everyone you know about everything to do with ticks: where they live, how they attach, preventative measures (read on for pointers) and how to remove them once they attach.

Don't Assume You Are Immune

If you have recovered from Lyme disease but get bitten again, please don't assume that you are immune. If anything, you are probably more susceptible to relapse with future tick bites.

Avoiding Tick-infested Areas

If it's possible, completely avoid areas that are known tick hot spots and any areas that are bushy, overgrown and leafy. After all, ticks do not fly or jump; they crawl! This being said, giving up bush walking or moving away from your dream home in the bush may not be the top of your priority list or even a possibility! If you are going to continue to live in or be exposed to bushy areas, then you need to learn some tips and tricks to prevent tick bites. In addition, check yourself and your pets regularly and know how to remove a tick if you get one!

Tips and Tricks to Prevent and Protect Yourself from Tick Bites

❖ Stephen Buhner (Forsgren 2010) believes the primary herb for prevention is astragalus. He recommends a minimum of 1,000 mg daily if you live in a Lyme-endemic area. It will keep the immune markers high that need to be high in order to prevent infection (but it can also be used to keep the disease symptoms as minimal as possible if you are infected). *After I had my son, I decided to follow this protocol to minimise any chance of him contracting Lyme disease post-birth* (astragalus is contraindicated during pregnancy).

❖ When in bushy areas, minimise the amount of skin exposed by wearing light-coloured, long clothing so you can have the best chance of noticing if ticks do crawl onto you.

❖ Tuck your long pants into your socks to prevent ticks getting under your pants and onto your skin (I know this sounds totally dorky, but anyone with Lyme disease will tell you that it's better to look a bit dorky than to get Lyme disease!).

❖ Wear a hat or beanie to protect your head.

❖ If you are in bushy areas, stick to cleared paths and trails to minimise contact with overgrown, leafy, bushy and grassy areas.

❖ Check your clothing regularly and ideally take off clothing before you go inside so you don't get any hitchhikers. (The neighbours will love you!).

❖ Place clothes that you wore outside in a HOT dryer for about 15 minutes. That way, any sneaky ticks will be killed (they can't survive the heat).

❖ You can use insect repellants on clothes and exposed skin, but sometimes these chemicals can be quite dangerous. You need to weigh up your risks. There are some natural repellants available on the market that you may want to look into and invest in.

❖ Some natural ways to prevent ticks include citronella oil, rose geranium oil and Palmarosa. If you put any of these oils on your skin (try adding them to your moisturiser or a base oil), they are supposed to repel ticks, as ticks are not attracted to the smell. Rub these on your beloved pets as well.

❖ I have also heard that ticks detest vinegar, so putting a teaspoon of vinegar in your water (and your pet's water) can make you less attractive to the blood-sucking ticks! Who knows? It may make you less attractive to mosquitos, too!

❖ Ticks don't like chlorine either, so although I don't really think chlorine is great for you, a dip in the pool if you have been in the garden or tick areas could be a good idea!

❖ The product permethrin can be applied to clothing and boots (NOT to the skin). I don't recommend this, but if you are in an epidemic area and severely allergic or sensitive to ticks, you may want to. It actually kills ticks that come in contact with the treated clothing and stays effective through several washes.

❖ Check your pets daily, especially if they are house pets.

❖ If exposed to tick areas, you need to check yourself thoroughly using a mirror. Be sure to check in all those places ticks love to get into including the backs of the knees, groin, between the toes, behind the ears, around the scalp and in the hair.

❖ Know the signs and symptoms of acute Lyme disease in case you don't notice the tick but get symptoms after being in bushy areas.

❖ Being a country girl, a farmer told me a great proactive suggestion for those that live in bushy areas: spray the lawn and surrounding areas with beneficial nematodes after it has rained. Nematodes love wet soil and as they burrow down they are supposed to not only kill ticks, but fleas, grubs, worms, fire ants or any other lawn and garden invaders, too!

❖ If you have bush turkeys on your property, then encourage them to stay. It's believed that they actually eat ticks!

❖ There are certain plants that ticks don't like. My aboriginal healer told me that ticks do not like lilly pillies, so plant these in your garden to repel the ticks!

Safe Sex

The jury is still out as to whether Lyme disease can be passed on via sexual intercourse. There is no strong evidence or studies to support this theory. However, that doesn't mean that it can't occur. What we do know is that spirochetes have definitely been found in seminal and vaginal fluids. If you have been diagnosed with Lyme disease, then it is my opinion that it is better to be safe than sorry and always have protected sex. The doctors at St. Georg Klinik in Germany believe it is unlikely that sexual contact is a major mode of transmission; otherwise, EVERYONE would have it, but they certainly believe that partners who have had continual sexual contact can pass Bb onto their partner. Of the families I know in Australia, both partners are often affected, but whether that is because they are both exposed to the same ticks or from sex is hard to determine. It is my belief that if the load of bacteria is great enough or the exposure constant enough, then sexual contact via seminal and vaginal fluids is a viable mode of transmission. If you actually have enough energy or libido to have regular sex, then keep it safe and use a condom!

Tick Removal Technique

1. Use a special tick removal tool (fine point tweezers or finger nails will suffice), and use a tissue to protect your fingers if you don't have a tool or tweezers.

2. Grasp near the tick's mouth as close to the skin as possible. Pull it out with steady, even pressure perpendicular to the skin.

3. Avoid squeezing or breaking the body or allowing any blood to remain on your skin after removal.

4. If parts of the tick are retained, see your local GP to have them removed ASAP.

5. Place the tick in a vial or plastic bag.

6. Wash your hands and disinfect the bite site and the tool or tweezers if used.

7. Put a damp tissue or some grass or leaves in the bag and label with the date, site of bite and how long it was possibly attached.

8. Keep the tick to be tested and consult your doctor as soon as you can (Diagnosis 2015).

If you don't have access to this book at the time of a bite but have access to a computer, you can log onto *www.lymedisease.org.au* and find Lyme-literate information about prevention and the removal of ticks.

Big No Nos!

There are many methods that people will tell you about to get the tick to unlatch without the aid of a tool or tweezers. Although these techniques may be successful in getting the tick off, they increase the chance of the tick transmitting infected bacteria into your blood as it becomes stressed. Under no circumstances should you do any of the following no matter what anyone tells you or what you read on the forums:

❖ Cover the tick in methylated spirits or alcohol

❖ Cover the tick in Vaseline®

❖ Cover the tick in any type of oil

❖ Put bicarb soda on the tick

❖ Put any other drawing agents on it

❖ Light a match near it or burn the tick in any way

A WORD ON TREATMENT

The most important thing to remember is that our bodies are self-healing. Having said that, our current environment is not in sync with the way our bodies are designed to function. We are born to be hunters and gatherers, eating off the land, living in well-supported communities and continually moving. Our only major stress should be animals higher on the food chain than ourselves! So, yes, we have evolved since then. However, it takes much longer than a generation or two to make huge evolutionary and genetic shifts. What hasn't changed is that the more physical, chemical and emotional stress we are exposed to, the harder it is for our bodies to adapt and the weaker we become. The word stress often evokes the feeling of emotional stress and many people who don't outwardly show signs of stress or are more laid-back often don't realise they are affected, too. Stress includes but is not limited to:

Physical – accidents, injuries, repetitive sports or movements, poor posture, ill-fitting footwear, tight clothing

Chemical – pollution, medications, drugs, alcohol, dehydration, pesticides, chemicals, food additives / colours / flavours, genetically modified foods, caffeine, sweeteners

Emotional – emotional stress from injury, illness, work, relationships, low self-esteem, harmful environment, being bullied, domestic violence, finances, moving house

When our body is exposed to many different stressors, it starts to break down and lose the communication pathways that allows it to self-regulate (know what's going on inside and outside), so our once, very smart body is no longer able to adapt to the environment or detect disease. Consequently, the ability to self-heal is affected.

WHAT TO DO IF YOU GET A TICK BITE WHILE YOU ARE PREGNANT

If you are pregnant, then most of the herbal and antibiotic treatments for Lyme disease and it's co-infections are contraindicated for use. *I had the unfortunate experience of finding a tick on me when I was seven weeks pregnant, and it sent me into a tailspin. I had been a bit tired that week, my muscles had been sore and all my glands were swollen. Because I had never been pregnant before, I assumed that I was experiencing normal pregnancy symptoms. I started getting back pain, but it wasn't until I started getting pain and numbness down my right leg that I suddenly realised it could be from a tick. Sure enough, there was a tick on my lower back near my right sacro iliac joint, exactly where I had been feeling the back pain for days and where the sciatic-like symptoms were originating. I had one of my work colleagues safely remove it, and I worked through the afternoon anxious and in extreme pain. I was extremely paranoid and thought that every pimple, mole and ingrown hair was a tick, and I was so itchy. I couldn't tell which symptoms were from my pregnancy, which were potential tick infection side effects and which ones were totally in my head. Speaking of heads, I felt like I had a tick in my head. The next night when my face went numb, I woke up my hubby and told him that I absolutely must have a tick in my head, as my face was numb and I had a headache. He looked but couldn't see anything, and even I couldn't feel any lumps in my head. I finally pinpointed a patch of numbness in my head, and upon closer inspection, Nick found a tiny nymph (smaller than a pin- head) on my head! (Please note that these symptoms all subsided once the tick was removed.) After fretting for 24 hours, I put my practitioner hat on and thought about what I would recommend to my clients. This is what I did.*

❖ Removed the tick from my head and sealed it in a plastic bag

❖ Had my husband and two colleagues use homeopathic vials to test for Lyme disease via the use of kinesiology. Babesia came up positive, so we harmonised the vial (this is a kinesiology technique to help the body become aware of what is happening and to supercharge healing)

❖ Contacted Australian Biologics the next day and made an appointment to have the bite site on my back biopsied and the tick tested with Dr. Peter Mayne

❖ Had a kinesiology session to clear the fear of ticks and the emotional overlay that came with that fear

❖ Had an acupuncture treatment to give my immune system the best chance of fighting any infection. I also had raw Chinese herbs made up specifically for me to address the spirochete and Babesia bacteria, and also the symptoms that were happening specifically in my body

❖ Had a 35g vitamin C IV and continued to take vitamin C powder until I reached bowel tolerance (diarrhoea) every day for four weeks

❖ Took a liver tonic that consisted of 100% cranberry juice, fresh lemon juice and apple cider vinegar to assist my struggling liver

❖ Rested and meditated twice daily to allow my immune system the best chance to fight the potential infection

❖ Closely monitored my symptoms each day using a modified Burrascano checklist given by Dr. Mayne

❖ Had Bicillin injections each week until the tick and biopsy results came back

Doctor Peter Mayne believed that Bartonella symtoms would occur within days to weeks, Babesia usually within 10–14 days and Borrelia often not until 3–4 weeks, hence, the precautionary measure of Bicillin to address the Borrelia (it is known that Bb can cross the placenta and affect the baby). I was very hesitant to take the Bicillin injections. The first time I had an injection back when I first started treatment, I fainted, and that set off a bout of blackouts that would last 2–20 minutes for months afterwards. I was very scared that it would happen again this time, but my husband (who is my voice of reason) believed that I was healthier and would handle it much better the second time around. Turns out he was right. Despite really struggling to come to terms with taking antibiotics during my pregnancy, I initially decided the risk of my baby contracting Lyme disease outweighed my concern over using the intra-muscular antibiotics, and the decision, although not taken lightly, was made. I was recommended to take the Bicillin injections until the end of the first trimester and then take Flagyl (type of antibiotic) for the rest of the pregnancy.

After the first few weeks of Bicillin and the extreme anxiety and pain that came with the injections, I reassessed and decided to stop the injections and rest while continuing to monitor my white cell count, symptoms and other blood markers. I had no symptoms and felt good, and all my blood markers were normal. I made the hard decision that I would not continue antibiotics through my pregnancy. I felt the risk of such strong antibiotics "just in case" outweighed the risk of contracting Lyme disease at that stage for baby and me. I now have a beautiful healthy baby boy, so following your intuition is very important if you are able to do this!

"In the middle of difficulty lies opportunity."

Albert Einstein.

Chapter 6 –
Physical Treatment

"If you take any activity, any art, any discipline, any skill—take it and push it as far as it will go, push it beyond where it has ever been before, push it to the wildest edges, then you will force it into the realm of magic."

Tom Robbins

PRACTITIONER-BASED TREATMENTS

The role of practitioner-based therapies is to assist the body, re-establish communication within the body, take off some layers of stress and support it to heal itself again. During my healing journey, I used many practitioner-based therapies but found there wasn't much information about why they are helpful. My husband and I own a group of natural health care clinics across Sydney, Australia and have some of the best practitioners in the world working together. We also have a wholefood store attached to the Potts Point clinic to make eating and living a healthy lifestyle more accessible and affordable for our clients (and of course our staff and selves). My hope is that the information that follows encourages you to choose one or more of these therapies in your healing journey (ideally working with your primary practitioner), and to be confident in your body's ability to heal itself. Some of the therapies cross over into biochemical and emotional healing too, so be aware of that when reading.

"Natural forces within us are the true healers of disease."

Hippocrates

BICOM Bioresonance Method

This method is a form of bioenergetic testing that works by reducing the total load of stressors on the body. It has been used for over 25 years and is a non-invasive therapy suitable for everyone including children, infants and even sensitive patients. Developed in Germany by Hans Brugemann, BICOM is based on homeopathy, electromagnetic acupuncture and quantum physics. It can be used to help diagnose and treat people with known diseases as well as those searching for answers, which is why it is particularly helpful for those suffering from chronic illnesses like Lyme disease and/or its co-infections.

With BICOM Bioresonance Therapy, homeopathic vials of viruses, bacteria, parasites, mould, metals, naturally occurring chemical compounds in foods (e.g., salicylates, phenolics) and foods are tested against the body to see what registers as a "stress" for you. Not only do you get an overall picture of everything that is going on in your body, but you discover the nutrients that may not be absorbing. The nutrient absorption can be corrected and the "stressors" can then be eliminated through BICOM treatment, which improves the body's own resistance in order to fight any infections / imbalances and assist the body back to optimal health.

The many benefits of this therapy for people suffering with chronic illnesses include supporting any organs that may have been affected, improving the detoxification process, helping to eliminate metabolic wastes, endotoxins and xenobiotics (substances foreign to the body), strengthening the elimination organs and boosting detoxification pathways to allow the toxins to be expelled.

There are now over 7,000 BICOM devices in Germany alone, and Health Space Clinics are the first in the Eastern Suburbs of Sydney to offer this therapy. Petra Behuliak is the Health Space BICOM practitioner and works at the Health Space Potts Point Clinic.

Kinesiology

What is Kinesiology?

Kinesiology is an advanced and holistic therapy that is based on the science of energy balancing. It uses muscle monitoring or biofeedback to identify imbalances in the body that may be causing health concerns. It looks at health as a whole, addressing not just the symptoms in the physical body, but the biochemical and emotional environment of each individual.

History of Kinesiology

In the 1960s an American chiropractor, Dr. George Goodheart, developed a system of evaluating body functions by testing specific muscles. He discovered that each muscle was related to an energy circuit and each circuit was connected to an organ. Since then, many different branches of kinesiology have evolved with the aim of restoring balance to three key areas of health – structure (muscular-skeletal), mental / emotional (psyche) and biochemical (nutrition). Kinesiology combines the knowledge of the Chinese acupuncture theory of chi (energy that unites body and mind), modern chiropractic, nutrition and psychology.

How Does Kinesiology Work?

Kinesiologists are able to assess how the body is functioning and can locate imbalances within the body by using a process of gentle muscle monitoring techniques to gain an insight into muscle patterns. The process indicates whether stress is directly related to the muscle or is linked to a particular organ / gland or energy pathway. Various methods may be employed during treatment including tapping, emotional release, massage, magnets, oils, crystals, homeopathic remedies, acupuncture, nutritional advice and/or affirmations depending on the practitioner and the style of kinesiology being applied.

Who can have Kinesiology?

Kinesiology is suitable for all ages and may help remedy a variety of health concerns, from musculoskeletal-skeletal issues to allergies, stress, fatigue and emotional problems. It is especially helpful for people with a chronic illness like Lyme disease as it can take the guesswork out of your treatment. Remember in the Treatment section when we talked about the body's ability to heal itself? Well, a skilled kinesiologist can ask your body if it knows what is wrong and what it needs to heal, so it can really fast track your healing time!

What Can Kinesiology Help?

Because kinesiology reveals the body's overall state of structural, bio-chemical and emotional balance, it may be able to help the body to heal a wide range of health issues. These may include:

PHYSICAL PROBLEMS such as headaches, migraines, ligament, muscle, bone, nerve or joint pain / strain.

CHEMICAL IMBALANCES such as food allergies / sensitivities / malabsorption, hormonal imbalances (e.g., PCOS, endometriosis, infertility etc.), nutritional toxicity or deficiency.

EMOTIONAL ISSUES such as anxiety, depression, and recovery from emotional overload .

What Does a Kinesiology Session Usually Involve?

You will be asked to provide detailed information about your health status, medical history, environment and goals. Avoid wearing perfumes and jewellery that can affect your energy circuit. Ensure you are well hydrated, as a dehydrated body often doesn't heal as quickly. You will be fully clothed and either sitting or lying on a treatment table. Sessions last from half an hour to an hour and a half depending on the style of kinesiology chosen.

Different Kinesiology Techniques

TBM (TOTAL BODY MODIFICATION)

My primary health care practitioner was a TBM practitioner. TBM is an advanced technique that only a small number of practitioners in Australia practice. It was developed by Dr. Victor Frank and has been fine-tuned and used all over the world for more than 50 years. In this day and age many people find their body can be affected by chronic stress (physically, chemically and/or emotionally), creating overstimulation of the sympathetic nervous system (fight or flight). Long-term activation of your sympathetic nervous system (due to stress) affects the way your body heals itself (or more likely how it doesn't heal itself), and particularly affects the systems that generally aren't required during a life-threatening situation (e.g., our reproductive, digestive and immune systems). Therefore, this technique is particularly effective when dealing with reproductive issues such as infertility and decreased libido; any digestive complaints such as IBS, bloating, constipation and malabsorption; deficiency syndromes such as iron or mineral deficiency; and, of course, anything where the immune system is affected, as in Lyme disease, chronic fatigue syndrome, lupus and autoimmune disorders.

TBM utilises kinesiology muscle testing to detect an organ or area of the body that is out of balance, determine the cause of this imbalance and correct the problem by restoring balance to the nervous system so the body can heal itself once again. TBM corrects the functional physiology (how the body works), which may then influence the body's structure. It involves a combination of gentle, low-force techniques including cranial work, acupuncture and acupressure points, chiropractic realignments, emotional tapping and releases, and nutritional advice.

Imagine the body is like a circuit. For a circuit to work, it must be plugged into a power source (e.g., the brain) and not be too overloaded (e.g., stressed). If a circuit is blocked or has too many things plugged into it, then at some point it will blow a fuse, affecting everything on that cir-cuit and, therefore, needing to be reset. So, too, if the body is blocked somewhere or too stressed (physically, biochemically and/or emotionally), and a particular neurone or pathway is overloaded, the brain essentially loses effective control over the afflicted organ or body part, leaving it with little or no information about its internal or external environment. Over time, your body loses its ability to heal itself and disease occurs.

A TBM practitioner using tried-and-tested reflex points and muscle testing can find the problem and stimulate specific reflex points on the spine or body to stimulate neurons in the brain to repolarise (like resetting a blown fuse). This allows the brain to fully connect and communicate with the body again so it can give important feedback to organs, muscles, skin, etc., in order to guide the body back to good health. Lifestyle factors must be addressed in order to keep the body in balance long-term, and a special eating plan called the Autonomic Recovery Program (which essentially balances the body's sugar metabolism) may be introduced for two or more weeks to assist this recovery.

TBM can be used in combination with many other natural health care treatments such as massage, chiropractic, physiotherapy, osteopathy, naturopathy and acupuncture.

TBM helped me get my blood sugar levels balanced, which eliminated my blackouts, dizziness, blood pressure issues, headaches and, of course, sugar cravings! It helped me balance my water circuits so I could rehydrate my body optimally and also detox better. It helped me start absorbing proteins again, which helped improve my energy and healing. It also worked on certain allergies / intolerances by harmonising my body.

The key work of balancing the body is to get out of sympathetic dominance (fight-or-flight mode) and return to parasympathetic dominance (rest–and–digest), where your body is designed to be most of the time so it can heal. This means that any anxiety, depression or suicidal thoughts all go away when the body is back in balance. Nearly all Lymies suffer from these things at some stage in their journey. Go to http://www.tbmseminars.com/index.php?route=information/practitioner to find practitioners worldwide.

NEURO-EMOTIONAL TECHNIQUE (NET)

NET was created by Dr. Scott Walker, who was inspired to take the emotional work of TBM one step further. NET uses kinesiology to detect links between current and stored emotional issues and how that expresses physically in the body. NET is based on a proven combination of the latest scientific research and century-old techniques used in Eastern healing to acknowledge the relationship between the body's emotional health, environmental toxicity, nutritional balance and structural integrity. It is a technique used by a variety of professionals, including chiropractors, physiotherapists, psychologists, doctors, naturopaths and dentists, to help improve physical and behavioural stress-related conditions. NET is particularly useful for anyone with emotional blockages (conscious or unconscious) that may manifest in any number of physical ways (such as addictions and/or phobias), or helping eliminate any symptom(s) that is / are chronic or won't shift.

NET does not claim to heal, cure or treat symptoms or the client as a whole, but rather it removes or helps the body integrate emotional blockages so the body can once again heal itself.

NET is known for its Home Run Formula that categorises and prioritises health into four areas. First base represents emotional and stress-related factors, second base represents the effects of toxicity on the body, third base represents nutritional requirements and fourth base represents the structural needs of the body. Although stress is quite often the overloading factor in disease, it is still very important to understand that any health concern may include multiple factors, all of which must be addressed to get to the cause of the imbalance.

I found this technique very useful when my healing had reached a plateau or when I had emotional outbursts that were hard for me to control. I became easily frustrated and even the littlest thing, such as my phone not working, no hot water for a shower or the printer not working, could set me off! Usually my husband was in the firing line, and later I would feel guilty for taking it out on him! I had recurring right neck pain that didn't seem to be mechanical in nature (regular massage and chiropractic would only help for a short while, so I knew there must be more to it). I asked my NET practitioner to do a body entry treatment (you find a physical problem or pain and see if there is an emotion connected to that problem), and we found an old stored emotion in my liver meridian that, once cleared and integrated, saw my neck pain gone for good.

NET helped me deal with the emotional overlay that not only exacerbated many of my symptoms, but were often the primary cause of those symptoms. Post-Germany treatment, as my body physically healed from Lyme disease, NET allowed me to clear and integrate the emotional trauma and shock from being sick for so long so I could move forward and enjoy my life. During my recovery I had a meltdown and felt the worst I had ever felt emotionally (despite being the healthiest I had probably ever been since my physical recovery). My naturopath explained to me that when the physical body heals, it is often then that the deep and dark emotions emerge because the body is physically strong enough to deal with them. It was the aftermath of emotions that was the hardest part of my recovery. I share this with you to encourage you to continually work through the underlying emotional issues throughout your whole treatment and recovery, and to keep clearing them and working through the emotional baggage well after your physical body is healed. Emotions are an indication of how you are healing, so use them to guide you in the right direction. There is no negative emotion, just an emotion to tell you that you are off course!

You can log onto www.netmindbody.com to find a practitioner near you. Keep in mind that only NET certified practitioners will be listed on this site. There are many more amazing practitioners who practice this technique but haven't gone through the certification process, so they won't be listed. Do a Google search for NET practitioners in your area and ask around as well. A personal recommendation is always the best.

Neurological Integration System (NIS)

NIS was developed by the global company Neurolink and is based, as the name suggests, on the principles of neuroscience that extend beyond the scope of mainstream medicine. Muscle testing, a technique which has been scientifically validated as an indicator of altered physiological function, in combination with the meridian system (a proven series of contact points used in Chinese medicine to enable access to information from glands, organs and muscles) has been used for over 20 years. The integration is the research specifically carried out by Neurolink based on the premise that by collectively stimulating both hemispheres of the brain (by tapping the top of the head), it reinforces the recognition and healing of the meridian points being contacted during the treatment. The three principles of NIS are unique and set this technique apart from other kinesiology modalities.

Principle 1 – All neurophysiology is governed by the brain and not the mind. Therefore, it is your brain that detects, evaluates and corrects all complaints (not the practitioner).

Principle 2 – One must look beyond "labelled" complaints or symptoms to the CAUSE of the problem. The underlying ROOT issues of the symptom(s) (which can be structural, physical, hormonal, emotional, neurological or pathological) are evaluated and identified using a series of scientifically validated protocols (the NIS system). Did you know that there are over 600,000 possible symptoms that the human body is capable of experiencing? These are all indications that the body is out of balance.

Principle 3 – The brain makes the corrections, NOT the practitioner. The practitioner's role is to facilitate the resetting of the neural circuitry so that the BRAIN becomes aware of what is happening in the body and can make the corrections required.

NIS specialises in acute pain and chronic illness, and the protocols use the latest scientific research at a cellular level to address CAUSES, not symptoms. ONLY by addressing your health at a cellular level can you achieve optimum sustainability. Your practitioner is accessing the brain's intelligence through a muscle test and proprietary integration method developed by Neurolink. This approach is safe, non-invasive and non-manipulative, so it is suitable for newborns to the elderly as well as for those who are very sick or injured. NIS is suitable for the whole family!

NIS is particularly great for helping people with Lyme disease, as it has specific protocols for bacteria, virus, fungus and parasites and can locate where they are in the body. You can log onto www.neurolinkglobal.com for more information or practitioners near you.

APPLIED KINESIOLOGY (AK)

AK stands for Applied Kinesiology and is founded on the belief that optimal biomechanics of the body, personal biochemistry and emotional balance are all essential for optimal health. All your bodily functions, both conscious and subconscious, are controlled and monitored by your nervous system. AK practitioners use muscle testing to assess the function of your nervous system in order to find imbalances and their causes, and then formulates a treatment plan to balance the nervous system so they body will heal itself. The theory of AK was developed by George Goodheart, Jr., a Michigan chiropractor, so you will see AK practitioners who are often chiropractors but may also be osteopaths, dentists or even doctors. Practitioners must first be trained in their respective fields before they can study AK in a postgraduate setting. (International College of Applied Kinesiology Australian Chapter n.d.)

I have used all of these kinesiology techniques with my clients and have also had treatments myself. I encourage you to find a skilled practitioner, and don't stop until you do! Kinesiologists make great primary health care practitioners, as they have a wide range of knowledge and always focus treatment on what YOUR body needs and wants! Pretty amazing!

Acupuncture and Traditional Chinese Medicine (TCM)

Acupuncture is an element of Chinese medicine that treats patients by inserting and manipulating very fine sterilised needles into the body in order to affect nerve impulses in the nervous system and restore energy flow or "Qi." It is based on the premise that energetic pathways or channels exist within the body and influence our internal organs and structures. Energy surfaces at certain points in the body called "acupoints," and these points are where needles are inserted. Diagnostic tools may include looking at the tongue, palpating the body or organs, and feeling the various organ pulses (found on both wrists), in combination with taking a history and examining signs and symptoms. It can also include the use of herbs, electricity, magnets, cupping, moxa and lasers. Acupressure (applying pressure to the acupoints) or lasers can be used instead of needles for those who don't like or respond favourably to needles.

It is well-known in Western medicine, with strong research to support it, that acupuncture and herbal medicine are effective at relieving pain, treating imbalances within the body, preventing disease and promoting general health and well-being. Those who haven't tried acupuncture are often surprised by how painless it is. Often people describe an overwhelming sense of calm and relaxation whilst the needles are doing their work!

I believe acupuncture can benefit everyone. Acupuncture may help improve your overall health and may be particularly effective if you have Lyme disease. TCM practitioners treat the body as they see it, not the disease. So regardless of whether you have been diagnosed with a chronic illness or Lyme disease (or anything else for that matter) clinically or via lab testing, it doesn't really matter. According to most TCM practitioners who treat people with Lyme disease, they believe the sick body has a latent pathogen. Acupuncture and herbal medicine are especially important for expelling the latent pathogen and getting the body back into balance.

Symptomatically, I found acupuncture and raw herbal formulas were great for relieving and healing many of my symptoms including rashes, pain, digestive issues (especially constipation and IBS), anxiety, depression, insomnia, night sweats and emotional instability. I felt instantly relaxed once the needles were inserted, and it was one of the few treatments where I felt significantly better afterwards. I usually felt really good after a session as opposed to feeling tired and Herxing all the time!

Technically, any TCM practitioner can treat the symptoms created by Lyme disease, but it is handy to see someone who has treated Lyme disease or at least chronic disease regularly, if possible, as they will have more knowledge and experience on how to better support you.

Acupuncture uses needles, lasers or acupressure points with great success, so if you are finding treatments uncomfortable, let your practitioner know! Acupuncturists have trained for at least five years, and I believe they should be considered doctors like they are in China. There, they are at the forefront of preventative health, even in hospitals.

Lyme Disease, TCM and Modern Chinese Medicine

Acupuncture was the first TCM modality introduced to the Western world, which is why in Australia (and most of the Western world), we know Chinese medicine practitioners more as acupuncturists. It is important to point out that in the literature, Chinese medicine generally pertains to the study and application of herbs in treating disease, with the use of acupuncture as more of a supportive therapy.

According to the Zhang Clinic, as outlined in the book *Lyme Disease and Modern Chinese Medicine* by the Zhang's (Zhang and Zhang 2006), TCM considers Lyme disease as bi zheng (numbness or stagnation syndrome) or toxic dampness-heat, which has a similar pattern to water retention, MS, rheumatoid arthritis, vasculitis, peripheral neuritis and encephalitis. The body's CNS (Central Nervous System) and neurological symptoms are categorised as TCM syndromes of jian wang (forgetfulness) and shen bin (mental fog).

The TCM principle for treating infectious disease is fu zheng qu xie, which means supporting the right immunity and expelling the evil pathogens. So the goal is to eradicate the pathogens naturally by supercharging the immune system. This is done with needling and Chinese herbs to clear heat, dry dampness and resolve the toxin load. Formulas are anti-pathogen, immune-regulating, anti-inflammatory and tissue-regenerating.

Zhang's book has a great treatment flow chart for treating Bb, Bartonella and Babesia and tips on how to distinguish between them. If you are working with a TCM practitioner (or herbalist or acupuncturist), I suggest you buy and read (and get your TCM practitioner to read and refer to)

Zhang's book, as it has some great herbal protocols and is very easy to read and follow.

Massage

Massage is no longer considered a luxury but an important part of regaining and maintaining your health. The many benefits of massage for health in general include easing tension and pain, improving blood flow and the healing properties of muscles, stimulating weak and tired muscles, aiding recovery, improving elimination of toxins from the body and relieving stress.

For those suffering from Lyme disease, there are many styles of massage available; it is just a matter of choosing a practitioner and a style that is right for you! Many people talk about the benefits of lymphatic massage for Lymies to improve detoxification, but a skilled massage therapist will be able to use various techniques to get the results you want. Techniques include remedial, deep tissue, myofascial, sports, shiatsu, relaxation, aromatherapy, acupressure, trigger point therapy, Swedish, Chinese tui na, lymphatic and anthroposophic, to name the main ones.

If you are sick, Herxing or weak, then pick a massage style that is relaxing and gentle like lymphatic, aromatherapy or anthroposophic. If you are more robust and still able to exercise, then you can try some of the deeper techniques such as myofascial, deep tissue or sports massage. For Lymies, I think the best massage practitioners are the ones who will know the right balance and tailor the massage to what they feel in your body that day. They won't use so little pressure that you feel like you didn't even get a massage, and they won't use so much that it takes you days to recover and leaves you feeling stiff, sore or tired. If you can find a therapist that works with Lyme disease, that would be ideal. Otherwise, those that do oncology massage or specialise in lymphatic or more balancing and healing types of massages are usually the best. Keep trying until you find the perfect practitioner for you.

Some of the many benefits of massage include:

❖ Improves lymphatic flow and detoxification

❖ Releases emotions / mental stress

❖ Enhances metabolism and circulation

❖ Increases blood's oxygen capacity by 10–15%

❖ Helps to loosen contracted, shortened muscles

❖ Stimulates weak, flaccid muscles

Be sure to drink plenty of water and rest after your massage to get the best healing effects. Remember, massage, even a gentle one, can increase detoxification, so it can help you if you are Herxing, but can also exacerbate or even contribute to a Herx.

Chiropractic

As you know by now, I am a chiropractor. I did kinesiology seminars in NET (neuro-emotional technique), TBM (Total Body Modification) and NAET (allergy elimination technique) whilst I was studying chiropractic, and that's where my love of kinesiology and holistic healing really flourished. I also studied musculoskeletal acupuncture and later became a doula (birth assistant), as I found this helped support my pregnant clients much better.

I think it is really important to keep your spine healthy all the time, but it's more important when you are sick, and even more so when you have any type of chronic disease. As many of you know, Lyme can attack any system in your body, and guess what controls and coordinates every system in your body? That's right. It's the nervous system. Although chiropractic is primarily known for neck and back pain, holistic or wellness chiropractors should also be known as nervous system doctors.

It is interesting to note that whenever I saw doctors, dentists, chiropractors or osteopaths, they were always really surprised to find that I was neurologically sound and musculo-skeletally functioning well, even though I had so many symptoms that were neurological (especially brain fog, memory loss and sight disturbances). I believe my body was functioning well from a neurological and musculoskeletal perspective due to having weekly chiropractic nervous system checks (and adjustments, if needed). I have been adjusted regularly (at least once a month) since my early twenties. I realised then that if my pelvis and spine were aligned, then my scoliosis and leg length issues weren't a problem and didn't cause me any pain.

In my teens I experienced seven years of constant low back and right hip pain, despite going to physiotherapy and massage often multiple times a week and stretching twice a day. I saw a chiropractor who prescribed foot orthotics (with a heel lift on my short leg side) and rehabilitation exercises for me, and did a series of adjustments (after x-rays were taken), combined with soft tissue work. This holistic approach not only alleviated all my pain, but improved so many other symptoms, like my digestion and breathing!

I think one of the biggest factors in healing is feeling loved and heard. Once I know someone, I can easily adjust and treat them in a few minutes, but if the client is rushing to the clinic, in the room for 2–5 minutes and being rushed out again, how relaxing or healing can that really be? Will I, or any of their practitioners have time to find out what's going on with them beyond a superficial level? Will the client feel loved and positive that we are helping them? So when you choose a chiropractor or any health care clinic / practitioner, how will you know when you are in the right place? You will walk in and the energy will feel right. You will be welcomed by someone who genuinely cares that you are there, your practitioner will know what's going on in your life and your treatment, and a care plan will be tailored individually for you.

If you are lucky enough to live in Sydney, then you will have access to our amazing Health Space Clinics and Lyme-literate practitioners. At Health Space our experienced and passionate chiropractors combine their 5-year training and skills, including a Master's of Chiropractic, with a range of other techniques to ensure you are getting the most up-to-date treatments and the most for your money. We have the most advanced digital gait scanning equipment (including orthotic prescription) and x-ray facilities at most clinics, including on-the-spot Medicare and private health fund rebates to make it easy for you. Many of the chiropractors have extra training and qualifications in a range of techniques including the rehabilitation skills of a physiotherapist, the soft tissue techniques of an osteopath and massage therapist, kinesiology (AK, TBM, NET and NIS) and dry needling / musculoskeletal acupuncture. These are combined to ensure that you have effective and enjoyable treatments every time! There are many chiropractors who work like this, so ask and shop around until you find the practitioner that is exactly right for you.

Each care plan at Health Space and many other chiropractic clinics around the world are individually designed and may also include other tests and choices of treatments aimed at increasing the value of each session and improving your overall quality of health including:

❖ PH testing

❖ Zinc testing

❖ Referral for blood tests

❖ Rehab exercises and stretch programs

❖ Functional injury prevention testing

❖ Pillow and bed advice

❖ Dietary advice – including recipes, supplement prescriptions & detox recommendations

- ❖ Gait scan and an orthotic prescription

- ❖ Soft tissue and trigger point techniques

- ❖ Dry needling / musculoskeletal acupuncture

- ❖ Hot and cold packs

- ❖ Strapping

Chiropractic may help Lymies with:

- ❖ Neck and back pain

- ❖ Headaches and migraines

- ❖ Neurological pain including sciatica

- ❖ Disc injuries and nerve pain / palsies

- ❖ Joint injuries – hip, knee, shoulder, elbow, fingers and wrist pain

- ❖ Repetitive strain injuries – e.g., carpal tunnel syndrome

- ❖ Tendinitis – Achilles, golfer's and tennis elbow

- ❖ Scoliosis management

- ❖ Postural correction

- ❖ Bell's palsy

- ❖ Improving sleep (by deactivating the sympathetic nervous system)

What Is the Difference Between a Chiropractor, an Osteopath and a Physiotherapist?

Honestly there isn't much difference between a well-trained and passionate practitioner in any of these fields. Did you know that chiropractors and osteopaths originally trained together for the same degree and Master's? That's why many of the older practitioners call themselves osteopaths and chiropractors; it's not because they have done two degrees and Master's programs, but because they have a choice under the grandfather clause to call themselves one or the other or both!

It's an age-old question, "Should I see a chiropractor or an osteopath or a physiotherapist?" It seems to be one of those things that everyone one way or the other will have an opinion on, usually based on previous success or sometimes lack of success with a particular technique or person. Or even just hearsay!

What works best for a particular injury or problem is dependent upon the type of injury and the causative factors of that injury. The aim of treatment and a rehabilitation program should be to ensure optimal healing in the fastest possible time but also to correct for any underlying causes and imbalances that may have contributed to the injury in the first place. Failure to address and fix the causative factors often results in re-injury, often multiple times in the future. When done properly, a good rehabilitation program should result in not just faster healing, but also more strength, more stability and less likelihood of re-injury.

In a nutshell, physiotherapists usually target a specific injury or pain and are trained in a pain-based model similar to medicine. Many doctors refer to physiotherapists more so than chiropractors and osteopaths, as they work in the same pain-based model. Basically, physiotherapists are trained to look at an injury or pain and treat what is occurring in that area; if someone has tendinitis in the knee, they treat the tendinitis in the knee. Treatment modalities include ultrasound, TENS machines, strengthening and stretching exercises, muscle release techniques and massage. Some physiotherapists even do manipulation now, although the amount of training in their course is significantly less than that of a chiropractor or osteopath.

Chiropractic and osteopathy, on the other hand, usually look at the body as a whole, no matter what the complaint / injury / pain that a client presents with. Their focus is to find the underlying cause of the problem and the factors that may be overloading the body and the injury as well as what's slowing or stopping the body from healing itself as it's designed to do. Chiropractors are well-known as the "back and neck doctors," but the real reason chiropractors look to the spine is to see how well the nerves are exiting between the spinal joints and communicating with not just the muscles, but the skin and the organs that control EVERYTHING we do! Once a cause is identified and x-rays are taken (if required), treatment will include techniques to adjust or correct these misalignments in order to take pressure off the nervous system so the body can heal itself. This may be done manually where you may hear a gas sound pop out of the joint when you're being adjusted or with gentler techniques such as an activator (a special implement that applies a measured and gentle force) or special tables that drop up and down to increase functional movement in the spine.

Chiropractors and osteopaths are generally trained more holistically. If someone presents with knee pain, they would look at the entire body to ascertain whether it was a primary knee problem or a secondary problem, such as inflammation in the knee due to issues elsewhere in the body (e.g., misaligned pelvis, feet issues, agluteal muscle not firing properly on one side). Chiropractors are trained to take, refer for and read x-rays, whereas osteopaths can only refer and read them, and physiotherapists are trained only to read them. In my opinion a good physiotherapist is the best at rehabbing injuries and post-operative care. Chiropractors and osteopaths are better at looking to the spine and the whole body for the CAUSE of the problem in order to correct it and prevent it from coming back rather than just treating symptoms every time they arise. Having said that, I know physiotherapists who are amazing at looking at the body as a whole for diagnosing and treating in that holistic model and many chiropractors and osteopaths who are very pain-based, only focussing on the area that hurts or, even worse, thinking they can adjust the neck and fix anything in the body.

So once again, ask around and even try different practitioners until you find a practitioner or, ideally, a group of various practitioners who can help you and you are happy with. At the end of the day, the treatment should be therapeutic and the experience enjoyable (most of the time anyway!). If you don't like the cracking sound when being adjusted, then go to a low-force practitioner who uses techniques like Sacro-Occipital Technique (SOT) or Thompson drop piece, activator, dry needling, kinesiology and/or soft tissue techniques. About 10% of my clients don't get adjusted manually because they don't like the clicking and cracking sounds. About 30% don't get their neck manually adjusted either because they don't like it or it's contraindicated. There are lots of ways to achieve the same outcome, so the more skills a practitioner has and the more seminars they have done, the more likely it is that they will be able to help you!

Common Myths Surround Chiropractic

It is important to understand what chiropractic is (and isn't) so you can make an informed choice of whether it is for you. Visit the Chiropractors' Association of Australia website (CAA) at www.chiropractors.asn.au for more information and research on the importance and validity of chiropractic care.

"CHIROPRACTORS CRACK BONES."

Contrary to popular belief, the cracking or popping sound you hear when you have an adjustment is not bones cracking or cartilage popping. It is actually a pressure change in the joint that causes the fluid surrounding the joint to move into a gaseous state (explained as a nitrogen bubble), which creates a sound as this pressure change occurs. Chiropractors believe that by aligning the spine and joints and relieving pressure off the nervous system, the body can then do what it was designed to do— heal itself.

"CHIROPRACTORS DEAL WITH BONES AND JOINTS WHEREAS OSTEOPATHS AND PHYSIOTHERAPISTS DEAL WITH THE MUSCLES."

This is a common comment I hear! "I tore my muscle or I have tendinitis so a chiropractor can't help me." Close your eyes for a second and imagine all the muscles in your body. What do they attach to? How do your muscles work? If you can't imagine it in your head, Google it! Your muscles attach to bones. Your bones create levers that help your muscles do their job. The muscles are fired by the nervous system! So looking at the muscles in isolation may help the pain short-term, but it is unlikely to fix the problem long-term! Without the whole bony structure and the nervous system, muscles are useless! Getting my drift yet? It's unlikely that you have a muscle problem without a joint and even a nerve problem.

For example, imagine you have a recurrent tight, sore hamstring that is constantly being strained or torn when you sprint. It is okay to jog, but as soon as you start doing agility work or speed work, it spasms and gets inflamed. If you continue to train when it's inflamed, it tears. So, why is only one hamstring the problem? If it was due to the training load, wouldn't they both be sore? If you stretch, ice, rest or massage the hamstring, it feels better, but as soon as you start training it hurts again. Have you fixed the problem? Probably not! Let's take a step back and think about what else could be causing a recurrent one-sided hamstring strain. Here is my immediate list of things to check:

Feet – are they hyper-pronating (rolling in too much), hyper-supinating (rolling out too much) or functioning the same on each side? What happens when the muscles and ligaments of the foot / ankle are fatigued? What are the three arches doing? Is the footwear fitted correctly? Are orthotics necessary?

Pelvis and sacrum balance – if one side of the pelvis is tilted, rotated or twisted, it will cause strain on the hamstring (as the hamstrings attach to the ischial tuberosity (sit bone) located on the pelvic girdle.

Lower back or sacrum – if there are misalignments in these joints, it can cause impingement on the nerves that supply the hamstring (i.e., the hamstring muscle is not getting the message from the nerve to contract, so the muscle does not activate properly and, therefore, fatigues too quickly. Long story short, the hamstring on that side becomes overworked, inflamed and strained.

Gluteal firing – if the glutes (butt muscles) aren't firing optimally and first (one side or both), then the hamstring has to fire too early; it is not designed to take that much strain, so it becomes overworked and injured (glutes are the biggest muscle in your body and should fire first when a person is running, not only because it's the most efficient way to run / move, but it protects the hamstrings).

You get the picture. Resolving injuries by looking to the entire body, including bones, muscles, tendons (where the muscle attaches to the bone), ligaments (structures that attach bone to bone) and your nerves, improves your chances not just of a quick recovery, but one that lasts! With Lyme disease, many muscles, tendons, ligaments and joints get inflamed. If you are always treating the pain, you will find that you will be chasing your tail. If you have a holistic practitioner who is treating the cause of the symptoms, you will not just save yourself a lot of pain, but also money!

"CHIROPRACTIC IS DANGEROUS – IF YOUR NECK IS CRACKED THE WRONG WAY, IT COULD PARALYSE YOU OR CAUSE A STROKE."

Spinal adjustments have been shown to improve mobility in the neck, restore range of motion, decrease or relieve hypertonicity (tight muscles), and relieve pressure and tension. As with any risk, you need to weigh up the risk of the procedure versus the risk of not doing it (or the risk of other activities that you do that may have a higher risk). For example, research shows that taking a Panadol® is 100 times more dangerous than having a cervical (neck) adjustment, but I am sure that many people have never even considered the risk of taking Panadol®. The safety and efficacy of the chiropractic adjustment has undergone significant scrutiny and been assessed extensively. Over the last 25+ years, at least five formal government studies from around the world have found spinal adjustments to be safe, effective and cost-effective. If you want more information and scientific evidence, go to http://chiropractors.asn.au/about-chiropractic/fact-sheets and download the Chiropractic Safety Fact Sheet. (Fact Sheet-Is Chiropractic Safe? n.d.)

At the time of writing this book, strokes are Australia's second biggest killer after coronary heart disease, and they're the leading cause of disability. Despite the fact that someone in Australia will have a stroke every 10 minutes or less, there is no reference to neck adjustment as a factor contributing to stroke in any of the Stroke Foundation literature in Australia, the UK or the US. Studies show the risk of a cervical (neck) adjustment causing a stroke to be between 1 in 1,000,000 and 1 in 5,000,000. In comparison, did you know that taking birth control pills has a risk of causing stroke in 1 in 24,000? NSAIDS (pharmaceutical anti-inflammatories) have a risk of 1 in 1,200 persons! How often have you slipped a Celebrex® or Mobic® tablet and, without realising it, significantly increased your risk of stroke? 1 in 145 cervical spinal surgeries end in stroke! The risk of stroke from playing soccer is 1 in 25,000! You do the math! If you want more information and scientific evidence, log onto www.chiropractors.asn.au and download the neck adjustment fact sheet, "Neck Adjustment: Benefits and Safety." I encourage you to do your own research beyond that if you still have concerns. (Fact Sheet-Neck Adjustment Safety and Benefits n.d.)

The other important point to mention is that in the few instances mentioned in the literature that report a "chiropractic adjustment" as the cause of a stroke, I have not found a study that indicated a chiropractor actually delivered that adjustment. It was usually a medical doctor. Remember that chiropractors do a much higher level of anatomy (they study neuro-anatomy) and complete, on average, about 5000 more hours of training in spinal manipulation than medical doctors. I know who I'd rather have crack my neck!

"CHIROPRACTORS HAVE A BAD REPUTATION."

Chiropractic sometimes does have a bad reputation, especially in the media. Like any profession, there are good and bad chiropractors. Every profession I can think of is like this! Think about it. If you went to the doctor and weren't happy with their diagnosis, what would you do? Go to another doctor, of course! If you had a massage that hurt you or wasn't very good, would you assume that all massage therapists are dangerous or useless? No, of course not! You would find another massage therapist. If you took your car to get serviced and they charged you a fortune and didn't fix the problem, would you say that you were never getting your car serviced again? That's ridiculous! You would ask your friends if they knew an honest mechanic and take your car there! So like anything else, the best way to find a good chiropractor (or any health professional for that matter) is to ask around and get a good recommendation.

"YOU HAVE TO GO TO THE CHIROPRACTOR FOR LIFE ONCE YOU START."

You don't have to do anything you don't want to do! Chiropractic is a lifestyle choice as well as a pain management and treatment option. Just like you brush your teeth everyday to prevent cavities and exercise to keep fit (hopefully), you also need to look after your spine and body. If someone told you that you only had to go to the personal trainer a few times and you would be fit for life, would you believe them? Of course not! We all know that fitness takes time to build up and that you need to exercise consistently to get the benefits. Our spines are no different. If we have an injury that builds up over time, then it takes time to get the body working optimally again. Is it reasonable to think that you can be exposed to physical stressors, such as sitting at school, the car or the office for hours a day; biochemical stressors such as food colouring / flavours / preservatives, pollution, medications; or mental stress such as relationship issues, low self-esteem, and financial troubles, and that your body will just function normally? We were designed to be hunters and gatherers, so the further you are from that lifestyle, the more time and money you'll need to spend to get your health back (at some stage anyway!).

"IF I DON'T HAVE ANY PAIN THEN THERE IS NO POINT GOING TO SEE A CHIROPRACTOR."

Just because you don't feel pain or have any symptoms doesn't mean you are healthy. For example, many people have no idea that a cavity is building in their tooth until one day it hits the nerve and BOOM, the pain is severe. Is it realistic to think that it was just what you did that day that caused the hole in your tooth and allowed the nerve to be exposed? No! It was all those times you forgot to brush your teeth or had a midnight snack or ate sugar. It was the accumulation of "letting things go" that broke down the enamel until the decay could reach the nerve. Many of our nerves are pain-sensitive, but if you have arthritis or mild decreased range of motion in your spine, you may never even know there's something wrong if you only depend on how you feel!

I believe everyone needs some sort of preventative health care treatment, whether it is physiotherapy, chiropractic or osteopathy. Other modalities will also help maintain and even optimise your health when everything is aligned. Most of my clients who work and exercise come in for monthly maintenance treatments regardless of how they are feeling. This is 12 treatments a year (as long as nothing else goes wrong!). If anyone injures themselves or gets sick, it's often going to take AT LEAST 12 treatments to fix it. So it's actually cheaper to have consistent maintenance care than to rehab yourself a few times a year when your body fails you! You will often heal quicker from an accident (e.g., a car accident) if your body was in good shape beforehand too. Have a think about it!

So How Does the Nervous System Actually Work?

The nervous system is broken into two categories: The Central Nervous System (CNS) and the Peripheral Nervous system (PNS), also known as the involuntary / autonomic / visceral nervous system. The CNS has two types of nerves: spinal nerves (which innervate most of the body and connect the spinal column to the spinal cord) and cranial nerves (which innervate the head and connect directly to the brain). The PNS connects the CNS to the organs, muscles, glands and blood vessels and it controls involuntary actions, such as the heart rate, digestion, salivation, perspiration, pupil dilation, micturition (urination), and sexual arousal, although we do have a degree of control over our breathing, swallowing, sexual arousal, heart rate and micturition.

To help you understand, imagine the nervous system as a map. The spinal cord is the main highway (a very quick, direct route) and the smaller nerves are the roads and back streets. These are coming to and from the brain. If you look at a nerve chart, you will see that exiting off the spinal cord are the peripheral nerves which end at the muscles, discs, tendons and ligaments, or an organ or group of organs. Nerves are either <u>afferent</u> (they carry information from sensory neurons in the periphery back to the CNS), <u>efferent</u> (they carry information from the CNS to motor neurons and target muscles and glands) or <u>mixed</u> (a mixture of sensory and motor information coming to and from the CNS). There may be physical / biochemical or emotional factors, such as swelling, infection, autoimmune disease, failure of blood vessels in the area, a pressure / injury to the nerve from muscle, bone and disc, or a direct injury, that can cause injury to the nerves and nervous system and, hence, affect the delivery of messages to and from the brain from the body.

Your nervous system is pretty amazing in that it singlehandedly coordinates EVERY function of the body. It is your nervous system that allows you to adapt and live in your environment, and it gives information to your body about what it needs to self-heal within that environment. Chiropractic is a holistic, safe and drug-free method of keeping your spine, nerves and immune system functioning optimally by removing interferences that cause disease (see Appendix E:9 for a chart summarising the nervous system).

Beyond Feeling Structurally Better, How Does Chiropractic Help People Heal Themselves?

So what does this mean for healing? If there are increased or decreased nerve signals going from our body to and from our brain, then the body can't communicate properly in order to keep you healthy; if the nervous system is impaired via nerve damage or pressure, then your immune system can't function optimally. That means invaders like microbes are more likely to pass by undetected or cause the body to work a lot harder to get rid of them. This is very important when you have a chronic illness like Lyme disease. Because the spirochetes can change forms and invade so many parts of the body, it's essential to be detoxing optimally and to have your immune system functioning at its best. Every time pressure is removed from a nerve or the nerve is stimulated via a chiropractic adjustment, it increases signals to the brain and helps the body (and immune system) to function optimally.

When you understand the philosophy of chiropractic, you will see that, although you do feel physically better after a chiropractic adjustment and treatment, there is so much more going on underneath. The original chiropractic philosophy was, "The power that created the body, heals the body." Our bodies are the most amazing creations in the world. How does a body heal a cut or create a baby in nine months? Innate intelligence is how. We all have innate knowledge inbuilt in us, with information on everything we need to grow and heal. Think about a simple cut. Do you need to think, "Ok, body, send clotting factors, send anti-inflammatories, right granulation tissue, start healing?" Of course not! Your body does it. I believe we have this power on a grander scale, too, but only if we give our body what it needs physically, biochemically, emotionally and spiritually to do its job.

Your body is robust and can withstand a lot of abuse as well as compensate and automatically make changes to adapt. Often health issues have been building for months or even years without pain or problems, although there may have been small warning signals, such as twinges, tiredness, rashes, and aches that we ignored or suppressed along the way. If someone kicks you in the shin, then it's an acute injury, and you know exactly how you developed that injury; the person who kicked you caused trauma. But some injuries and illnesses build up over time, so it can be difficult to determine and understand the cause. For example, you may have back pain that comes and goes over time. The pain could be attributed to many factors including birth trauma, years of heavy weight lifting with poor technique or many years sitting at a desk. What you may not realise is that the nerves causing the back pain are also affecting the organs that they are connected to. So, many people with back pain also have digestive issues and, consequently, impaired immune system function (as over 70% of the immune system is located within the digestive system). Your take-home message: If you always judge your health on how you FEEL, then you will never know how your body is really FUNCTIONING.

With any chronic illness like Lyme disease, you need your body to work and function at its best, and chiropractic can help with that in so many ways, for example, physically (improves blood flow, biomechanics, nerve flow), biochemically (assists balancing of hormones, digestion of nutrients, detoxification) and emotionally (release of endorphins which are your natural happy hormones). Many chiropractors have other skills they implement such as kinesiology, so if your chiropractor also does some kinesiology, then you can address even more physical / biochemical and emotional imbalances with that combination.

There is a lot of evidence now to support the mind-body connection. Believe it or not, there are people who have healed themselves just through the power of thought. I highly recommend reading *Dying to Be Me,* an inspiring book about a lady who had a four-year battle with cancer and when admitted to the hospital was pronounced physically dead by the doctors. According to the author (Moorjani 2012), she was *out of her body* but made the conscious decision to return to her body... and she lived! Once she *returned* to her body, she healed within just three weeks! The amazing thing about this lady is that she had all the medical reports, scans and blood tests both pre-and post-cancer, so it's a phenomenal story to see that the tumours that were detected many years ago, literally disappeared within three weeks! Though it's scientifically documented, it can't be explained! The book is a testament to the importance of the mind-body connection. Unfortunately not all of us have tapped into that power, so the best we can do is to utilise all the tools we have in our power right now in order to give our bodies a fighting chance to heal us. Adjustment anyone?

Naturopathy / Nutrition (including Bioimpedance Scans such as VLA and Live Blood Analysis)

A good nutritionist or naturopath is worth their weight in gold. If you can't get your nutrition right, it's unlikely that you will have a good functioning GIT (gastrointestinal tract), which means your immune system and detoxification capacity will be poor. If these are poor, it really doesn't matter what treatments or supplements you take because they are not going to work as effectively. In my opinion, steer clear of dietitians, as their advice is counterintuitive to healing. They still focus on the "healthy" food pyramid that I and many other health professionals agree is not the healthiest way to live. However, some dietitians do practice more like a naturopath / nutritionist, so finding out their beliefs before making a booking is important. I will discuss diet and nutrition more in the Biochemical Treatment chapter, but the following sections include some great tools that naturopaths and nutritionists use (other health care professionals can also have training in nutrition) that are very useful for diagnosis and objectively measuring your health.

Live Blood Analysis (LBA)

WHAT IS LBA?

LBA is a diagnostic test that is used to detect certain health conditions and diseases within your body and can give you an accurate idea about your overall state of health. A drop of blood is taken from your fingertip and immediately put on a glass slide to be observed under a special microscope called a dark field microscope. The image from the microscope is then projected onto a screen to be studied. The practitioner will look at the size, shape, ratio and finer structures of the red blood cells, white blood cells, platelets and other structures. You are present during the analysis, so the practitioner will explain and show you the findings. It's fascinating!

WHAT INFORMATION CAN LBA PROVIDE?

Information that can be gleaned from observing your blood and the shape and size of your blood vessels includes: immune system function, possible vitamin deficiencies, toxicity, pH imbalances, mineral imbalances, fungus and yeast (mine showed huge amounts of Candida), poor nutritional status (e.g., malabsorption), oxidative stress and free radical damage, inflammation, health of the liver, heavy metal toxicity and whether your diet is too high in fats and acids.

WHY USE LBA?

LBA is a great tool to monitor your progress objectively and gain extra information about your health so you can be proactive, not reactive. LBA is designed to detect functional imbalances in the body (often before symptoms arise or show on blood tests) that can be potential precursors to disease. Changes to diet and lifestyle can be implemented and supplements tweaked or prescribed to reverse these changes and assist your body back to optimal health. Many medical practitioners will tell you that there is no research supporting LBA, but that doesn't mean it doesn't work. At the end of the day, you are looking at YOUR live blood and determining what should and shouldn't be there! The more skilled the practitioner, the more information you will get; it's hard to make things up when the information is right in front of you! Live blood picked up my Candida infection and my husband's heavy metal's load (which we had tested in the lab to confirm), so I believe it is a great tool.

Bioimpedance and VLA (Vitality, Longevity and Healthy Ageing) Screening

At Health Space we use a bioimpedance machine called VLA.

WHAT IS BIOIMPEDANCE?

Bioimpedance is the response of a living organism to an externally applied electric current. It is a non-invasive way of objectively measuring the internal body such as blood flow and body composition.

WHAT IS VLA?

VLA stands for Vitality, Longevity and Healthy Ageing and is a bioimpedance device that generates a living record of the patient's key physiological and biological markers of ageing. It is quick and painless.

HOW IS VLA USED?

First, measurements such as height, weight, wrist and waist circumference are taken (It is best to rest for a few minutes before the scan and to do the scan lying down). Then, two electrodes are placed on the wrist and ankle on one side of the body. Once they are in place, a current is run through the body and a reading is transmitted to a hand-held device. This reading along with the other data is entered into a special program that calculates your results within seconds. This is all very quick and painless.

<u>WHAT INFORMATION DO I RECEIVE FROM THE VLA SCAN?</u>

You'll receive information on <u>active tissue mass quality</u> (quality of the muscle, cellular function and general energy levels), <u>active tissue mass</u> (amount of metabolically active tissue including nerves, organs, visceral and skeletal muscles), <u>fat distribution index</u> (can predict the risk of a range of conditions including cardiovascular disease and metabolic syndrome), <u>cellular fluid balance</u> (indicates the body's ability to regulate fluids), <u>phase angle</u> (quantity / quality of active tissue and is the key to health and ageing), and <u>bio age</u> (the age your body thinks it is due to its function and lifestyle rather that chronological age!)

<u>WHY USE VLA?</u>

The chronic degenerative diseases of ageing are now known to be partly due to genetic inheritance but mostly due to our lifestyle. By adopting a particular pattern of activity and eating, it is possible for anyone to positively or negatively affect the ageing process and, subsequently, their functional capacity and vitality. VLA will help identify areas in your body that are under stress and give you guidelines to change your lifestyle in order to minimise or eliminate these effects on your body. The effectiveness of implemented lifestyle changes, such as nutrition, hydration and exercise, can be seen on subsequent scans. As VLA is quick, cheap and easy, it's a great tool for monitoring and motivating yourself to make the changes and sustain them.

Bowen Therapy

History of Bowen Therapy

Bowen Therapy is known by lots of different names including the Bowen technique, fascial kinetics, Smart Bowen, Neurostructural Integration (NST), Fascial Bowen and Bowenwork. Bowen is named after an Australian practitioner called Thomas Ambrose Bowen, who died in 1982 as an unrecognised practitioner of manual therapy (he did not document his technique). However, years later the technique was named, officially used and popularised by six men who had observed him work. If you can't find a good Bowen therapist, I suggest you try NST, another technique which was inspired from Bowen. (Nixon-Livy 2015)

What Is Bowen Therapy?

It is a holistic and multidimensional approach to pain relief and healing that requires finding and correcting problems in the soft tissue or fascia, a specific type of connective tissue that surrounds every tissue in the body in a three-dimensional structure (including nerves, bones, muscles and veins). Therefore, any adhesions or dysfunction in the fascial layers can disturb or affect any structure, muscle, nerve or organ within the body. Fascia is believed to be the largest sensory organ in the body due to its abundant range of receptors and can, therefore, powerfully influence neuromuscular physiology.

What Does Bowen Therapy / Treatment Involve?

As with any profession, the technique can be used with a variety of personal interpretations. Generally, each session involves the practitioner using their hands to apply gentle, rolling motions along the muscles and tendons in order to affect the fascia. Distinctive features include the gentle nature of the technique (often you feel like it is so gentle that nothing could possibly result from it!) and the distinct pauses incorporated into the treatment. It is believed that these pauses allow the body to reset itself. (Bowen technique 2015)

How Does Bowen Therapy Help Lymies?

Through specific soft tissue and fascial releases, specific receptors are stimulated that allow the body to correct dysfunctions and restore homeostasis (balance). It is particularly helpful for those affected by muscle and joint pain, and decreased lymphatic flow. The therapy is also very gentle; even if you are in a lot of pain, the sessions are tolerable and even enjoyable. Bowen treats the whole body, and its healing effects often go above-and-beyond pain relief to include increased energy, decreased stress, improved sleep, and emotional release and healing.

Rife Therapy

Rife therapy is based on the premise that all living organisms have a frequency. Energy healing medicine works on a similar premise: if the various frequencies within the body are disrupted (physically, chemically or emotionally) and not restored, then this can lead to imbalance and disease. Frequencies are hard to understand because they can't be seen. For example, you can hear your radio playing, but you can't see the radio waves. Just because you can't see the radio waves doesn't mean they don't exist. Another example is where certain pitched sounds that you can't see have the ability to shatter glass.

The body is more subtle. While no one disputes radio waves exist or work to produce sound, there are many people who express doubt as to the efficacy of vibration within the human body and whether this vibration affects your overall health. However, your body, including your organs and the living organisms inside your body, all have their own ideal frequency or vibration. Microorganisms (including bacteria, yeast and viruses) have their own frequency, so for example Rife therapy works by exposing unfavourable microbes to a MOR or *mortal oscillatory rate* that either deactivates or kills them.

The Rife machine was developed by Dr. Royal Raymond Rife in the early 20th century. It is believed that many doctors were using Rife as a therapy during this time, and there was scientific research validating the efficacy of the Rife machine to rid the body of infectious microbes. Unfortunately, there is a lot of missing information and missing records that are believed to have been hidden or "lost" by those (notably in the drug companies, as this was around the time penicillin was first discovered) who did not want the Rife machine rivalling their drug treatments. Whether this is true or not, there is very little documented information as to what sorts of Rife machines or frequencies were used to treat or even cure the body of pathenogenic, microbe-driven diseases.

About 50 years later, Doug Maclean, a Lyme sufferer, stumbled upon the knowledge that certain frequencies have the ability to disable and kill infectious microbes. With conventional medicine failing him, he created his own makeshift lab and Rife machine, and using a dark field microscope studied the effects of different frequencies on Borrelia spirochetes (which he had obtained from a friend who worked in a biomedical research lab). Maclean showed that applying certain electromagnetic fields to the spirochetes could kill them! While he was completing this study, he started having Herxes. He eventually realised that by being within the vicinity of the testing and exposing himself to the frequencies, the frequencies produced a die-off effect within his own body! Long story short, he continued to experiment, build bigger machines and eventually developed frequencies that are known today as the modern Rife machines we see and use. And he cured himself!

Types of Rife Machines

There are many types of Rife machines, but according to Bryan Rosner (Rosner 2005), there are five that he would recommend as effective for fighting infection. They are the Doug machine, the Experimental Electro-Magnetic machine (EMEM), the High Power Magnetic Pulser, the AC Contact machine and the Resonant Light PERL machine. Learn more about Rife machines at www.royalrife.com. It's a private site, so you have to become a member first.

My main concern with Rife is that you are submitting yourself to electromagnetic radiation. However, I believe that the benefits I gained from the treatments outweighed the risks and side effects from the exposure. Read the book *Lyme Disease and Rife Machines* by Bryan Rosner to get the full picture. Visit this website for a list of frequencies that can be used with a Rife machine to treat Borrelia: http://www.lymeprotocol.com/assets/pdf/rife%20freaks%20appendix.pdf

Ozone Therapy

Ozone Therapy is the use of ozone gas (O^3), a molecule that contains three oxygen atoms, to help alleviate or treat the symptoms of certain medical conditions. Ozone therapy has been used for a long time and dates back at least as far as World War I. German soldiers who had severe gangrene were treated by having the affected body part placed in a plastic bag filled with medical ozone. The first ozone machine was developed in the 19th century by Dr. Joachim Hansler, and ozone was first inserted into the bloodstream around the 1940s by Dr. H. Wolff (now known as autohemotherapy). Ozone is even being used in pool systems now.

How Does Ozone Therapy Work for Lyme Disease?

Ozone therapy is believed to deactivate microbes, such as bacteria, yeast, fungi and protozoa, whilst also fuelling oxygen metabolism and boosting the immune system. Ozone therapy is believed to be helpful for people with Lyme disease for the following reasons:

❖ Potential to deactivate the Bb bacteria and co-infections

❖ Assist with the treatment of opportunistic infections such as candidiasis (yeast)

❖ Oxygenise the environment, as it is believed that Bb do not thrive or even survive in high oxygen environments

❖ Boost an already depleted immune system by stimulating white blood cell production and releasing cytokines that assist the body to fight the infection

❖ Facilitate the elimination of free radicals and neurotoxins caused by the die-off of the bacteria!

❖ Aid and support a number of vital functions in the human body

How Is Ozone Therapy Administered?

The most common applications of ozone can be broken down into systemic methods (direct, intra-arterial or venous, rectal insufflation, and major and minor autohemotherapy) or topical applications. The most widely used application for Lyme disease is major auto-hemotherapy, which is used by the St. Georg Lyme and Cancer Klinik in Germany.

MAJOR AUTOHEMOTHERAPY (MAHT)

MAHT involves the use of a butterfly needle to extract blood into a glass container. Ozone and oxygen are carefully infused into that blood, and then the blood is fed back into the body using an IV drip method. As long as your veins are not compromised, the process can take anywhere from 20 minutes to an hour. (Viebahn-Haensler 2002)

Exercise Physiology and Rehabilitation Programs

According to Wikipedia, "Exercise physiology is the study of acute responses and chronic adaptations to a wide range of physical exercise conditions." Exercise physiologists may be able to help Lyme disease sufferers because they understand "the effect of exercise on pathology and the mechanisms by which exercise can reduce or reverse disease progression" (or, alternately, how exercise can make people sicker if they are not doing the right thing). (Exercise Physiology n.d.)

It is my belief that no matter what treatment protocol people are using, it will be hard to fully recover without a properly implemented exercise and rehabilitation program. Enlisting the help of an exercise physiologist or Lyme-literate, exercise-related practitioner will not only help motivate and support you, but will also play a pivotal role in your recovery. If you can't afford an exercise physiologist, see your local doctor. In Australia your GP can refer you for five visits under the Allied Health, Enhanced Primary Care program (EPC – covered 100% by Medicare) and at least get you started.

Important Points to Remember About Exercise and Lyme Disease

❖ Bb (and many infectious bacteria) do not like heat, so raising your body temperature can be helpful in more ways than just fitness!

❖ Bb can die if exposed to oxygen (even small amounts), and exercising increases oxygen levels in the body (including the tissue).

❖ Exercising increases lymphatic flow and circulation which assists detoxification.

❖ There is T-cell suppression for 12–24 hours after anaerobic exercise (which then rebounds), so never exercise two days in a row if you are immunosuppressed.

❖ It's best to start with one session a week and build up as your stamina and tolerance increase. Progressively overload your program, as it's better to do too little than overdo it and put yourself in a fatigue hole again. Then you won't be able to do anything!

❖ Avoid aerobic activity as this will suppress your immune system further (this can be implemented when fully recovered).

❖ If you are too tired or weak to exercise, then you could try using a TENS machine (electrical stimulation) and/or have someone perform passive physical therapy on you, such as massage, stretching, range of motion exercises for the joints, heat and ultrasound.

❖ Always have a rest or sleep after exercise so your body can recoup and recover quicker.

❖ Don't exercise if you are Herxing.

❖ Ideally, exercise sessions should last an hour – decrease intensity in order to reach an hour, if necessary.

❖ Remain hydrated before, during and after exercise.

Magnetic Therapy

The St. Georg Klinik in Germany, where I went for treatment, used magnetic therapy. In Australia, you won't hear much about it, but it's definitely something to look into. A great website to check out, which includes articles about electromagnetic therapy as well as the use of magnetic mattresses and overlays, is http://www.shokos.com/science.htm created by Dr. Dean Bonlie. He has some great information and research on how magnetic therapy can assist the repair of nerves and stem cells, which can really help Lymies who have a lot of neurological symptoms. Magnets have been used for 1000s of years and, whilst there are a lot of gimmicky ones for sale, there is no denying the amazing results of good quality magnets. They've been used to decrease swelling, improve the oxygen-carrying capacity of the blood, improve blood flow and circulation, increase the uptake of nutrients into the cells and supercharge cell repair and regeneration. Magnets are definitely not going to hurt you, so it's worth giving them a try. They are also implicated in grounding and offsetting the harmful effects of EMR.

SUPPORTIVE TREATMENTS

Far Infrared Sauna

I bought an infrared sauna for personal use and put it in my clinic at Mona Vale so everyone could enjoy it. They are not as expensive as you would think either, and not too expensive to run. As our clinics grow and expand, we are adding more infrared saunas, including now in the Potts Point and Bondi Junction clinics. In the following sections, I have summarised some information from *The Holistic Handbook of Sauna Therapy* by Nenah Sylver, Ph.D. (Sylver 2003)

So What Is an Infrared Sauna Compared to Any Other Sauna?

Traditional saunas are basically a room with a heater. The heat is generated by burning wood, a gas stove, hot rocks from a fire, an electric coil or a gas heater. These saunas operate at high temperatures but only heat the surface of the body, mainly by convection. They were originally designed for drug and alcohol detoxification.

Far infrared heaters, on the other hand, are heated by metallic or ceramic elements that emit a narrow spectrum of mainly far infrared energy. They were introduced in the early 1980s and use radiant energy that heats the body from the inside as well as the surface. Research shows that the infrared can penetrate about 3.5–4cm into the body, and for this reason, they get great results at much lower temperatures. Not only is the cooler temperature more comfortable for people, but far infrared also cleanses the tissues more effectively. The heat is not just effective for bacteria die-off (by creating an artificial fever) but has a whole host of other detoxification effects, as it allows the skin to detoxify toxins (including heavy metals) more effectively, essentially taking pressure off the internal detoxification organs.

In many infrared saunas, there is the option to turn on the colour therapy, which is an ancient and often highly effective healing modality. Different spectrums of light provide different healing qualities, including the nourishment of vital organs, emotional release and the movement of chi / vital energy from the head down the body (where we are often deficient) to improve one's healing capacity.

How Does an Infrared Sauna Help Your Health?

Saunas provide many benefits. In Australia, saunas are not used as regularly as in other parts of the world to improve health. In many

European countries, there are health recovery centres that include saunas to improve healing, recovery and the optimisation of health. Some of the many benefits include:

❖ Releases heavy metals, chemicals, radioactive particles and other toxins via the sweat

❖ Improves circulation

❖ Enhances immune system function

❖ Relieves internal congestion

❖ Destroys pathogenic microbes (bacteria, viruses, tumours, fungi, parasites)

❖ Gives the body the effect of gentle exercise without the exertion

❖ Relaxes tight muscles

❖ Cleanses the skin

❖ Heals infections

❖ Improves alkalinity of your system

❖ Improves your DNA

❖ Decreases swelling in the body

❖ Normalises enzymatic function

❖ Assists weight loss programs

❖ Fights ageing by boosting the metabolism and releasing toxins

❖ Reduces stress by inhibiting the sympathetic nervous system (fright / flight system)

❖ Balances the autonomic nervous system to enhance parasympathetic activity (rest / digest) which is essential for healing

Phases of Healing in an Infrared Sauna

The effects occur in two phases:

PHASE 1 – the body temperature remains at basal level and sweating is minimal to light. Although tissue heating occurs, the body is able to dissipate the extra heat by increasing circulation and shunting blood to the skin in order to release heat instead of increasing body temperature.

> **Phase 1 sauna effects** – *inhibition of sympathetic nervous system (stress), light sweating, pain relief, improved circulation due to dilation of blood vessels, improved oxygenation, muscle relaxation, improved flexibility of tendons and ligaments, internal organ congestion relief.*

PHASE 2 (AFTER 10–30 MINUTES*) – the body can no longer dissipate the heat of the sauna which causes the body temperature to rise. Heart rate and sweating increase, and blood is shunted to the surface more forcefully. It can recreate the feeling of a fever including the lightheadedness and labored breathing. Start slow and build up your tolerance, as the greatest effects occur in Phase 2 (*Note – Phase 2 begins at different times for different people and depends on your health and your acclimatisation to the sauna. If you want to know when *your* Phase 2 starts, you can measure your temperature, as basal temperature jumps up quite quickly once your body can no longer deal with the heat!). Most people have a basal or resting temperature around 37.5° C. Once you see your temperature jump above your resting temperature, then you know you have gone into Phase 2.

> **Phase 2 sauna effects** – *all the benefits of Phase 1 plus increased body temperature which hastens the death of weaker cells, increased heart rate and circulation, and disabling of pathogenic microorganisms.*

Do the Effects of the Sauna Continue Even After I Get Out?

Your temperature can stay elevated for up to 15 minutes after your sauna. If it suddenly drops back down to basal level, you may feel lightheaded or tired for 10–15 minutes. Therefore, resting for 10–15 minutes post-sauna is important to give your body a better opportunity to gradually return to normal functioning.

What Does Sauna Therapy Mean?

It means that you are following set protocols to achieve a specific healing goal, which is usually associated with regular use. Although you can use saunas any time, once a week is good for maintenance. To release toxic loads, a year of sauna therapy is often required, but intermittent use still has its benefits, of course. Those who are chronically ill often need a therapy program of at least 1 to 2 years.

How Do I Prepare for a Sauna Session?

❖ Ideally wait until 1–2 hours after a meal

❖ Drink at least half a litre of water BEFORE starting your sauna

❖ Bring multiple towels with you to sit on and wipe your sweat

❖ Bring your swimmers to wear if you are sharing the sauna

❖ Bring a bottle of water to sip on during the sauna

❖ Some saunas have a CD player so you can bring CD's with music / meditation / visualisations

❖ Remove all jewellery and as much of your clothing as possible to get the maximum effect of the infrared rays

Please note that you are detoxing even as the infrared sauna is heating up; you don't need to be uncomfortable or have the infrared sauna at the maximum heat to get the full benefits. Remember, the heat is NOT as hot as an air sauna, but the benefits are believed to be as good, if not better.

What Do I Do During a Sauna?

1. Ideally, move around every few minutes so different parts of your body are directly exposed to the infrared and colour panels.

2. Keep your hands open as much as possible, as many of the acupuncture and reflex points are on the palms of the hands.

3. If you feel lightheaded or dizzy, or your body releases odours that are unpleasant, open the door slightly or sit outside until it passes.

4. Relax and focus on your breathing at all times. The sauna is a great place to meditate and positively visualise.

5. Keep sipping your water throughout the session to remain hydrated.

What Do I Do After I Have Finished My Sauna?

1. Brush your skin, including the face and scalp, with a body brush or loafer if you have one.

2. If it is possible to shower, do so as soon as you get out in order to wash off any lingering toxins. Ideally, the shower should be cool to warm but preferably not hot (if you can't shower, just wipe yourself down with a wet towel).

3. Ideally, avoid using any soap, shampoo or moisturiser after your sauna as it can block up the lovely open pores of the skin and stop the post-sauna detox effect.

4. Drink another 500ml of water over 10–30 minutes.

5. Ideally try and rest for 10–30 minutes after your sauna. This helps transition the body back to homeostasis (balance) and decreases the chance of lightheadedness or fatigue later in the day / night.

6. You may need to replace vitamins and minerals, such as magnesium, potassium, zinc, omega-3 fatty acids and calcium, when you first start doing sauna therapy. See your health care professional for further information and testing.

7. Many health practitioners recommend taking kelp after a sauna to provide electrolyte and trace mineral replacement as well as assistance for internal detoxification processes.

When Is the Best Time to Have a Sauna?

Anytime is fine. However, research supports having a sauna first thing in the morning or just before bed to be more effective. This is because the autonomic nervous system is usually less stressed so the healing effects are often greater during these times.

Can I Have a Sauna on My Own?

Yes, it is safe to have a sauna on your own. However, if you are chronically ill or feel nervous, then it's best to bring a friend or family member with you. They can join you!

Are There Any Cautions or Contraindications for Sauna Use?

Not really, but young children and the elderly as well as those with the following conditions require extra care when using a sauna:

❖ Hypertension

❖   Dental amalgams

❖   Past use of LSD or other psychotropic drugs

❖   Multiple Sclerosis

❖   Respiratory conditions

❖   Acute infections

❖   Lymph node removal

❖   Diabetes

❖   Prostheses, silicone implants or metallic pins

❖   Sensory nerve damage

❖   Pregnancy and breastfeeding

❖   Chronically ill

❖   Anyone taking pharmaceutical medications

*Saunas are not recommended during pregnancy

Am I Likely to Have Any Reactions After the Sauna?

Healthy people generally don't have too many reactions. Anyone that is toxic in any way (surprisingly, most of us are) or sick can have what we call a healing reaction. Symptoms include but are not limited to:

❖   Fatigue

❖   Aches and pains

❖   Rashes

- ❖ Bowel symptoms (usually increased)

- ❖ Odours – can be from your breath, sweat or vaginal / seminal discharge

- ❖ Computer sensitivity

Are Their Specific Protocols for Sauna Use?

The key is to determine your goal before you start a sauna therapy program. Using a sauna sporadically will help, but you aren't going to achieve any long-lasting results that way. Anyone who has a chronic illness, a very stressful lifestyle, or is undergoing weight loss or detoxification will particularly benefit from a regular sauna program. Combining sauna use with other health care modalities, such as massage, chiropractic, naturopathy, acupuncture, counseling, herbal medicine, Pilates and yoga is ideal.

General Protocol for Lyme and Chronic Disease

1. Start with 20–30 minutes 3–7 times a week for 3–12 months (if you're really sick, then start with 5–15 minutes).

2. Slowly build up to 60 minutes for each session.

3. Once you can do 60 minutes (ideally daily), you should start doing saunas twice daily if you have the access and the time.

4. Resting or sleeping after you have had a sauna is recommended.

Hyperbaric Chamber Treatment (HBO, HBO2 or HBOT)

Oxygen in optimal quantities (if you have too much or too little, you will die) is one of the elements necessary for life, and it is also a key factor in healing. At sea level, the air we breathe is about 20% oxygen and 80%

nitrogen (that includes trace amounts of other gases, including carbon dioxide). It is then circulated throughout the body and exhaled before the next breath is taken. This is why hyperbaric treatment can be really effective for healing and promoting optimal health.

What Is a Hyperbaric Chamber Treatment?

Hyper means "increase" and *baric* means "pressure." So, hyperbaric simply means an increase in pressure. Hyperbaric oxygen therapy (HBO2 or HBOT, for short), which is believed to supercharge the body's natural self-healing capacity, is a system that delivers oxygen under high pressure. This system mimics the effect you get at altitude (above sea level) where there is increased atmospheric pressure. In other words, more oxygen is breathed in and saturating the body.

What Is HBO2 Used for?

HBOT is used for biologically repairing and regenerating human tissue and is approved for use in acute medical emergencies, such as carbon monoxide poisoning, decompression sickness (which occurs when deep sea divers rise to the surface too quickly and is also known as the bends), gas gangrene, and air embolism (when a blood vessel is obstructed by an air bubble, which can happen in IV therapy). Mild hyperbaric therapy is still being researched but is used in hospitals to treat nervous system and neurological issues such as stroke and brain injuries.

Athletes often travel to high altitude locations during the off-season to train in the increased oxygen in order to improve their training outcomes. Often, athletes are known to use HBO2 for similar effects without having to travel to high altitudes (although sitting in high altitudes via HBOT versus training in high altitudes is not believed to be as effective). HBO2 is also believed to decrease healing time for injury and illness and create a feeling of well-being, which is great for athletes, the general public and, of course, the chronically ill.

Why Is HBOT Treatment Recommended for Lyme Disease Sufferers?

In America HBOT is FDA-approved for a long list of treatments, including Lyme disease. In Australia HBOT is not TGA-approved (Therapeutic Goods Association) for Lyme disease, so clinics and hospitals with hyperbaric chambers CAN'T advertise their use for the treatment of Lyme disease (which is why you won't see much literature on it), but that doesn't mean you can't use it as part of your treatment plan. Increased oxygen, whilst having a positive healing effect on the body, is especially important for Lyme disease sufferers, as it is well-known that Bb cannot survive or replicate in an oxygenated environment.

IT IS BELIEVED THAT HBOT WORKS BY: (Lombard 2008)

❖ Increasing and driving oxygen into infected cells which creates an oxygen rich environment that is not conducive for the Bb spirochete.

❖ Reviving and helping the cells regenerate.

❖ Helping the cells to function optimally.

❖ Providing antimicrobial action for co-infections, as many other "non-beneficial" microbes can't survive in a high oxygen environment (including viruses and mycoplasma).

❖ Assisting regeneration of neurological function (hence, why it's used for that purpose in hospitals).

❖ Increasing oxygenated plasma, which allows oxygen to be distributed at very high levels within muscle and body tissues where blood flow is often compromised. This not only disrupts Bb reproductive cycle but creates a die-off effect.

❖ Producing natural free radicals that create an antibiotic effect.

❖ Increasing new capillary formation to up-regulate the distribution and perfusion of antibiotics, anti-microbials and other anti-Bb treatments.

How Long Are HBOT Sessions?

Most sessions will last an hour. If you are really sick, then I suggest you start with a much shorter session and see how you tolerate it.

How Much Does HBOT Usually Cost, and How Often Would I Need to Go?

The cost for a session will vary, but it will usually be $90–$100/hr. To really get the benefits, you will need to go regularly. The schedule is ideally 2–3 times a week for a few months, and then at least once a week during remission and beyond, or for as long as possible whilst symptomatic. As Bb has a long life cycle, many experts agree that at least 40 treatments are necessary for HBOT to be effective. HBOT is very expensive, so it is not in the budget for everyone. However, most places will offer discount packages to help keep the costs down. The other option is to buy a hospital grade unit and use it at home.

Whilst many sessions are recommended to aid full recovery, initially doing a few weeks in a row and then having sporadic treatments when you can afford it will still help.

What Is the General Treatment Protocol?

It is best to work with a professional to design a treatment protocol specifically for you. However, many Lyme-literate practitioners who recommend HBOT agree that the protocol for Lyme disease should be between 1.8–2.4 ATA (atmospheres absolute) for an initial series of 40 treatments. This is in conjunction with antibiotic regimes if you are taking them and can tolerate the two together. A repeat series of 6–8 weeks is recommended if symptoms persist or reoccur, and a further 40 treatments may be required for those who are chronic.

Will I Herx Using HBOT?

Often you will experience a Herx as the increased oxygenation of the cells is likely to kill Bb, which creates an endotoxin release as their cell wall breaks down. The better you are detoxing and methylating, the less severe the Herx will likely be. If the Herxing is extreme, it's an indication that your Bb load is high and also that you have done too much treatment too quickly, so decrease the amount or length of the HBOT sessions and implement some detoxification assistance with your primary practitioner.

How Long Will It Take to Feel Improvements?

Some people will feel results straight away, but generally, it will take about three weeks to three months in order for the buildup of endotoxins trapped in fat soluble tissues to be released. I personally recommend doing HBOT in combination with infrared saunas if you have the time and money for faster results (once again, if you can tolerate it).

Are There Other Options If I Can't Afford HBOT?

Yes! You can rent or purchase a portable mild hyperbaric chamber for use at home. They are simple, pressurised enclosures that mildly increase atmospheric pressure. This increased pressure in combination with purified, ambient air of 89–93% helps the oxygen to dissolve into the body's fluids (including plasma, lymph, synovial and cerebrospinal fluids) to increase oxygen throughout the body. They are safe and drug-free and can be used regularly without danger of oxygen toxicity. There are many different brands, but most have enough room to sit up or lie down, so you can read or work on a laptop if you want. (humanERGETIC THERAPIES 2015) A personal use HBOT is not believed to be as effective as a hospital grade HBOT. I don't have any personal experience with these chambers, but you can Google the *Hypo2 Mild Hyperbaric Oxygen Chambers*, which are available in Australia, for more information. The QLD distributors can be contacted on 07 5535 1859 or 0458 500 001, or http://www.hypo2hyperbarics.com/our-company.html.

Are There Any Studies Supporting HBOT?

Yes, there are plenty, and even some for Lyme disease. You can Google *Lyme disease and Hyperbaric research* and find lots of case studies and research papers. At Texas A&M University, William Fife, Ph.D., treated 91 Lyme disease patients with HBOT at 2.36ATA (atmospheres absolute) with 85% of those treated showing significant improvement, including improvements in pain reduction, return of clarity of the mind, and reduction of depression. (Fife 1998) Charles Pavia, Ph.D., also did a study that showed spirochetes exposed to an increased partial pressure of oxygen could not survive. (Pavia 2000)

Epsom Salt and Detox Baths

If you don't have a lot of time or money but have a bath, then you can still do wonders for your body and muscles. Many people are aware of the amazing benefits of Epsom salts, especially for your muscles. The salts help replenish your muscles with much-needed minerals, especially magnesium. Buy a box (or many boxes) of Epsom salts from your supermarket (you can also buy in bulk), pour them into a warm bath and soak away. For maximum results, skin brush before you get in and then soak for up to an hour. Make sure you have a water bottle with you so you can stay hydrated.

Another great trick I use is the detox bath. Put 2 cups of Epsom salts, 1 cup of baking soda and a few drops of ginger essential oil into a warm bath and soak for an hour. It's a great way to release toxins, absorb magnesium and relax! These baths are great for people who aren't detoxing well, have aches and pains or aren't sleeping soundly.

Float Tanks

In my opinion, float tanks (aka isolation tanks) are one of the most amazing things you can do for yourself to get healthy and stay healthy! They are undervalued, and I find very few people who know of or have tried floating. I was introduced to floating as an athlete. With all the training I did, I used to get sore muscles and sometimes found it hard to recover between training sessions and when traveling for races. The float tanks helped infuse magnesium and other important minerals back into my tired and often aching body as well as gave me much-needed relaxation. I recovered faster, felt better and trained harder as a result! A float complements other treatments, such as massage, acupuncture and even yoga, so don't be afraid to team a float with other therapies for even better results.

What Are Float Tanks Used for?

Anyone can benefit from floating, but the tanks are especially used for decreasing stress, anxiety and jet lag, increasing relaxation, and improving recovery from intense exercise. It even improves the healing time of injuries. Anyone with magnesium deficiencies, those having problems with sleep, those who exercise a lot or people under huge amounts of stress will particularly benefit.

Are There Any Other Names for a Float Tank?

It is also known as an isolation tank, think tank, sensory attenuation tank, floatation tank, sensory deprivation tank and REST tank.

What Is So Special About a Float Tank?

The tank contains water that is saturated with magnesium salts at body temperature (water is usually 35.5 °C). The density of the salt solution, very similar to that of the Dead Sea, allows you to float face up on top of the water. The tanks are designed to subdue the senses by blocking out all light (although if you are claustrophobic, you can leave the door / lid open), minimising sound (although some tanks do play relaxation music for part of the session), ensuring very little smell and decreasing skin sensation by having the water, air and body at a similar temperature. This helps to decrease stress in the body and the mind, assist muscle relaxation and improve blood flow. The high density salt mixture at body temperature also means that there is an uptake of magnesium into the cells via osmosis (which is hugely advantageous for Lymies and anyone who gets sore and tight muscles!).

How Do I Use a Float Tank and What Should I Expect?

Most places that provide float tanks will explain everything to you and orientate you with floating. The key things to remember are:

❖   Have a cold shower before you get in the tank. That way, it will feel warm when you get in, and your body temperature will adjust back to your normal basal body temperature quite quickly and comfortably.

❖   Use ear plugs and a blow up neck pillow so you can fully relax your head in the water.

❖   Put Vaseline on any cuts or open wounds so they don't sting (the salt is very good for these things but not so pleasant!)

❖   With most tanks, if you are claustrophobic, you will be able to leave the door / lid open slightly or keep the inside light on (over time you will often be able to close the lid and turn off the light).

❖   Let your mind and body relax, and don't be surprised if you fall asleep.

❖   The first float can be a bit weird (I didn't like it the first time I did it, but I felt so great afterwards that I kept it up and became addicted!).

❖   Most sessions last 60–90 minutes, but often people get out early on their first one, as it's an unusual experience.

❖   Often you can feel twitchy and itchy but it subsides, so just relax (be careful of scratching your face as the salt will sting your eyes if it gets in them!)

❖ It takes multiple sessions to get used to the sensation of floating as well as get the maximum benefit. Like anything, floating just once is great, but to get results, you need to do it regularly if you can.

❖ In the last 20 minutes or so of an hour float your brain will usually transition from beta or alpha brainwaves to theta, which is known to assist creativity, relaxation and problem solving, and improve learning.

Is There Any Research to Confirm the Benefits of Floating?

Yes, there is. Most of it comes from Europe and America, but a basic Google search will turn up some great case studies and research.

Skin Brushing

Most chemists, health food stores, department stores and your local supermarkets (like Woolworths and Coles) sell skin brushes for just a few dollars. However, it is worth investing in a good quality one if you want it to last and work optimally! Removing dead skin cells helps the body's detoxification pathways, which is essential when you are suffering from any chronic disease. Always start at the extremity, and using light, brisk strokes, brush towards your major lymph glands, which are located on the inside of your ankles, behind your knees, in your groin, under your arm pits and in your neck. For example, start at the foot and brush up the calf and shin towards the back of the knee, up the thigh to the groin (repeat on other leg), then brush down your tummy to the groin. If you have digestion issues, rub the brush in a clockwise direction on your stomach. Next, brush from your fingertips up the arm to the armpits (remember the palms), across the chest / breasts to the armpits and up the neck, front and back. Do this at least 1 to 2 times a day, ideally, just before you jump into the shower. It's simple and easy, and in my opinion, it doesn't just help detoxification but also improves skin appearance.

Parasite Zapper

Based on the published research by Dr. Hulda Clark and Royal Raymond Rife, Zappers use a specific frequency / harmonic pulsed through the body to boost the immune response and kill parasites, bacteria and viruses.

They are often used by travellers to purify drinking water when clean water is not readily available. The Zapper is not approved for use on humans. However, I learnt to use the Zapper on myself with great success as part of the TBM kinesiology protocol (see TBM in the Treatment section for more information on this type of kinesiology treatment) to target parasites in the body. I share this information for you to use guided by an experienced practitioner and to be used at your own risk. Often people find it hard to rid their body of the parasite Babesia and this protocol has been found effective by many.

To use the Zapper*, hold the copper rods for 7 minutes, rest 20–35 minutes, repeat for 7 minutes, rest for 20–35 minutes and then repeat for 7 more minutes. This takes at least 61 minutes, so it's best done in the evening. It's recommended to continue this protocol daily for four weeks, as the total length of the parasites life, death, and egg hatching cycles are usually around 3–4 weeks.

*If you are going to use this protocol, I suggest that you work with someone who has used a Zapper before.

Castor Oil Packs

Castor oil packs are age-old remedies and continue to be a great supportive therapy, especially for decreasing pain and inflammation, up-regulating the lymphatic system, improving colon function and supporting liver and gallbladder functions. They are especially great to use if you have high liver enzymes on blood test because it's believed that the packs can help stimulate the production and flow of bile from the gallbladder. This moves toxic build up more efficiently, which takes pressure off the liver. They can also help with symptoms caused by toxic build up (they stimulate the detoxification and elimination process) such as headaches, digestive pain, constipation and inflammation (especially joint pain).

Contraindications for Using Castor Oil Packs

Castor oil packs stimulate detoxification, so use them for short periods of time and increase that time if your body can tolerate it. Check with your doctor before using if you are pregnant or have any bleeding disorders, ulcers, chemical intolerances or skin lesions.

How to Make a Castor Oil* Pack

1. Get a cotton or woollen cloth / material 50–100cm x 60–120cm and wash and dry it before using

2. Fold it so that it's a few layers thick but still fits over most of your stomach

3. Soak the material in castor oil, making sure it does not drip once wrung out

4. Put the material soaked in castor oil in a glass, microwave-proof dish and heat in 30 second lots until the material is comfortably warm (you can heat in a saucepan if you have no microwave)

* Coconut oil can be substituted for castor oil

How to Use a Castor Oil Pack

1. Heat up a heat bag (like a wheat bag or its equivalent) to a comfortable level of heat

2. Find somewhere you can lie comfortably for an extended period of time and put plastic or an old towel down so any castor oil that might drip off doesn't stain

3. Place the castor oil-soaked material on your stomach

4. Put an old towel or some plastic over the material and place the heat bag on top of that

5. Wrap yourself in a warm blanket (especially if it's cold)

6. Ideally, you want to leave the castor oil pack on for 40–60 minutes, but if it's your first time, start with 10 minutes first and then see how you feel (you can build up from there)

The castor oil pack is reusable, so just add more castor oil and heat up each time. If you store it in a Ziploc or sealed bag in the fridge, you should be able to use it for a few months. Ideally, use daily or every second day if you are Herxing too much.

Yoga / Pilates / Tai Chi / Chi Gong

Aerobic exercise is not recommended when you are sick with any chronic illness, including Lyme disease, especially if your white cell count is suppressed. Any exercise can be challenging when you are not well. However, it is important to keep your body active and moving. Yoga, Pilates, Tai Chi and Chi Gong are the perfect way to keep your muscles activated and your lymphatic system flowing without too much exertion. Yin, or restorative yoga, is very relaxing yet energising. Tai Chi and Chi Gong are ancient forms of healing and breathing, and although not so well known in Australia, these classes can be found all over the world. You can also download apps or watch YouTube videos if a class isn't in the budget (money or energy-wise).

DENTAL CONSIDERATIONS

Root Canals

I have learnt the hard way that not all dentists are the same (surprise, surprise!). They don't all use the same material to fill your cavities or recommend the same procedures. I had my first filling done at a random dentist who I believe drilled too far and hit the nerve. The pain I had from that day continued to get worse and worse until I finally went to another dentist who agreed with me that she had likely drilled too far and hit the nerve (which had slowly degenerated). I was told I would now need a root canal procedure done. The dentist said the only option was to drill the tooth, take out the nerve and sterilise it, and then seal the hole in my tooth where the root had been. At the time, it sounded like the normal thing to do. Because he told me it was the only option, I didn't even think to get a second opinion.

The more I learnt over the years, the more I wondered whether my root canal could possibly be harbouring infection. After three separate kinesiologists told me the tooth was a problem energetically for me and that I needed to have it removed, I began the process of dentist shopping! I went to dentist after dentist, and they all told me the same thing: the tooth was fine and all the rumours and research linking root canal to disease were not true. They also said that if there were an abscess (infection), they would be able to see it on the x-ray.

The first four dentists I went to all refused to remove the tooth. The fifth dentist I consulted was Dr. David Howard, a holistic dentist in Sydney. He showed me the research and explained why he believed root canals should never be done for most people in the first place as well as why they should be removed if they had been done (especially if someone was sick). Everything he told me made perfect sense and was what I had thought all along. He agreed that the tooth needed to be extracted and gave me three options for the gap: leave it as a gap, get an implant (fake tooth drilled into the gum) or get a bridge (fake tooth hanging in the gap attached to the two teeth on either side). The implant and bridge cost was about the same, so I opted for the bridge. It meant less dental visits, it looks totally natural (I even forget which one is fake sometimes!) and I didn't want to have a gap (not just for aesthetic reasons, but my teeth are quite crowded and I didn't want to undo all the years of orthodontic work I had to make them look nice and straight!). You have to buy a special floss for cleaning above / around the fake tooth (although it looks like the fake tooth attaches at the gum, it doesn't), but I don't find it takes any longer than normal flossing.

My Miraculous Root Canal Story

The reason I added this section to the book and why I'm sharing this information is because the day my root canal was removed, miraculously, I felt so much better. It was pretty instantaneous but even more noticeable the next day. I woke up at 7 am ready to get up and actually felt rested (at that time, I was usually dragging myself out of bed, even as late as 9–10am, with big black circles under my eyes!). When my tooth was pulled out, it DID have a HUGE ABSCESS on it and lots of little ones, too (contrary to what the previous dentists had told me about the impossibility of having an infection without being able to see it on an x-ray)!! I'm sure the infection from the abscess combined with my already struggling immune system from the Lyme disease was dripping infection into my system through the tiny canals in the mouth and continuously setting off an immune response. From that day forward, I slept better and had more energy than I had had in a long time. It didn't cure me, but it was a significant step in my journey.

Amalgam Fillings

There are two schools of thought on amalgam fillings. One is to leave them in until they need to be replaced, because removing them releases more mercury into the system which is even worse than leaving them in. The other theory is to remove them totally. Because I don't have any amalgam fillings, I have not been forced to jump off my fence perch and make a decision as to what I believe or what I would do, though I can see the argument from both sides.

Leaving in Amalgams

If you are leaving your amalgams in, I think it's important that you have regular check-ups and have them removed immediately if they are cracked or damaged in ANY way. There is a kinesiology technique used by TBM practitioners that uses a light and a magnet to seal amalgam-filled teeth. Just shine a torch in your mouth over the affected tooth (or teeth) and hold the north end of a magnet on the outside of the cheek over the same tooth.

Taking out Amalgams

The holistic dentist who extracted my root canal tooth believes amalgams should be taken out and that how it is done is VERY important. He believes that ALL mercury must be removed before the body will show signs of detoxing. So only after the last piece of mercury is taken out of the last tooth, will the body then detox (hence, he leaves a mercury piece in the mouth deliberately until the end and then allows the body to detoxify after the procedure is finished). To me, this theory makes sense. Our bodies are very smart, so it's unlikely that the body will try to rid itself of something toxic (like a mercury-filled tooth) if it knows the effect of mobilising that mercury is likely to be more than the body can efficiently handle at that time. It is important that your dentist uses the correct supplements to assist and support this process or you can get very sick. This is obviously not my area of expertise, so if you wish to have your amalgams taken out, consult a holistic dentist who knows what they are doing.

WHAT ELSE CAN I DO TO HELP MYSELF PHYSICALLY?

Exercise

Exercise is a hard one for people who are sick. There are so many factors to think about. Exercise increases endorphins, which help you feel mentally and physically better. It also increases circulation, improves joint mobility and promotes lymphatic flow, all very important factors in healing. However, someone suffering with fatigue can find it hard to get out of bed some days let alone exercise, and anyone who over-trains can also significantly suppress their immune system function. So, getting the type and length of the exercise with the right recovery is going to be different for everyone. Although there is little scientific basis to go by for what sort of exercise is best when you have a chronic illness like Lyme disease, I have compiled some information from my own journey and from speaking to health professionals (and of course, other Lymies) to help you along your way.

"It is quite possible to leave your home for a walk in the early morning air and return a different person – beguiled, enchanted."

Mary Ellen Chase

Why Is Exercise Important in Recovery from Lyme Disease?

Exercise is important not just for your mental state of health, but also to increase your core body temperature and the perfusion of oxygen into the tissues. Bb, as you have probably realised by this stage, are heat sensitive and can die if exposed to even small amounts of oxygen.

What Should I Do if I Don't Have the Energy or the Strength to Exercise?

If you feel like you couldn't possibly exercise, then you need to find a way to replicate exercise. Examples include stretching, getting a massage, acupuncture, ultrasound and hot / cold therapy (alternating hot and cold packs or hot / cold in the shower). Anything that can stretch or improve circulation and lymphatic flow is going to be advantageous. If you are really sick, you can have someone mobilise and move your joints whilst you are still in bed, or you can use a TENS machine.

Why Do Many People Say You Shouldn't Do Aerobic Exercise if You Have Lyme Disease?

Most exercise will cause a suppression of the T-cell function (immunity) for 12–24 hours post-exercise before it then rebounds back to normal. However, aerobic exercise, especially if strenuous, tends to have a greater effect on the T-cell suppression and an increased rebound effect (i.e., the immune system can potentially be suppressed for days afterwards before it returns to normal). Anyone suffering a disease that already causes suppressed immune system function, as seen in Lyme disease, will generally not recover and even get sicker if exercise is too strenuous or if too much aerobic exercise is done (especially if it is on consecutive days).

As I Start to Feel Stronger and Have More Energy, What Are the Best Types of Exercises to Do?

Once your immune system starts to recover and your white cell levels climb into the optimal range on blood tests, choose an exercise that you enjoy. Whether you take a light walk, a gentle swim, spin your legs over on an exercise bike, join a Yin yoga class, use a resistance band or swing some kettlebells, be sure to start slow and light. You can also try an exercise app or a YouTube video at home.

How Will I Know if I Have Done Too Much?

Hopefully you will not overdo it, as that can really set you back. Always progressively overload yourself and finish BEFORE you are tired. Better to finish and wish you had done more, then finish and realise that you have overdone it! Exercise should only be every second day at the most until you have fully recovered. If you listen to your body, it will tell you what you can and can't do. If exercise tires you out during or after, then you have done too much.

Tips and Tricks for Beginning an Exercise Program

❖ Always warm up and cool down and include stretching

❖ Start with non-aerobic exercises such as light weights, Swiss ball exercises, TRX straps, or medicine ball work

❖ Try to work one muscle group at a time before moving to the next one

❖ A whole body conditioning program is required, so make sure you are working on all the different muscle groups

❖ Build up to sessions of an hour. This is enough time to work the body but not too much time that the immune system will be severely compromised

❖ Always plan to rest or sleep after your exercise session to assist recovery

❖ Start with one session a week and then build up to every second day (it's important to have a rest day between each session)

❖ Keep a diary of the exercises you did, how long it took, and how you felt before, during and after (and how you recovered)

❖ Do not start even light aerobic exercise until your immune system (especially white cells on a blood test) and adrenals are ready (salivary cortisol test). You don't want to do too much too soon or you could relapse

❖ Get the help of a personal trainer (PT) and/or exercise physiologist to help you design your program. Be sure to find a PT who either specialises in or is aware of the requirements to train someone with a suppressed immune system, or give them this book if they are willing to learn!

Joseph Burrascano has some recommendations for how to progress your exercise (he calls it the Rehab-Physical Therapy Prescription) in his e-book *Advanced Topics in Lyme Disease: Diagnostic Hints and Treatment Guidelines for Lyme and other Tick-borne Illnesses*.

Working

I recommend taking as much time off of work as you can, or at least significantly cutting back your work hours so your body can heal while you attempt any type of treatment. At first I didn't feel that bad physically.

I thought I could be super woman and work through the treatment, so I worked until I literally couldn't lift my head off the pillow. I believe this drained my reserves and slowed my long-term healing progress. Some people don't have the luxury of owning their own business with income protection insurance like I did, but it gave me the flexibility to take time off (and it was still stressful!). I totally understand that working is a necessity for some people. However, if you work yourself to the bone and end up having to take time off anyway, then it's likely in the long-term that this will be more costly, not just financially, but personally. If you ask anyone who has been sick or had a near-death experience what the most important thing in the world is, they will say health and/or family / friends (which is essentially love). It doesn't help to have money if you don't have your health or someone to share it with. It's hard, but sometimes you have to ask for help, move back in with your parents or take out a loan. There is no right or wrong way, but listen to your body and try to get the balance right. The longer you push yourself, the harder the road to recovery will usually be!

Sleep

People who are highly stressed or have a chronic disease will often experience sleepless nights. Sometimes this is intermittent, and for some, it's constant. Sleep disruption can come from many sources including pain, anxiety, nervous system interference, hormonal imbalance (especially adrenal fatigue), digestive disorders, detoxification issues and electromagnetic disturbances. Identifying the cause(s) of sleep interference is an important step. If you can't sleep, then it's very hard to heal, as most of our healing and regeneration is done during sleep. If you fail to establish the cause of your sleep problems or are finding it hard to make any changes, there are some supplements and even drugs that you can take (as a last resort) to assist sleep. Please know that any pharmaceutical drug you take will consciously "knock you out" so you feel like you have slept, but it will detrimentally affect your normal sleep cycle so you are not truly healing or recovering.

Sometimes it's stressful being awake, as you think and stress about everything when you just need to sleep. In these cases, having a sleeping tablet might be a good option. However, just know that this is only a short-term solution for a long-term problem. Another option is to supplement with melatonin for a short period (speak to your doctor before trying this, of course), as it is sleep-inducing rather than a knockout pill! Another option is to supplement with L-Tryptophan, the precursor to melatonin, so speak to your doctor about the best options. If you don't find the cause and reestablish your sleeping patterns, it is near impossible to heal. That is why you often feel groggy after a sleeping tablet and sometimes wake up feeling even more tired than before. Sometimes understanding how sleep works gives you more power to control and implement healthy changes.

The Sleep Cycle

There are two different types of natural sleep cycles, the outer cycle (also known as the circadian rhythm) and the inner cycle. Both have an effect on the quality of sleep.

OUTER CYCLE = CIRCADIAN RHYTHM

Your body's circadian rhythm is like your body clock. It's your internal system for knowing what time it is without having to look at a clock and is predominantly controlled by light. It can be externally influenced by things like travel to different time zones (jet lag), shift work, daylight savings clock changes, the temperature or anything that can wake you from your sleep (e.g., noises from cars, a partner snoring or a baby crying). Changes to the circadian rhythm directly affect the inner sleep cycles.

INNER CYCLE = 5 STAGES OF SLEEP

The sleep cycle moves through different stages repeatedly when you are asleep. Most people complete 3–5 sleep cycles per night if they are sleeping well. The five stages are:

Stage 1 Light sleep – the doorway to sleep.

Stage 2 Light sleep – where you can still easily be awakened.

Stage 3 Deep sleep begins – where immune system healing is at its greatest and delta brainwaves occur once you are totally unconscious.

Stage 4 Deep sleep – it is difficult to wake someone in this stage with over 50% of brainwaves being delta, which decreases cortisol levels (stress hormones), stimulates the pituitary gland to release melatonin, creates deep states of relaxation and healing, and triggers the release of anti-ageing hormones as well as HGH to repair the musculoskeletal system (amongst many other functions).

Stage 5: REM (rapid eye movement) – where most dreaming occurs and many people believe that stored negative emotions can be integrated and released during this phase.

The sleep stages cycle through every 1 to 2 hours. It is important to understand that Stage 1 is not repeated unless your sleep is broken; therefore, if your sleep is unbroken, you get extra time in the deep sleep and REM cycles, which means extra healing time! So, if you can't get to sleep or your sleep is broken, then you must start all over again in Stage 1. This can prevent you from having enough time in the latter stages or possibly not reaching the healing stages of sleep at all. The immediate effects of poor sleep are noticed physically and mentally. Over time, if sleep is continually disrupted, then it can have long-term physiological effects.

If your circadian rhythm is affected externally and the body does not go through the inner sleep cycles at night, then it affects how your body heals and feels. For example, human growth hormone (HGH) is released during deep sleep and helps the body to repair and build muscle, slows down the ageing process, switches your metabolism to burn fat and boosts immunity. Stage 4 sleep is required at least once per night to heal and takes about 3.5 hours of unbroken sleep to achieve. So you can see how important sleep is for you, not just so you feel mentally refreshed, but so your physical body can regenerate and function optimally.

Tips and Tricks for a Good Night Sleep

❖ Go to bed and get up at the same time each day to support your circadian rhythm.

❖ Avoid overstimulation before bedtime (avoid TV, computers, phones, bright lights) especially blue light (you can buy special goggles that block out this light and put programs on your electrical devices to minimise blue light at night, like F.Lux if you use a Mac).

❖ Eat low carbohydrate meals during the day and especially at night.

❖ Avoid stimulants (e.g., caffeine, sugar, processed foods, and nicotine), especially after lunch and never within three hours of bedtime. If you do need to eat close to bedtime, eat high protein and high fat.

❖ If you have adrenal fatigue or wake up hungry during the night, try the TBM autonomic recovery meal just before bedtime (½ banana, ⅛ cup full fat cream, ¼ cup natural yoghurt and 1 raw egg blended together just before sleep time). This works well to relieve nausea (including nausea from morning sickness during pregnancy!)

❖ Keep your sleeping quarters cool (21–23 °C is believed to be ideal), but try not to have fans or air conditioners blowing directly on you.

❖ Exercise during the day but not too close to bedtime.

❖ Maintain positive thoughts with meditation, affirmations, gratitude, and prayer.

❖ Ensure you have a good mattress and contour pillow (if your spine is not supported, it can create tension and wake you up).

❖ Unplug all power points within three metres of the head of your bed to decrease electromagnetic radiation exposure that may disrupt sleep.

❖ Make sure your room is as dark as possible (use a face mask if it is not possible to block out all light), as light inhibits melatonin secretion which is your sleepy hormone.

❖ Seeing the sun rise and set is a great way to reset / maintain your circadian rhythm and assist with sleep, so get outside during these times wherever possible.

❖ Minimise noise as much as possible (even if that means using ear plugs) so your sleep cycle is not disturbed.

❖ If you sleep with a restless sleeper or someone who snores, then it may be best to move to your own bed for awhile until you can re-establish your sleep cycle.

❖ If you do need to get up in the night, use a torch rather than turning on the lights and fully waking yourself up, and ideally warm light (so have red cellophane over your torch or a red bulb in your night light).

❖ Try some herbal remedies such as magnesium to promote muscle relaxation, valerian root to induce sleep and chamomile to relax you.

❖ Treatments such as chiropractic, massage, acupuncture, Bowen therapy and kinesiology are great for finding the cause of the sleeping / insomnia issues.

❖ Tai Chi, Chi-Gong and yoga are all based on centring your energy, which are great for relaxing the body and promoting sleep.

❖ There are meditation techniques and even apps you can try that claim to promote a delta brainwave state and improve your sleep.

❖ If you have tried all the tips and tricks and are still having problems getting or staying asleep, then talk to your doctor about a trial of melatonin or tryptophan for a short period to assist in inducing sleep.

TBM Exercises to Help Program the Body to Improve Sleep

AT BEDTIME

To activate your body's sleep mechanism, rub both mastoid bones (the bumps just behind the ears) until you feel a wave of sleepiness, which usually occurs in 10 to 15 seconds (if after 90 seconds you're still not sleepy, it probably won't help, so you'll need to look at calming your body and/or your mind through reading, stretching, sexual intimacy, conscious breathing or meditation). Rub the mastoid bones each night at bedtime until you find your body's rhythm has adjusted. Do this any time you lie down but are finding it difficult to go to sleep. Also do this if you wake during the night and are having difficulty going back to sleep.

UPON RISING

To program your body to sync with the current time, rub the Spleen 21 point (left rib cage halfway between the armpit and the bottom of the rib cage) for 30 seconds. Immediately following, rub both ears beginning at the bottom of the ear lobe and working toward the top of the earlobe as if you were trying to uncurl or flatten the ears (use the thumb on the front of the ear and the index finger on the back of the ear). Do one pass up and one down. NOTE: This works to program infants' sleep cycles, too.

People who are sick need MORE sleep than the average person. So don't feel bad if you are sleeping more than usual.

Rest and Relaxation

Please don't underestimate the benefit and importance of rest and relaxation. If you are not sleeping, then you need to increase the amount of rest and relaxation time that you get during that day. Ideally, rest is taking time out and giving your mind and body a break. If you are like me and find it hard to slow down without your mind driving you crazy, then rest could be reading, watching TV or a movie (which can be overstimulating, so never before bedtime!), creating art, colouring in, stretching, meditating, creating a dream board, planning a holiday, chatting on the phone or cooking. Rest ideally needs to be physical and mental relaxation, so watching a scary movie would not count as relaxing whereas watching a comedy or a love story would be. For some people, meditating may be boring whereas others may love it. Find things that make your heart sing. Give yourself the gift of rest, relaxation and the permission to enjoy it.

EMR Exposure

EMR Symptoms and Effects

There is no doubt that EMR (electromagnetic radiation), EMF (electromagnetic frequencies / fields) and RF (radio frequency) negatively affect the body. Some of the symptoms in even healthy bodies can include sleep disturbance, headaches, fatigue, memory or concentration issues, depression, skin disorders, nausea, digestive issues, lowered immunity, irritability, pain, reduced libido and fertility problems. Sound familiar? People with chronic disease often already have a lowered immunity and tolerance, so it is easy to see how EMR could not only exacerbate their symptoms, but slow or even hinder their recovery process. More and more research confirms the adverse effects of EMR such as genetic damage, cell damage, and the disruption of important hormones and neurotransmitters. Research also shows that EMR can affect brainwave patterns and even disrupt the blood-brain barrier. Government authorities have yet to agree on the long-lasting effects EMR has on your health, but I for one am not going to sit around and be a guinea pig.

What Can Emit EMR and EMFs?

INCLUDED BUT NOT LIMITED TO:

Power lines, substations, metre boxes, computers, electrical appliances, conductive pipes and wiring, mobile phones, cordless phones, WiFi, baby monitors, smart metres, iPads, mobile phone towers, other wireless equipment including neighbours' wireless equipment.

For further information log onto http://www.emraustralia.com.au/emr_ meters.html (Home Test Kit 2014)

EMR and Lyme Disease

When your body is already sick and rundown, you become more susceptible to changes in energy. I knew EMR was affecting me once I realised that I would get a headache if I put my mobile phone next to my head for even a minute. I couldn't even have my mobile phone next to my bed at night! Not everyone is this sensitive.

What Are Some Easy Steps I Can Take to Decrease My EMR Exposure?

I made a few small changes that made a huge difference. I stopped plugging my phone in to charge next to my bed, and I turned off and unplugged all power points within three metres of my bed (ideally, unplug everything in your room). If you have WiFi at home, turn it off when you're not using it. Throw your microwave in the bin (if you haven't worked that out already!). Avoid using or installing dimmer switches that can cause "dirty energy." I also bought an Earthing kit for my home, work and sleep (see more information in the Earthing section).

What if That Is Not Enough or I Want to Do More to Decrease My EMR Exposure?

If you are in Australia, log onto http://www.emraustralia.com.au/EMR_ symptoms.html (Do you experience symptoms from EMR? 2014) and follow the steps on their website. First, you can take a quick survey to see how much EMR could be affecting your health. Then, I highly recommend hiring a do-it-yourself EMF and RF metre to measure the EMR in your home and workplace. These metres come with step-by-step information on how to measure EMR and RF and then interpret the results. They also include handy hints on how to remedy the issues in order to create a safer environment for you and your loved ones. You can also pay someone to do this for you.

There is a great book called *The Force,* by Lyn Maclean, which gives you information on how to live safely in a world of electromagnetic pollution.

If you want to go whole hog, you can Google *Peter Sullivan* and/or *Faraday Cage* to learn how to protect yourself from EMF on a larger scale!

Earthing / Grounding

What Is Earthing and Grounding? With earthing (also known as grounding), you connect and bond with Mother Earth with your bare skin in order to receive a negatively charged surge of energy that grounds you. The negatively charged electrons help to neutralise the positively charged free radicals that affect your body's natural healing capacity. Earth possesses an unlimited and continuously renewed supply of "free" or "mobile" electrons as a result of a global atmospheric electron circuit. What this means is that the earth has a greater negative charge than your body, so your body absorbs these negative electrons which have a potent antioxidant-like effect as well as anti-inflammatory properties, too! (Mercola 2012) Check out Mercola's website for more information (http://articles.mercola.com/sites/articles/archive/2012/09/20/barefoot-on-electron-deficiency.aspx).

A study in the Journal of Alternative and Complementary Medicine demonstrated that connecting the human body to the earth during sleep (earthing), helped normalise daily cortisol rhythms (balances stress hormones), improved sleep, reduced pain and decreased inflammation. Subsequent studies have confirmed these earlier findings. (Oschman 2007)

Why Do We Need to Earth Ourselves? Earth provides you with air, water and food as well as the ground you live on. Being grounded keeps you balanced and healthy, which can help your body do the job it was designed to do. If your body becomes unbalanced with positively charged ions, then it disrupts your normal bodily functions creating issues such as increased inflammation, hormonal imbalance, tissue damage and impaired immune function. So, just like you need sunshine to naturally synthesise vitamin D, you need bare skin contact with the earth to remain grounded and healthy.

Why Don't People Talk Much About Earthing? I believe that information passed down to us from our ancestors slowly gets lost over the years. Our ancestors earthed themselves naturally every day, whether from walking barefoot or cultivating the earth with their hands. It was so natural and simple to them that maybe they never even spoke of it. Who knows! With advances in technology, our world has become modernised, so much so that now we nearly always wear shoes, we sleep off the ground on beds, our houses are often built off the ground, and we are exposed to frequencies that are all positively charged (mobile phones, microwaves, radio waves, wireless frequencies, etc.). We are so far away from our grounded roots.

How Often Should I Earth? As often as possible. You can't "over earth" yourself! If your immune system is challenged like it is with chronic infections such as Lyme disease, then the more you earth yourself, the quicker you will heal and the better you will feel.

Are There Other Ways to Earth Without Going Outside? Whilst getting out on the ground and earthing naturally is ideal, it's not always practical. There are many companies that now provide earthing equipment such as sheets, foot pads, computer mats, and blankets. These are either plugged into the earthing point of your power point (bottom hole in Australia) or connected to a grounding rod that is put in the ground outside and run into the home. I bought an earthing kit from Barefoot Healing that included an earthing sheet for the bed, two earthing mats, a book, audio and the adapters and sockets that attach the grounding products to the power point. So, if you work a lot at the computer or drive a lot, these are great! Log onto www.barefoothealing.com.au for more info.

What Benefits Can I Experience from Earthing? Earthing will help the body to internally neutralise free radical damage. Not only will it decrease inflammation, improve immune function and decrease organ and tissue destruction, but you will often feel symptomatically better. You may notice increased energy, decreased pain / muscle tension / headaches (due to decreased inflammation), improved sleep (which, in turn, super charges healing), decreased stress levels (due to a more balanced nervous system), improved healing time from injuries / illness, better concentration, and less hormonal symptoms such as PMS or mood swings. The list could go on forever!

Earthing is easy and essentially free, and can make a huge difference to your health whether you are sick or not. So try it and continue it even after you are well again!

Breathing

How can breathing help you get rid of disease, you ask? As with anything, there are lots of pieces to the healing puzzle that can help. Breathing optimally is one piece of that puzzle that is quick, easy and free. There are specialists who teach proper breathing, which I highly recommend if the information that follows hits a spot with you! I have also included some information and exercises you can do from the comfort of your own home.

Why Do We Breathe? Quite simple, right? Oxygen is one of the vital ingredients for life, so you need to get oxygen into the lungs and expel carbon dioxide in order to live. It makes sense then that if you are not getting optimal oxygen into your body, your body will not function optimally!

What Affects the Way I Breathe? Breathing is a function of the autonomic nervous system, which is controlled by the brain. When your body is stressed, your nervous system switches from the parasympathetic mode of rest-and-digest to the sympathetic mode of fight-or-flight which automatically changes your breathing patterns. In our busy world, people have forgotten how to actually breathe properly. Many people use their accessory breathing muscles, such as the scalene muscles in the neck and their shoulders, to take small, shallow breaths into the upper part of the lungs. This style of breathing limits the uptake of oxygen, and the balance of gases in the body is disrupted.

Does It Really Matter How I Breathe? Yes, it does! When you deep breathe, not only do you get more oxygen circulating throughout your body, but it sends a message to your brain that is then relayed to the body to calm down and relax. If your body is continuously in a stressed state (which is directly affected by your breathing), it thinks it has to be super alert and in the fight / flight mode, in which case, extra blood and oxygen are sent to the areas that need to be ready to fight or flee. Constantly being in this flight / fight state decreases your immune function, slows digestion and affects your libido / fertility (this occurs because you really don't need to have an optimally functioning immune system, digest your food, or reproduce in a life-threatening situation, do you?!) All versions of stress affect the body in this way, so you can see how important it is to address stress and, of course, breathe!

How Do I Breathe Properly Then?

There are various techniques you can use to improve your breathing. Initially, you will need to consciously learn how to breathe properly, but with practice and time, these techniques should become subconscious. Fortunately, breathing is an automated action of which we have conscious control. The key is to breathe as deeply as possible into the abdomen so that your tummy expands on the inhalation as opposed to your chest expanding and your shoulders rising up! Sit or stand up tall; if you are slouched over, it limits the amount of air that you can physically breathe in!

What Are the Signs or Symptoms of Someone Who Isn't Breathing Properly?

Anything from physical postural issues / pain to anxiety, panic attacks, chest pain / tightness, fatigue, breathing problems, sleep issues, fainting, dizziness and, of course, the feeling of being stressed!

What Are Some Exercises I Can Do at Home to Improve My Breathing?

You can set <u>My Calm Beat</u> (a free app) to guide you through this very basic exercise, or you can do it on your own.

<u>EXERCISE 1</u>

❖ Find a quiet place and lie down on your back (this can be done sitting or standing, but it's easier when lying down).

❖ Place one hand on your stomach and one hand on your chest.

❖ Take a few deep breaths in through the nose and out through your nose, and take note of which hands are moving up and down with your breath (chest hand or stomach hand?)

❖ As you breathe in, bring your conscious awareness to breathing air deep down into the abdomen so the hand on your stomach rises.

❖ As you breathe out, squeeze the air out of the abdomen as much as possible.

❖ Over time, you can start to slow down your breathing (which can be really hard at first!)

<u>EXERCISE 2</u> For a total of 8 minutes a day, breathe in for 4 seconds, hold for 1 second, breathe out for 4 seconds, then hold for 1 second.

I have used this breathing method myself and with my clients. At first, you may not be able to last a minute, but as you get better, you should be able to continue this pattern easily for eight minutes. This will greatly increase your sense of calm. If you get anxiety or are in a stressful environment, you will find that it makes a huge difference. This breathing technique combined with diet and lifestyle modifications may even totally eliminate anxiety.

EXERCISE 3

Use a 10-second breath in and 10-second breath out pattern. This was taught in the Calm Birth class I attended when I was pregnant, and when practiced over time (even for a minute at a time), can increase parasympathetic function (rest-and-digest). This technique is great not just for childbirth, but for when you are in pain or stressed in any part of your life!

What Other Health Professionals Can Help Me to Improve My Breathing If I Find It Hard to Do on My Own?

If you live in Sydney, a great place to start is www.breathingwell.com.au. (The Breathing Well Program: Re-learning Breathing and Posture 2015) They have designed a breathing program that targets the cause of the breathing dysfunction. The typical symptoms of faulty breathing that they see are asthma, snoring, high blood pressure, bladder issues, digestive disorders and, of course, anxiety and stress-related symptoms such as hyperventilation and panic attacks. Other sources of help include chiropractors, physiotherapists, GPs and stress management specialists such as psychologists. Yoga, Pilates, Tai Chi and Chi Gong practices also focus hugely on the breath, so if you prefer a more active form of breathing, try one of these. You can also Google *Buteyko breathing* to learn more and find practitioners who specialise in it.

What Benefits Could I See from Improving My Breathing?

The list is endless but includes decreased stress levels (this can be measured with a cortisol test), improved sleep, increased energy, decreased pain, lowered blood pressure, better immune function, decreased anxiety and, overall, a feeling of being more calm and relaxed.

Smiling and Laughing

Believe it or not, smiling plays a huge role in improving and maintaining good health—physically, biochemically and emotionally. Life throws you challenges, and you can either let them get the best of you or you can look at life as a game. By playing with your problems, you disconnect from them. This often allows you to transform them into opportunities for learning and growth. Easier said than done, you say? I agree! Look at children (or remember when you were a child if you can) and watch how they deal with problems. They turn them into games in order to gain a sense of control and the opportunity to experiment with solutions. As adults we are often programmed to look at life seriously, so when things go wrong, it's hard to laugh at ourselves. Detach from the situation and tell yourself, "Life is a game, and I am a player," and see how much better you feel and function!

With Respect to Your Healing Journey, Here Is How Smiling And Laughing Can Help You Heal:

- ❖ IMPROVED IMMUNE SYSTEM FUNCTION – laughter decreases your stress hormones, which improves your immune function, allowing your body to more effectively fight disease.

- ❖ DECREASED PAIN – smiling increases endorphins and the neurotransmitter serotonin which help to suppress pain signals.

- ❖ INCREASED RELAXATION – laughing decreases stress by slowing breathing and heart rate, and increasing endorphins (feel-good hormones).

- ❖ A NEW PERSPECTIVE – humour can help you see things for what they really are and help you feel less overwhelmed.

- ❖ A POSITIVE OUTLOOK – a smile sends a message to the brain that everything is okay, so it's very hard to have a negative thought while you are smiling!

- ❖ A LONGER LIFE – there is evidence to suggest that smiling can help you live on average seven years longer!

Tips and Tricks to Help You Laugh and Smile

❖ Laugh at yourself (don't take yourself too seriously)

❖ Laughing with others is even more powerful

❖ Surround yourself with happy and positive people, places, things and memories (such as photos or music that remind you of good times)

❖ Keep things in perspective (remember, life is a game and you are a player!)

❖ Play with your kids and pets regularly (or someone else's if you don't have any)

❖ Tell jokes or ask people to tell you some jokes

❖ Be grateful and count your blessings

❖ Be spontaneous and try new things

❖ Watch a funny TV show or movie

❖ Go to a comedy club

"Life is playfulness...
we need to play so that we can discover the magic all around us."

Flora Colao

Chapter 7 –
Biochemical Treatment

NEVER SELF-DIAGNOSE OR SELF-TREAT

If there is one thing I can drum into you, it is to NEVER self-diagnose (and yes, that includes Dr. Google) and definitely do not self-treat. I don't even recommend treating yourself if you are a doctor or health care practitioner; you need an objective person who isn't attached to the symptoms and outcomes to measure your progress. Many of the treatments, supplements and advice I give here are to HELP you work with your primary care practitioner, NOT to encourage you to buy them on your own and start dosing yourself. Many supplements / herbs / diets / drugs have research supporting them, but please remember that they are often tested in ISOLATION from other supplements / herbs / diets / drugs. What may be harmless when taken in isolation may be very dangerous when taken in combination with another product / supplement / drug / food (even if it is natural!). So make sure you are working with someone who has good nutritional and supplementation knowledge. It is even better to work with a Lyme-literate practitioner, as they are going to know what treatments work best for Lyme disease, what order to implement them and what combinations are safe.

MEDICATIONS

A Note on Drugs and Medications

I am not a medical doctor and, therefore, do not have thorough enough knowledge to give advice on the use of the antibiotics listed in this book. I have included an outline of the types of antibiotics available, what antibiotics are designed to do and also the regime of antibiotics I used. This will arm you with enough information to do your own research, speak to your doctor or read some of the available Lyme books written by Lyme-literate doctors and naturopaths. Dr. Horowitz, MD, (Horowitz 2013) and Dr. Nicola McFadzean, ND, both have books with useful antibiotic information. Dr. Burrascano (Burrascano 2008) and Dr. Klinghardt (Klinghardt 2009) also have articles with their protocols that are readily available.

Antibiotics

WHAT ARE ANTIBIOTICS?

Antibiotics are substances that stop, limit the growth / multiplication of, or destroy bacteria that cause infection (not viral infections). The word *anti* means "against" and *bios* means "life," so antibiotics are designed to be "against life" in the context of fighting a bacterial disease. Originally antibiotics were made from live organisms, but now many are synthetically developed (either in part or full).

HOW ANTIBIOTICS WORK

The body's balance between optimal health and disease is called homeostasis, which believe it or not, is dependent on the balance of bacteria in it. Did you know that in a healthy human body, there are ten times more bacteria than skin cells? So, in reality, we are more bacteria than we are cells! Crazy! Chris Kresser has some great podcasts on bacteria with information that is backed up by research. (Kresser 2015) There are many types of antibiotics and they each act in different and unique ways to destroy particular strains of bacteria. Some of their actions include disturbing the cell wall, interfering with the essential protein production and interfering with the metabolism of the substances found in the cell. It is essential that the right antibiotic is dosed for the appropriate illness or condition.

Dosage of Antibiotics

Much research has gone into testing the action of an antibiotic in order to see how much exposure to the drug is necessary to either decrease replication or eradicate the bacteria being targeted. Although a large dose of antibiotics may be effective to kill the bacteria responsible for the disease, in most cases, it's not feasible because they often cause severe side effects. A big part of the side effects is the ability of the body to detox the endotoxins released as the bacteria die. If the die-off is too large, our body can't handle the toxic load; it can be very dangerous and, in extreme cases, fatal. That's why antibiotics are usually given in smaller doses (and often with food) to offset these side effects. On the other hand, however, if too little a dose is given, the wrong type of antibiotic is given, or the course of antibiotics prescribed is not finished, the bacteria may survive and replicate. Those bacteria will now be immune to the antibiotics, as they have developed sufficient methods to protect themselves. Some people think that because they feel better, it's not necessary for them to finish the course of antibiotics, but this is not only dangerous for you, it is exactly how the "superbugs" (which then become immune to the antibiotic) are created.

If you decide to take the antibiotic route, it's EXTREMELY important to follow the instructions that your doctor gives you. Often various antibiotics are prescribed to target Lyme disease and its co-infections. They may be prescribed one type at a time and then changed, multiple types cycled at different times of the day / week or multiple types at once. Often the antibiotics are prescribed at very high doses for long periods of time, and it's essential that you have a good doctor managing these protocols to ensure they are as effective and safe as possible.

TYPES OF ANTIBIOTICS

The choice of which antibiotic(s) to use needs to be monitored by your doctor (ideally, a doctor who is Lyme-literate) and should be tailored to your specific needs. It's not just a one-size-fits-all approach when deciding which type (or types) of antibiotics to use. Your program should take into consideration your age, skin type (some antibiotics like doxycycline make you sun-sensitive, so if you have very fair skin, this may not be a good option for you), age, symptoms, body composition (especially weight), severity and longevity of the illness, past experience of your toleration to medications and which infections you are targeting (different types of antibiotics will target different co-infections and opportunistic infections more effectively and efficiently).

Side Effects of Antibiotics

The main side effects from taking oral antibiotics are GIT (gastrointestinal) symptoms, which can cause stomach irritation, irritable bowel syndrome, nausea, constipation, diarrhoea, fungal infections such as Candida (often known as thrush) and recurrent bladder infections. If you experience any of these side effects, see the Treatment section for specific remedies.

WHY DO ANTIBIOTICS FAIL SOME AND WORK FOR OTHERS?

There are many reasons why the antibiotic regime will work beautifully for some and not for others. In my opinion, if you haven't seen notable changes within three months, you need to keep changing the type / dose of antibiotics (and supportive therapy) until you get it right, or just stop and try something new.

Some of the reasons for antibiotic failure include: how long the Bb (and/or co-infections) have been in your system (the longer they have been there, the harder they are to get rid of), incorrect types or doses, noncompliance, incompatibility with your genetics, counteractive supportive treatments, incorrect combinations, immune system dysfunction, methylation issues, and the presence of multiple or undiagnosed co-infections / opportunistic infections.

Antibiotic Key Points

The key thing to remember about antibiotics is that they don't just attempt to wipe out the "bad" bacteria (they are generally not super selective); they attempt to wipe out any bacteria in their path. Our bodies are delicately balanced with "good" and "bad" bacteria. "Good," or beneficial bacteria, are very important to create a harmonious internal environment in the body. About 75% of our immune system is located in the GIT, so not only does an imbalance in gut flora cause digestive system issues, but it also hugely impacts the ability of the immune system to function optimally. It is important to have some "bad" bacteria in the body in order to challenge the immune system. However, when the balance of "good " and "bad" get out of whack, which is seen with antibiotic use (especially if probiotics are not used in combination), many other health concerns are initiated or exacerbated. Antibiotics are life-saving in many situations but must be used with extreme caution, care and understanding, and should always be taken with a good probiotic and under the guidance of a skilled practitioner.

My Antibiotic Schedule

Azithromycin – 250mg per day, 1 week on and 1 week off for 8 weeks (targeting Mycoplasma pneumoniae as well as Bb)

Doxycycline – After 8 weeks, I started with 100mg of doxycycline twice daily, building to 200mg twice daily for 6 months (beware that this drug makes you extremely sun-sensitive. You'll need to cover up your entire body when outside, especially your hands). *I swapped doxycycline for minocycyline after five months, because I was sick of being so sun-sensitive. The doxycycline made me extremely nauseous all of the time, and my doctor and I thought it would be good to change anyway.*

Tinidazole – After 2 months, I added 500mg tinidazole twice daily, 2 weeks on and 2 weeks off for 4 months (in combination with the doxycycline)

Bicillin LA – After another 2 months (4 months after starting doxy-cycline), I added 0.9 million units bicillin LA injections once weekly (in combination with the docyclycline and pulsed tinidazole). *I was supposed to build up to two bicillin injections per week but blacked out the first day I had an injection, landed on the cement and concussed myself. That started a string of blackouts (that would last for up to 20 minutes at a time), so I ended up only having three injections in total. The injections are extremely painful, so I have included some tips to help you administer them more effectively.*

Tips for Bicillin LA injections

1. Use an ice pack on the gluteal muscle for 20 minutes before the injection.

2. Make sure the syringe with the bicillin is out of the fridge for at least 30 minutes (I would hold it in my hand to warm it up, as it's way more painful if injected cold).

3. Make sure you are lying down or have no weight on the leg when the needle is inserted into the gluteal.

4. Inject very slowly, over at least five minutes. *The first time I had a bicillin injection, the nurse administered the whole dose in under 30 seconds, and not only was it excruciating, but I couldn't walk properly or sleep on that side for over a week. Insist the injection is done slowly. The second time, I asked again if they would inject it slowly, but the nurse was not very cooperative and injected it over a minute. It was still way too fast!*

5. Have a heat pack ready. Lightly massage and add heat to the injection site to help it disperse over the following hours.

6. If you are up to it, go for a light 20–30 minute walk and stretch after the injection. This also helps the bicillin disperse and prevents your butt from feeling like you have the biggest corked muscle of your

life! (A cork is a deep rupture of the underlying muscle tissue as it's compressed against the bone, caused from direct blunt trauma).

In total, I took antibiotics for six months. I'm sure that they did some good, but I kept getting sicker and sicker during those six months. I have a general rule that I use with my Lyme clients: if you aren't improving after three months, you should either change regimes, or stop and try something different. You will usually know within three months if the antibiotics are effective. Rotating different drugs so the bacteria don't have a chance to adapt is also a really good idea. Do not make these decisions on your own. It is important that this part of your treatment is overseen by your primary health care practitioner and/or doctor.

I also had IV flagyl and rifampicin whilst I was in the St. Georg Klinik in Germany (see the information about this clinic later in the book for more information on this regime).

TEAMING NATURAL THERAPIES WITH ANTIBIOTICS

Biochemical natural treatments work well in isolation or in combination with antibiotic therapy. It is super important that natural therapies are always used in conjunction with antibiotics in order to offset some of the side effects caused by the antibiotics. The biggest reported side effects of antibiotic use are nausea and gut disturbance (especially diarrhoea or constipation).

Nausea – use ginger (tea, capsules, in food, raw), peppermint (tea, drops in water, oil burner or diffuser)

Diarrhoea – eat fibres such as apple pectin, husks, chia seeds and ground flax seeds; binders such as activated charcoal; or a probiotic such as SB Floractiv (Bioceuticals® has a good one)

Constipation – increase vitamin C, magnesium, water, and/or slippery elm

OVERVIEW OF MEDICATIONS AND SUPPLEMENTS FOR LYME DISEASE

Please note that the supplements in bold are the ones that I used and found to be the most important or most effective for me.

Abbreviation Key

PB = Professional Botanicals brand

BIOC = Bioceuticals®

MG = Metagenics

NM = NutraMedix® (Cowden protocol)

RN = Researched Nutritionals

LYME DISEASE	Dr. Nicola's RestorMedicine & Research Nutritionals (RN)	Byron White	Drugs	Other
Spirochete			Penicillins and cephalosporins e.g., bicillin, cefuroxime	Guaiacum
Intracellular/ cell-wall deficient/L-Form		A-V	Tetracyclines and macro-lides, e.g., doxycycline, minocycline. azithromycin, clarithromycin Tinidazole Metronidazole	

LYME DISEASE	Dr. Nicola's RestorMedicine & Research Nutritionals (RN)	Byron White	Drugs	Other
Cyst			Tinidazole, plaquenil or metronidazole	Grapefruit seed extract Lactoferrin Xylitol
Biofilm	**Lumbrokinase** Nattokinase Serrapeptase	A-BIO	Vancomycin Diflucan Getamycin	Proteolytic enzymes (rec. Vitalzyme) T.O.A. Cat's claw Otoba bark extract LGG probiotic (MG) Other: berberine, artemesinin, citrus seed extract, black walnut hulls, echinacea, goldenseal, genetian, tea tree oil, fumitory, galbanon oil, oregano oil, neem, Phellodendron amurense, stem bark dry (Phellodendron) Greater celadine, NAC (N-Acetyl cysteine), Bromelain – from pineapple or BioHawks Pine Crush extract

LYME DISEASE	Dr. Nicola's RestorMedicine & Research Nutritionals (RN)	Byron White	Drugs	Other
General	**Fresh Teasel Root** **RN Transfer Factor** **LymPlus**	**A-L Complex**	Amoxycillin for kids	T.O.A. Cat's claw (NM Samento) Japanese knotweed Guaiacum Banderol Quinoa

OVERVIEW OF MEDICATIONS AND SUPPLEMENTS FOR OPPORTUNISTIC AND CO-INFECTIONS

OPPORTUNISTIC & CO-INFECTIONS	Dr. Nicola's Restor-Medicine & Re-search Nutritionals (RN)	Byron White	Drugs	Other
Babesia	**RN Artimisinin**	**A-BAB**	Malarone + Plaquneil +/- Septrin or Wellvone	Cryptolepsis Neem Noni fruit Artesunate (derivative of artemesia herb) Ozonated rizol oils containing artemesia Sida acuta Enula Mora

OPPORTUNISTIC & CO-INFECTIONS	Dr. Nicola's Restor-Medicine & Research Nutritionals (RN)	Byron White	Drugs	Other
Bartonella		**A-BART**	Doxycycline/ Minocycline + Rifampicin/ Azythromycin/ Septrin or Ciprofloxacin, Bactrim DS Plaquenil	**Dr. Zhang'sHH2 (Houttuynia)** **NM –** Cumanda **NM–** Banderol Japanese Knotweed Polygunum (resveratrol MG – Resveratrol Healthy Ageing)
Mycoplasma		A-MYCO	Azythromycin	
Fungal Infections	Dr. Nicola's Antifungal Formula	A-FNG		Loalsan Mollecular Products – Candicid Forte Grapefruit seed extract Tea tree oil Garlic Olive leaf extract Caprylic acid Herbs- cinnamon, clove, peppermint, rosemary Oil of oregano Probiotics NM: banderol and cumanda Pau d'arco

OPPORTUNISTIC & CO-INFECTIONS	Dr. Nicola's Restor-Medicine & Research Nutritionals (RN)	Byron White	Drugs	Other
Parasite(s)	Dr. Nicola's Anti-parasitic Formula			Garlic Genetian Olive leaf extract Black walnut Wormwood Clove Black seed
Ehrlichia			Rifampicin, Ciprofloxacin, Bactrim DS	
Rickettsia			Rifampicin, Ciprofloxacin, Bactrim DS	
Herpes		A-V	Valtrex	L-lyceine Mushrooms – reishi, maitake, shitake
Epstein-Barr Virus		A-EB/H6		Any viral support MG – Super Mushroom Complex Chinese mushroom blends Mushrooms – reishi, maitake, shitake
CMV (cytomegalovirus)		A-CM		

OPPORTUNISTIC & CO-INFECTIONS	Dr. Nicola's Restor-Medicine & Research Nutritionals (RN)	Byron White	Drugs	Other
Helicobacter Pylori		A-HP		Essential oils Lemon grass, oregano, melaleuca

OVERVIEW OF SUPPLEMENTS FOR SPECIFIC SYSTEMS DIRECTLY AND INDIRECTLY AFFECTED BY LYME DISEASE, AND OPPORTUNISTIC AND CO-INFECTIONS

This table includes a summary of supplements and supports (some of these are in more detail later in this section).

OTHER	Dr. Nicola's Restor-Medicine & Research Nutritionals (RN)	Byron White	Other
Detox Support	**Dr. Nicola's Smilax** Dr. Nicola'sDetox Formula 1 or 2 RN Liposomal Glutathione	Detox 1 (whole body)	**Vit C** P2Detox Heel galium Cell-Logic's DefenCELL® Dr. Ron's Ultra-Pure™ Fresh liver capsules Dandelion root Milk thistle Glutathione Phosphatidylcholine (PC) – caps/liquid/IV Binders – psyllium husks, flax seeds, apple pectin, chorella, activated charcoal

OTHER	Dr. Nicola's Restor-Medicine & Research Nutritionals (RN)	Byron White	Other
Immune Support	**Dr. Nicola Lyme Support Formula**	A-INFLAM	Olive leaf extract Garlic capsules Echinacea Zinc Iodine Colostrum Mushrooms – reishi, maitake, shitake Colloidal silver PB – ImmuneGuard and Attack (goldenseal) BIOC – Armaforce MG – Andro NK LDN (low dose naltrexone) – *need a script
Adrenal Support	Isocort		MG – Adrenotone BIOC – Adrenoplex PB – ADR Dr. Ron's – adrenal capsules (with cortex and liver) Adaptogens include Ginseng (Siberian and Korean), Ashwagandra, Rhodiola Rosea, Withania Other Adrenal Supportive Herbs – liquorice root Adrenal Precursors – DHEA and/or pregnenolone

OTHER	Dr. Nicola's Restor-Medicine & Research Nutritionals (RN)	Byron White	Other
Thyroid Support			Iodine (excluding Hashimoto's) Kelp Tyrosine Zinc and selenium (support natural T4–T3 conversion)
GIT Support		Detox 2	**BIOC – Intestamine®** **Probiotics** – e.g., BIOC Ultrabiotic 45 BIOC – SB Floractiv Multigest Enzymes (hydrochloric acid and betaine) Slippery elm (if constipated)
Inflammatory Support			MG – Inflavinoid (or anything containing curcumin) MG – Kaprex Liquorice Root Turmeric/Curcumin White willow Proteolytic Enzymes – e.g., bromelain, protease, papin, rutin, amylase, lipase, serrazimes (rec. Vitalzyme – www.worldnutrition.com) or PB Di-Aid Arnica

OTHER	Dr. Nicola's Restor-Medicine & Research Nutritionals (RN)	Byron White	Other
Sleep Support	Dr. Nicola's Sleep Support		BIOC – RestoraCalm® Magnesium Valerian root Chamomile Lemon balm Passion flower 5-HTP (supports serotonin) Melatonin (sleep-inducing) L-Tryptophan (precursor to melatonin) Withania
Energy Support	RN ATP Fuel		CoQ10 Ribose
Nutritional Support			**Juice Plus** (or any whole food supplement)
Viral infection Support		A-V	PB – ViralAid Olive Leaf extract Lauricidin Mushrooms – reishi, maitake, shitake
Neurological Support		NT-Detox	Any of the natural anti-inflammatory supports St. John's wort Lemon balm
Lymphatic Support	Dr. Nicola's Lymphatic Support Formula	BT-Detox	MG – Lymphatox Poke Root Cleavers Red Root Sarspatilla Deseret Biologics - Lymph Drainage

OTHER	Dr. Nicola's Restor-Medicine & Research Nutritionals (RN)	Byron White	Other
Alkalising Support			**Fresh wheatgrass, Spirilina (e.g., Good Green Stuff), Barley Greens** **MG Detox Express**
Mood Support			BIOC – RestoraCalm® MG – Neurocalm Innovative Therapies; Proxan St. John's wort 5-HTP (supports serotonin) Tyrosine (used for thyroid but also good for the brain) BABA/L-theanine (good for anxiety)
Cognitive Support			Phosphatidylserine Omega-3
Reproductive Hormonal Support			Chaste Tree (Vitex) to support menstrual cycle & decrease PMS Fertility Herbs – Shataran and false unicorn root from MediHerb, maca Menopausal Herbs – Liquorice root, red clover and black cohosh (also good for bladder symptoms)

OTHER	Dr. Nicola's Restor-Medicine & Research Nutritionals (RN)	Byron White	Other
Heavy Metal Detoxification			Binders = psyllium husks, flax seeds, apple pectin, chorella, activated charcoal Heavy Metal Chelators = DMSA, DMPS, EDTA, Cilantro, NDF, Zeolite HP Natural Heavy Metal Binding Support – ALA, high dose vit C, glutathione
Other			**Magnesium** **Organic Whey Protein powder (e.g., Isagenix, Raw, Bare Blends)** **B Complex** **Omega 3** Calcium Zinc (pincollate if you have pyrrole disorder) Vit D3 LDN (low dose naltrexone) – pain, inflammation, immune system

"Let food be thy medicine."

Hippocrates

NATURAL PROTOCOLS – ANTIMICROBIALS, HOMEOPATHICS, SUPPLEMENTATION

Byron White Formulas (BWF)

The company Byron White Formulas™ was created by Dr. Byron White when he was unable to find a company that would mass produce his products at the level he desired (VOC-free, potent and with the correct energetic herbal formula). This is how his private manufacturing company was born. Now he can produce the same high quality formulas for the rest of the world to use that he had made on a smaller scale to treat Lyme disease in his clinic.

To take Byron White formulas, you must have a consultation with a practitioner trained in using and dispensing these formulas, as they are extremely potent and not to be self-prescribed. It's important that someone can manage your dose in order to avoid negative reactions and side effects (also known as Herxing), and to help you if this reaction should occur. Health Space Clinics, which my husband and I own and run, have practitioners in every clinic who can have a consult with you and dispense either in the clinic or over the phone (postage applies). You can also log onto the Byron White Formula's website for more information (www.byronwhiteformulas.com) or contact the Australian distributor John Coleman via email (pdfree@returnstillness.com.au).

Always follow the instructions given to you by your Health Practitioner. These recommendations are general in nature and intended only to help you care for and take the formulas with ease.

What Are the BWFs Used for?

RESEARCH GROUPS AND CLINICAL RESULTS HAVE SHOWN THAT BWFS:

❖ Support the immune system response to current issues – most people feel a response to the formulas immediately

❖ Increase emotional well-being

❖ Decrease anxiety and depression, improve responses to stress and improve symptom relief (reported by a large percentage of clients)

❖ Improve sleep and energy

❖ Improve pulse diagnosis and Chi flow when assessed pre- and post- by acupuncturists (Horowitz and Corson, Byron White Formulas Brochure n.d.)

Getting Ready: When to Take BWFs

❖ The BWFs should ideally be taken before or after other oral medications by at least 2 hours, if possible. If this is not possible, then allow at least 30 minutes.

❖ The BWFs are best used on an empty stomach or at least 30 minutes before eating.

How to Take BWFs

1. Shake well before each use (this helps combine the micronised herbs with the liquid extract and enhances the activation of the formula's powerful effects).

2. Succuss the BWFs by hitting the bottle on the palm of the hand six times before taking.

3. Put the amount of drops you are taking in a small amount of filtered water (10–15 ml is sufficient) in a glass or ceramic cup. Swish the glass (do not stir it with anything metal). Do not mix with juice.

4. Take the formula into your mouth and hold it there for 30–60 seconds. This allows the formula to absorb into all the energetic pathways and increase absorption. (Return to Stillness n.d.)

Continue to increase your dosage (per your health practitioner's recommendations) as long as you are not Herxing (in which case, contact your health practitioner immediately).

Generally, it's recommended that clients start with 1 drop 1–2 times a day. Extremely sensitive people or those with heavy microbial loads and toxins may need to dose 1 drop over a day or require K dilutions (where the formula is diluted to less than one drop a day), which must be supervised by the prescribing practitioner. Always start each BWF one at a time. (Horowitz and Corson, Byron White Formulas Brochure n.d.)

Most people start a remedy at one drop only per day and observe their response before increasing the dose. Always follow your practitioner's instructions and advice.

Other Useful Information

❖ The Byron White Formulas are highly viscous. To keep the stoppers flowing properly, please shake thoroughly to prevent a buildup. If there is a blockage, you may use a clean pin or toothpick to clear the tip, or remove the rubber bulb and flush the tube with clean water.

❖ Formulas are gluten-free. Organic grape alcohol is used in the formulas, so if you need to decrease the amount of alcohol due to sensitivity, put the drops in WARM, filtered water instead to help dissipate the alcohol. NEVER use in hot or boiling water, and don't use a microwave to heat the water.

❖ You MUST continue to take your max dose for at least two months past symptom resolution and then slowly taper.

❖ **Note:** Each 1 ounce (30 ml) bottle contains approximately 900 drops. (Return to Stillness n.d.)

There are many Byron White Formulas available. An overview of their application can be found in table form in the previous section Overview of Medications and Supplements for Lyme Disease, Opportunistic and Co-Infections.

Dr. Nicola's Products – RestorMedicine

Dr. Nicola Mcfadzean is an Australian-born naturopathic doctor work-ing predominantly in the USA. Nicola does not believe in using antibiotic protocols without the support of natural therapies. Naturopaths in America are known as naturopathic doctors (NDs), and unlike naturopaths in Aus-tralia, they CAN prescribe antibiotics. Her preferred approach is a combina-tion of antibiotic and natural therapies (McFadzean, The Lyme Diet: Nutri-tional Strategies for Healing from Lyme Disease 2010), and she has created a range of products to support and enhance Lyme disease treatment. She has her own website, RestorMedicine, where you can buy these and other products online. The following products have worked well for my clients and I for the treatment of Lyme disease, its co-infections and opportunistic infec-tions (RestorMedicine 2015). They are also good for many other conditions. Please visit her website for further information or read her books.

The following information is reprinted with Dr. McFadzean's permission:

Dr. Nicola's Smilax – A tincture for binding neurotoxins, reducing inflammation, and supporting detoxification and Herx reactions. Contains: Chinese Sarsaparilla (Smilax glabra) Dose: Build up to 30–60 drops twice daily.

Dr. Nicola's Lyme Support Formula – A blend of herbs with antimicrobial, anti-inflammatory and immune-supportive properties. Contains: Cat's Claw (Uncaria tomentosa), Lignum-vitae (Guaiacum officinale), Astragalus (Astragalus membranaceus), Andrographis (Andrographis paniculata). Dose: Build up to 5–10 drops twice daily.

Dr. Nicola's Fresh Teasel Root – A high quality teasel extract helpful in the treatment of Lyme and other tick-borne illnesses. Contains: Teasel Root (Dipsacus sylvestris) Dose: Build up to 10–20 drops twice daily.

Dr. Nicola's Lymphatic Support Formula – A tincture for cleansing the lymph system and clearing waste from the body. Can help reduce toxicity in the body and combines well with the Detox Support Formula. Contains: Cleavers (Gallium aparine), Red Root (Ceanothus americanus), Burdock (Arctium lappa), Queen's Delight (Stillingia sylvatica), Poke Root (Phytolacca americana), Blue Wild Indigo (Baptisia), Prickly Ash (Zanthoxylum), Ocotillo (Fouquieria splendens). Dose: Build up to 30–60 drops, 1 to 2 times daily.

Dr. Nicola's Detox Support Formula #1 – A low-alcohol blend of liver cleansers and tonifiers. Detox #1 does contain Milk Thistle, which should not be taken by those on Mepron or Malarone. Contains: Astragalus (Astragalus membranaceous), Burdock (Arctium lappa), Dandelion Root (Taraxacum officinale), Goji Berry (Lycium chinensis), Lemon Balm (Melissa officinalis), Milk Thistle (Silybum marianum), Wu-Wei-Zi fruit (Schisandra chinensis), Thorowax (Bupleurum falcatum), Oregon Grape Root (Mahonia aquifolium), Liquorice root (Glycyrrhiza glabra). Dose: Build up to 60 drops, 2 to 4 times daily.

Dr. Nicola's Detox Support Formula #2 – A low-alcohol blend of liver cleansers and tonifiers. This formula does not contain Milk Thistle, which makes it appropriate for use by individuals taking Mepron or Malarone. Contains: Astragalus (Astragalus membranaceous), Burdock (Arctium lappa), Dandelion root (Taraxacum officinale), Goji Berry (Lycium chinensis), Lemon Balm (Melissa officinalis), Wu-Wei-Zi fruit (Schisandra chinensis), Thorowax (Bupleurum falcatum), Oregon Grape Root (Mahonia aquifolium), Liquorice root (Glycyrrhiza glabra). Dose: Build up to 60 drops, 2 to 4 times daily.

Dr. Nicola's Sleep Support Formula – Nerve-calming herbs and a gentle, nourishing sedative to help promote restful and consistent sleep. Contains: Milky Wild Oats (Avena fatua), California Poppy (Eschscholzia californica), Catnip (Nepeta cataria), Passionflower (Passiflora incarnata), Yan Hu Suo (Corydalis hanhusuo). Dose: 1–2 teaspoons ½ hour before bed, up to 4 times per night, not to exceed 3 teaspoons per night.

Dr. Nicola's Anti-Parasite Formula – A potent blend of herbs to support the body in ridding parasites, amoeba and helminths (worms). Contains: Wormwood (Artemesia absinthium), Sweet Annie (Artemisia annua),

Garlic (Allium sativum), Epazote (Chenopodium ambrosioides), Yellow Gentian (Gentiana lutea), Goldenseal (Hydrastis canadensis), Black Walnut (Juglans nigra), Oregon Grape Root (Mahonia aquifolium), Quassia bark (Quassia amargo), Pau D'Arco (Tabebuia impetiginosa), Tansy (Tanacetum vulgare), Ginger (Zingiber officinalis), Clove (Syzygium aromaticum). Dose: Build up to 60 drops, 2 to 3 times daily.

Dr. Nicola's Anti-Fungal Formula – Good for combating yeast overgrowth and combines well with the Anti-Parasite Formula to promote balanced intestinal flora. Contains: Garlic (Allium sativum), Curlycup Gumweed (Grindelia squarrosa), Oregon Grape (Mahonia aquifolium), Wild Bergamot (Monarda fistulosa), Pau D'Arco (Tabebuia heptaphylla), Eastern Arborvitae (Thuja occidentalis), Cinnamon (Cinnamomum cassia), Fennel (Foeniculum vulgare). Dose: Build up to 60 drops, 2 to 3 times daily.

Dr. Nicola also uses essential oil protocols to target Borrelia. Here is an example of one of these protocols:

❖ Every day – cinnamon and melaleuca – 1 drop of each twice daily

❖ 10 day cycles (10 days on / 10 days off) – oregano, clove, thyme, peppermint. Mix 1 drop of each oil in a capsule, and then swallow (build to 4 drops of each oil).

* Please note that, as always, I do not recommend self-prescription and dosing. You can have a phone consultation with Dr. Nicola McFadzean or book in with any of the Health Space Lyme-literate practitioners for help with products and dosing. You can also use this book with your primary health care practitioner.

The Cowden Protocol (CSP)

The Cowden Support Program (CSP) is a protocol developed by Wm. Lee Cowden, MD, who is board certified in internal medicine, cardiovascular disease, and clinical nutrition. The protocol was initially designed for the treatment of late-stage Borrelia and Lyme co-infections. According to Dr. Cowden, the protocol helps to resolve the majority of the root causes of most patients' symptoms and can also be used to treat Post-treatment Lyme Disease Syndrome (PTLDS) as well as many other chronic health conditions of unclear cause. Dr. Cowden continually collects data and information from patients who are using his protocol with the aim of educating and keeping doctors up-to-date, so they can implement less toxic and more effective treatments for Lyme disease.

I have taken a summary of this protocol and products from the website www.nutramedix.ec/ns/lyme-protocol. (COWDEN SUPPORT PROGRAM: Protocol for Borrelia and Lyme Co-Infections & Most Chronic Conditions 2011)

The Cowden Support Program utilises 13 different NutraMedix® products including six Microbial Defense herbals (three pairs of herbals) that are taken rotationally. The first pair, Banderol and Samento, were studied in vitro by Eva Sapi, PhD, and her group at the University of New Haven in Connecticut and found to eliminate all forms of Borrelia burgdorferi (spirochetes, round-body forms and biofilm forms). In that study, the antibiotic doxycycline was not nearly as effective against biofilm and round body forms of Borrelia burgdorferi. Richard Horowitz, MD, in New York State, has found the Cowden Support Program to be effective in markedly improving the condition of 70–80% of the advanced Lyme Borreliosis patients with co-infections over 4 to 6 months time, even if the patients had previously failed to improve on multiple courses of antibiotics. Dr. Horowitz presented his findings at the ILADS conference in autumn of 2007. More recently, a nine-month observational study of the Cowden Support Program was conducted by the Borreliose Centrum Augsburg, Germany. Completed in 2012, this study resulted in 80% of patients showing symptomatic improvements (via questionnaire) and 90% of patients showing improvements via lab blood tests.

One reason for the success of the CSP is that the Microbial Defense products have broad-spectrum action against bacteria, fungi, parasites and even viruses, and they are natural anti-inflammatories that are non-toxic. Pharmaceuticals often have a much narrower spectrum of action than the broad-spectrum herbals, so many late-stage Lyme patients fail to get well or remain symptom-free if they only use pharmaceuticals such as antibiotics. The pharmaceutical drugs are often not able to resolve the various remaining microbial infections or deal with the immune dysregulation and gut dysbiosis. Toxicology studies at the University of Guayaquil in Ecuador show that herbs from the CSP can be given to animals at thousands of times the recommended doses without changes in animal behavior or in organ histopathology.

The CSP is also so successful because of the other eight constituents of the program. These include: Zeolite and Zeolite-HP supplements used to detoxify most heavy metals, various biotoxins and several other man-made toxins from the body; Pinella, which appears to remove toxins from the brain, spinal cord and nerves; Burbur Detox and Parsley Detox, taken rotationally, help detoxify the liver, gall bladder, kidneys, lymphatics, and interstitial spaces (the space between cells); and Sparga, which helps detoxify the Sulfa antibiotics and other sulfa drugs that block the body's sulfation and glutathione toxin-conjugation pathways.

Most chronically ill patients are magnesium deficient. The Magnesium Malate is the most highly absorbable and highly utilisable form of magnesium. Approximately 50% of the metabolic enzymes that ultimately cause ATP energy production for the cells require magnesium as a co-factor. Magnesium is also necessary for normal heart rhythm, normal blood pressure, normal nerve and brain function, normal contraction and relaxation of the skeletal muscles as well as the smooth muscles in the gut, bile ducts, pancreatic ducts, etc.

Serrapeptase, taken 30 minutes before food, gets absorbed and breaks down biofilm and fibrin in the body. When fibrin that covers the microbes is stripped away with Serrapeptase, the immune system can more effectively attack and remove those microbes underneath. When fibrin that has adhered to capillary walls is stripped away by Serrapeptase, oxygen moves more easily from the red blood cells into the tissues, thus converting the predominantly anaerobic metabolism back into aerobic metabolism. This results in a shift from a microbe-friendly lactic acidosis tissue environment to a normal acid-base environment.

Adult patients taking the CSP are urged to drink 2–3 litres or quarts of water per day (proportionately less for children based on weight). Patients are urged to practice stress reduction techniques, such as deep-breathing while visualising and using all five senses (e.g., imagining a relaxing vacation / holiday spot), for four minutes before each meal and before bedtime. Patients should rest in bed (whether they fall asleep or not) in a dark bedroom with minimal electromagnetic pollution, from 11pm to 6 or 7am each night. Patients are urged to eat more raw, organic, (mostly vegetarian) foods that are NOT genetically-modified and avoid sugars, excessive starches, processed foods, fried foods, peanut products, canola oil and hydrogenated oils. Patients who also avoid all wheat products and all cow and dairy products seem to improve much faster.

Patients on the CSP are encouraged to find ways to laugh each day, to avoid unnecessary stress and bad relationships, to pray or meditate each day, and to find a way to give and receive love each day, even if that means having a dog or a pet. Unconditional love is one of the most powerful healing sources in the universe.

ATTENTION: Binders such as activated charcoal and calcium bentonite clay should be avoided as much as possible while using the CSP, as it is believed that activated charcoal always binds to the active ingredients that are in the herbal remedies and pharmaceuticals, and often makes them ineffective. These binders should only be considered on the rare occasion when you have been severely affected by a Herxheimer reaction that does not resolve with Burbur Detox, Parsley Detox, Pinella, or water.

Researched Nutritionals

Researched Nutritionals is an American company (I was introduced to their products by Dr. Nicola McFadzean). Their website https://www.researchednutritionals.com has online products as well as great information and research. Once again, I do not recommend self-diagnosing or dosing, so work with your Lyme-literate practitioner to decide which products are right for you. I have used the following products and have included information about them taken straight from their website to save you time looking it up yourself. (Researched Nutritionals: solutions for life 2015)

Tri-Fortify*™ *Orange Liposomal Glutathione – provides the preferred reduced L-glutathione, the major intracellular antioxidant essential for detoxification in the body, plus vitamin C, in an absorbable liposomal delivery system. The unique liposome structure allows it to combine effectively with the body's natural fluids and penetrate its protective membranes, bypassing the digestive system and directly entering the blood stream. By avoiding the process of digestion, nutrient absorption and utilisation is much quicker and more complete. Dose – 1 teaspoon before breakfast.

***ATP Fuel*®** – is designed to support the Krebs Cycle of cellular energy production. The Krebs Cycle takes place inside the mitochondria or "power plant" of the cell, and it is the body's primary energy producer. ATP Fuel® is formulated for athletes and fatigued patients seeking optimised energy. ATP Fuel® offers the top three energy nutrients and cofactors synergistically combined for maximum mitochondrial performance and energy production: NT Factor Energy™, NADH and CoQ10. Dose – 5 caps 30 minutes before breakfast and 5 caps 30 minutes before lunch for 2 months; 5 caps 30 minutes before breakfast from month 3 onwards.

***Artemisinin SOD*™**– combines pure artemisinin for immune support, green tea extract to promote healthy levels of SOD (superoxide dismutase), curcumin and quercetin for their healthy impact on inflammation and resulting inhibitory affect on NF kappa B, and black walnut hull to arm the body's anti-parasitic arsenal. Dose – 1 cap per day building up to 2 caps twice a day.

Transfer Factor LymPlus*™ *Specific Immune Support – provides the physician with a targeted formula developed to support the body's immune system. As with all targeted transfer factors, it is recommended that the health care professional confirm the patient's condition with the appropriate lab tests prior to administering the targeted transfer factor. Dose – build up to 2 caps per day.

Beyond Balance

Beyond Balance, Inc. was developed in 1990 and is the exclusive distributor of many unique herbal extracts that were developed by herbalist / formulator Susan McCamish. I had the honour of meeting this brilliant lady at a conference where she explained that her son had been so debilitated by Lyme disease that he was in a wheelchair. With nowhere to turn, she created her own herbal products in order to help him recover. And help him she did! When I met Susan, she was traveling with her son and he was very much thriving.

The Beyond Balance range of products includes both capsules and extract formulas that are made in a glycerin base (as opposed to alcohol which many Lymies are sensitive to). They have various formulas for detox support, inflammation reduction, environmental detox (including heavy metals) and organ support. They have a huge range of immune support products specifically for Lyme disease, including two different formulas to target Borrelia, two for Bartonella and three for Babesia. They are practitioner-dispensed products, so you must work with a health professional trained in using these products.

Salt / C Protocol

This protocol can be used as an adjunct therapy and uses sea salt and vitamin C (as the name suggests!). I don't suggest doing this method on your own but am adding it, as I have had multiple people say they have had good results using it. It is hypothesised that the protocol has a broad action antimicrobial effect and that it's unlikely that the microbes can or will develop a resistance to the salt or vitamin C. Vitamin C is used as a supportive therapy for most Lyme treatments. Once you reach bowel tolerance, it induces diarrhoea, which can be a helpful detox method in itself when monitored closely. There are lots of varying salt and C protocols, but the key is to start slowly and make sure you are well-hydrated.

Salt Protocol

Add pure sea salt (e.g., Celtic, Himalayan) to a glass of purified or distilled water at a ratio of 1 teaspoon per 1200ml. Allow the salt to dissolve over a few hours before drinking. Once the salt has dissolved, drink the 1200ml of salty water followed by the vitamin C protocol, and then refill the glass and drink another 1200ml of purified water over the next hour. Start with a ¼ teaspoon of salt and increase every few days until you reach one teaspoon (if you start Herxing, stay at that level or decrease the amount). Once you reach one teaspoon per day, do the protocol in the morning and at night (build the second dose from ¼ teaspoon to 1 teaspoon again every few days).

Vitamin C Protocol

Mix vitamin C with 1200 ml of water at a ratio of 5000mg per 1 teaspoon of salt. For example, if you are starting with ¼ teaspoon of salt, you will use 1250g of vitamin C. Drink this right after the salt drink as explained before.

Example Protocol

1. Day 1–3 = ¼ teaspoon salt in 300ml water, 1250mg vitamin C in 150–250ml water, 300ml plain water over the following hour.

2. Day 4–6 = ½ teaspoon salt in 600ml water, 2500mg vitamin C in 150–250ml water, 600ml plain water over the following hour.

3. Day 7–9 = ¾ teaspoon salt in 900ml water, 3750mg vitamin C in 150–250ml water, 900ml plain water over the following hour.

4. Day 10–12 = 1 teaspoon salt in 1200ml water, 5000mg vitamin C in 150–250ml water, 1200ml plain water over the following hour.

5. Day 13–15 = AM: 1 teaspoon salt in 1200ml water, 5000mg vitamin C in 150– 250ml water, 1200ml plain water over the following hour; PM: ¼ teaspoon salt in 300ml water, 1250mg vitamin C in 150– 250ml water, 300ml plain water over the following hour.

6. Day 16–18 = AM: 1 teaspoon salt in 1200ml water, 5000mg vitamin C in 150– 250ml water, 1200ml plain water over the following hour; PM: ½ teaspoon salt in 600ml water, 2500mg vitamin C in 150– 250ml water, 600ml plain water over the following hour.

7. Day 19–21 = AM: 1 teaspoon salt in 1200ml water, 5000mg vitamin C in 150– 250ml water, 1200ml plain water over the following hour; PM: ¾ teaspoon salt in 900ml water, 3750mg vitamin C in 150– 250ml water, 900ml plain water over the following hour.

8. Day 22–25 = AM: 1 teaspoon salt in 1200ml water, 5000mg vitamin C in 150– 250ml water, 1200ml plain water over the following hour; PM: 1 teaspoon salt in 1200ml water, 5000mg vitamin C in 150– 250ml water, 1200ml plain water over the following hour.

You can increase the doses from here if you are tolerating the treatment, you can continue this dose or you can pulse the treatment one month on and one month off. Listen to your body, and don't attempt this protocol on your own.

I have summarised some of the plausible reasons why this protocol can work well for Lyme disease and chronic fatigue (from the forum entry at http://curezone.org/forums/am.asp?i=478977(linkin 2005):

❖ The Salt/C elevates blood salinity short-term, which may cause osmotic shock (dehydration leading to death) to certain vulnerable bacteria.

❖ Salt up-regulates white blood cells (which assists the immune system) by allowing them to use the salt to kill certain bacteria.

❖ Salt causes mild blood alkalinity, which is believed to make the environment less favourable for "bad" bacteria to survive.

❖ On a cellular level, salt can assist with the detoxification process. As salt gets into the cell via the osmotic process, it is believed that it may help destroy bacteria such as Bb and mycoplasma.

❖ Salt helps absorption of water, which assists the lymphatic system to get rid of toxins, therefore decreasing microbial load. Salt helps absorption of water, which assists the lymphatic system to get rid of toxins, therefore decreasing microbial load.

❖ Salt assists in the destruction of pathogens in the gut that contribute to dysbiosis in the gut. Improving the GIT function assists immune function and allows for more favourable conditions to get the bacterial balance right.

❖ Some parasites, particularly nematodes (as shown on www.LymePhotos.com), are known to be sensitive to salinity levels and will move away from salt doses to areas of the body with more 'optimal' salinity.

❖ Salt increases salinity, which is believed to repel or even paralyse unwanted parasites (particularly nematodes), making them more vulnerable to immune system destruction.

❖ A salt shock activates the adrenals, which then signals the kidneys to try to balance the salt burst by desalinating, hence dumping excess microbes. Once the blood returns to its ideal salt balance, the adrenals are signalled to rest, which is beneficial for healing.

❖ The adrenals often work harder when the body is salt deficient (which is common in chronic bacterial infections), so increasing salt can assist adrenal function as well.

❖ When someone has an infection, it affects their electrolyte balance. An increase in salt may help reverse that imbalance. Often other components also need to be addressed to achieve this balance.

❖ Vitamin C is a well-known immune booster (boosting white cell production), and that, in combination with the salt up-regulating the white cells, creates strong antimicrobial action.

❖ Many body functions rely on salt, and due to the low intake of salt in most people's diets, detoxification via sweat, lymphatics, blood, etc. is adversely affected (I'm talking about mineral salts such as Celtic and Himalayan salts, not iodised salts).

❖ Supplementation with good mineral salts, displace the bad salts and minerals, and the toxins that may have contributed to poor health even before the chronic infection (e.g., like putting clean petrol in your car after putting dirty fuel in it for years).

❖ Increasing salt improves sodium-potassium pump action and therefore cellular function.

❖ Salt helps relax the muscles.

❖ Salt is corrosive by nature and so may assist to thin the blood and other buildups that are common with Lyme and related illnesses.

❖ Salt improves digestion by improving stomach acid, which is often compromised in chronically ill patients.

❖ Salt provides sodium bicarbonate which is known to increase antimicrobial action and possibly boost neutrophil function.

❖ Salt/C may be used as a natural version of the Marshal Protocol with salt providing the antimicrobial action of minocycline and vitamin C the anti-inflammatory action of Benicar®.

❖ Salt increases the enzyme elastase in your tissues making microbes and parasites more vulnerable to the immune system.

❖ Heavy metal toxicity often leaches minerals from the body so increasing salt can help to balance minerals.

❖ Salt improves blood volume. Dr. Paul Cheney, who is a CFS expert, recommends drinking sodium / potassium drinks (he recommends Recup) at least twice a day to increase blood volume in order to improve diastolic heart dysfunction. Many people with Lyme disease and CFS report cardiac symptoms. Here is a link to Dr. Cheney's home brew version of the recipe (previously called *gookinaid* and now called *hydralyte*) – http://www.dfwcfids.org/healing/gokhmbrw.htm.

❖ Salt is an electrolyte, and there are theories that a salt deficiency can disrupt the body's natural electromagnetic field making it more sensitive to electromagnetic and radiofrequencies (EMF and RF). It's also theorised that when this energy field is disrupted, it can cause dys-regulation of the immune system and, in fact, many of the body's systems. So the Salt/C protocol may then have the ability to protect the body from harmful EMF and RF as well as improve or even restore the natural biological processes of the body.

❖ Salt water alkalises the fluids of the body, which slows the excretion of vitamin C. This means that vitamin C is in the system for longer and has a greater ability to enhance immune function without increasing the dose.

❖ Salt and water are believed to increase blood volume and, hence, lymphatic flow. Toxins are often processed and eliminated via lymphatic fluid, so by increasing lymphatic flow, you are essentially improving detoxification of microbes.

Natural Antibiotics

There are some very powerful natural herbs that have antibiotic actions. Just because they are natural does not mean that they can't have very potent effects (and these can have both positive and negative side effects just like antibiotics can). For example, the International Congress on Natural Medicine in 2014 presented research that supported previous findings that grapefruit seed extract is NOT selective for certain bacteria and is actually more detrimental in wiping out gut flora ("good" and "bad" bacteria) than most antibiotics! (The 2014 International Congress on Natural Medicine Conference (Metagenics) n.d.) Due to the fact that Bb is hard to eliminate, an option may be to wipe out the majority of bacteria ("good" and "bad") and then rebuild using various strategies. However use extreme caution and work with a health practitioner who knows what they are doing when using natural antibiotics.

Olive Leaf Extract

Olive leaf extract has many antimicrobial properties including antiviral, antiparasitic, antiprotozoan and antifungal (believed to work against Candida). It is also a very powerful immune stimulant, and it's my go-to when I feel like I am getting the flu! Bioceuticals® has a fermented olive leaf extract that I believe is the best product available in Australia.

Colloidal Silver (aka Silver Colloid)

Colloidal silver, a natural antibiotic, has been used for centuries. Hippocrates described it as an antimicrobial back in 400 BC. There is clinical research to support that colloidal silver can make antibiotics 1000 times more effective and even eradicate antibiotic-resistant microbes. (Morones-Ramirez, et al. 2013) Other studies (Barwick 2008) showing that colloidal silver can enhance the action of pharmaceutical antibiotics include:

- Brigham-Young Clinical Study – If colloidal silver was used in conjunction with certain drugs, it up-regulated the effect of the drug, even against multi-drug resistant (MDR) pathogens.
- Taiwanese Clinical Study – This study showed that colloidal silver could single-handedly eradicate MDR's such as MRSA and *Pseudomonas aeruginosa.*
- Czech Clinical Study – This study also showed that colloidal silver was effective against MRSA.

However, not all colloidal silver products are equal. According to Dr. Mercola, there are tips and tricks you can use to distinguish if the product is true colloidal silver, silver protein or an ionic silver solution. True colloids will contain about 50–80% silver particles with the remainder consisting of silver ions. Due to the high concentration of silver particles, they are NEVER clear like water, as the silver particles block the light from passing through; hence, the liquid appears darker. Ionic silver solutions are generally clear like water or have a slight yellow tint, and if you put regular table salt (sodium chloride) into the solution, it will become white and cloudy. Whilst ionic silver is not bad for you, it is not as effective as true colloidal silver. Silver proteins, on the other hand, are not absorbed safely or effectively, so you want to avoid these types of products. The giveaway that a product labelled colloidal silver is actually silver protein is that when you shake the bottle, white foam will form and stay on the surface for a few minutes. The colour will also usually be yellowy or as dark as black. If your colloidal silver has these qualities, throw it in the bin and search for some true colloidal silver. (Mercola 2009)

Grapefruit Seed Extract

Grapefruit seed extract has antibiotic and antifungal properties, and it's believed to particularly target the cyst form of Bb. However, it is a very potent herb and not particularly selective, so it can also wipe out a lot of the beneficial bacteria in your body in the process. Dr. Cowden warns that it can make antibiotics less effective, so it is not a good microbial to use in combination with pharmaceutical antibiotics. It is a powerful antimicrobial and needs to be prescribed by an experienced practitioner. Note: do not confuse it with grape seed extract, which is a different product.

TOA-free Cat's Claw

TOA stands for tetracyclic oxindole alkaloids. Cat's claw with TOA is not only believed to have a much more powerful antibiotic action than plain cat's claw, but also has better anti-inflammatory and immunomodulating effects. Dr. Lee Cowden tested TOA-free cat's claw on 28 diagnosed Lyme sufferers with amazing results, which led to its acceptance as a natural antibiotic to use in combination with other therapies in the treatment of Lyme disease. Unfortunately, just like antibiotics, the bacteria do eventually develop a resistance to TOA-free cat's claw, so its use is only recommended for a short duration or in a pulsed dose. In my opinion, the best brand to purchase is Dr. Cowden's product Samento, which is part of his Nutramedix® range of products. (COWDEN SUPPORT PROGRAM: Protocol for Borrelia and Lyme Co-Infections & Most Chronic Conditions 2011)

WATER, WATER AND MORE WATER

Most people know that our bodies are about 72% water, but did you know that your skin is 80% and your blood 90% water? All our physiological processes, such as temperature regulation, digestion, respiration and detoxification, require water to function. Did you know that a 5% drop in body fluids can cause a 25–30% drop in energy? If you are hungry, that can sometimes be a sign that you are dehydrated, so if you are watching your weight or trying to lose weight, then staying hydrated can keep your satiety under control, too! To put it bluntly, water is one of the most important things you can ingest if you want to be healthy and stay alive. Water works optimally to hydrate in its natural form. The only thing you can really do to improve water is purify / filter it (which I also recommend). Even if you have a rainwater tank, the water still hits the roof and runs through the gutters and pipes before it reaches your tap and your glass. This means that it can be contaminated by whatever is on your roof, or in your gutter, tank or pipes (this includes dead animals, rust, chemicals, copper and other heavy metals, to name a few things!). Altering water by adding anything to it (including lemon, vitamins, minerals, sweeteners or alkalising) changes the way water is processed, and in most cases, changes water from life promoting to a diuretic; instead of the body using the water to support vital physiologic functions, the kidneys excrete most of it instead!

Do We All Need the Same Amount of Water?

I have always found it interesting (even before I came across the water formula I believe to make the most sense) how eight glasses of water was the standard recommendation for everyone. How big should the glass be? What if you don't sweat or, alternatively, sweat a lot? What if you are sick and have a higher toxin load? Shouldn't your size, health status, lifestyle and activity level have an influence on how much water your body needs to function optimally? The answer to that question is a resounding YES! YES! In my opinion, it does matter how much you weigh and what activity you do and how stressed you are! The more toxic you are, the more water you'll need to consume!

> *"If there is magic on this planet, it is contained in water."*
>
> *Loren Eisley*

The Water Formula

So who is right when it comes to how much water we should drink? Who knows!! But one thing is for sure: we all require different amounts of water to be healthy. Besides calculating your water requirement specifically for your body, health and lifestyle, you can also check your urine colour. If you are well-hydrated, your urine should be clear or close to it (Please note: if you are taking supplements and medication, especially those with B or C vitamins, they can often turn your urine bright yellow!).

I recommend using the TBM (Total body Modification) formula for water recommendations:

43ml of water per kg per day if you sweat a lot or are injured, ill, exercising or stressed.

35ml of water per kg per day for maintenance of your hydration if you are generally well.

If you are not good at maths (like me), another way to quickly calculate this is to allocate 1L of water for every 25 kilograms of body weight.

Ideally, you should have an extra 500ml of water for every coffee, alcoholic beverage and processed piece of food you consume (especially processed sugar and sweeteners).

What Are the Main Sources of Water You Need to Know About?

According to Dr. Mercola (Mercola 2010), the main sources of drinking water are:

Tap Water – Test your water to see what contaminants are lurking before trusting it as a clean source. To make your water supply "safe" to drink, many treatment plants add chemicals like chlorine, chlorine dioxides or chloramines.

Bottled Water – More than 40% of bottled water is actually tap water, and Australians spend more than $385 million dollars a year on bottled water! Not only that, bottled water is not subject to the same EPA standards as tap water is. Check on the bottle to ensure you are drinking natural spring water. Remember, most plastic bottles contain BPA and other nasties, not to mention the energy it takes to produce the bottles, obtain the water, and then transport, refrigerate and recycle the bottles. The huge environmental impact is often overlooked. Did you know that in Australia, only 35% of plastic water bottles are recycled whilst more than 67 million plastic water bottles are thrown out each DAY in the US alone?!

Distilled Water – It's believed that long-term use can be detrimental to our health due to the lack of minerals in the water which may be leached out of our body to maintain overall mineral balance, not to mention that contaminants in the water are more concentrated!

Alkaline Water – If you are really sick or acidic, then alkaline water may be useful as a short-term health aid, but beware that alkalising does NOT necessarily filter water of other nasties. If your body is already alkaline, it can actually upset your natural body pH causing you to crave acidic foods to balance it out. *I put on 4kg in two weeks, craved carbohydrates and felt awful drinking alkaline water! My theory is that my body craved the sugar (which is acidic) to try and get my alkaline-acid levels balanced again.*

Vitamin Waters – I'm sure you realise that vitamin water is not really water, but just in case you didn't know, it often contains high fructose corn syrup (HFCS), artificial additives, preservatives, colouring and caffeine, not to mention that it's made with distilled water (which you now know is not ideal!).

What is the Best Container for My Water?

Glass wins hands down, as it is does not leach ANY contaminants into your water. I'm not sure if it's just me, but water tastes soooo much better out of a glass, too! Your next best option is stainless steel. No matter what type of water bottle you use, please make sure you wash your bottle regularly so no mould or microbes start growing in it; you don't want to ingest them!

If You Are Going to Use Plastic, Here Are Some Tips:

❖ Buy a reusable plastic drink bottle

❖ Do not ever reuse bottles that are used to sell bottled water (as soon as they get hot, they leach all sorts of contaminants)

❖ Use high-density polyethylene, labelled as *#2 HDPE*

❖ Use low-density polyethylene, labelled as *#4 LDPE*

❖ Use polypropylene, labelled as *#5 PP*

❖ ***Avoid all plastic bottles labelled* Nalgene, PVC #3, or Polycarbonate #7** (Mercola 2010)

What Are the Most Common Water Contaminants?

❖ *Microbiological* bacteria, protozoa (E. coli, cryptosporidium, giardia and their cysts), viruses, faecal coliform

❖ *Inorganic compounds and chemicals* pesticides, herbicides, nitrate, nitrite, fluoride, arsenic, heavy metals (especially aluminium, copper, and lead)

❖ *Radionuclides* alpha, beta and photon emitters, combined Radium 226 / 228, radon gas

❖ *Volatile Organic Compounds (VOCs)*

❖ *Disinfectants and their byproducts* chlorine (and chlorination byproducts such as chlorine dioxide and chloramines), total trihalomethanes, haloacetic acids, bromate, chlorite (EPA 2014)

How Do I Choose a Water Filter?

The four main things to consider:

Value for Money: Look at the ongoing cost of running it (and factor in how much you will save if you buy bottled water instead) rather than the initial outlay of money. A cheaper filter may not actually filter what you want it to either.

Effectiveness: Make sure that all the nasties can be filtered, including fluoride.

Ease of Use: Make sure you ask and understand what is involved to install, clean and change the filters. Otherwise, you may find you don't actually make the most use of it!

Certification: Get a filter that is certified to ensure that the filter is filtering what is advertised.
(Mercola 2010)

What Types of Water Filters Are There?

❖ *Jug or Water Bottle Style Filter* – These are the least cost-effective and least effective filters as they are only designed to filter five or less contaminants. The filters need to be changed regularly (which most people don't do, rendering them relatively ineffective) and the bottles need to be filled regularly. They are generally used to make water look, taste and smell better (but not necessarily better for you!)

❖ *Reverse Osmosis (RO) Filter* – These are the most expensive but generally remove the most impurities. Water is passed under high pressure through a thin membrane where contaminants are either physically blocked or washed away. Unfortunately, it also filters many of the essential minerals from the water, minerals which will need to be replaced (easy, if you are organised!)

❖ *Ion Exchange Filter* – These filters remove dissolved salts such as calcium from the water, soften the water (softening) or exchange natural forming mineral ions in the water with ions from the filter (deionisation).

❖ *Distillation Filter* – These filters boil the water, which creates steam that cools and condenses to form mineral-free water droplets that are then collected in a container. This is then combined with a carbon filter for 99.9% contaminant-free water. However, all the minerals are removed.

❖ *Granular Carbon and Carbon Block Filters* – These are the most common filters and can be used on the countertop or under the counter.

GRANULAR ACTIVATED CARBON FILTERS – They are recognised by the EPA as the best available technology to remove chemicals. However, due to the loose material inside, some of the contaminants can escape filtering through the channeling in the carbon.

CARBON BLOCK FILTERS– These filters can selectively remove a wider range of contaminants because they are made of more solid material that eliminates the channeling and escaping of contaminants. They also have the added benefit of cyst reduction, which makes it more effective at removing organisms like cryptosporidium and giardia. (Mercola, The Most Dangerous Types of Water You Can Drink 2010)

"Ideally, you want a filtration system that offers a variety of methods to remove different contaminants. Most systems do not address a combination of organic, inorganic, cyst, sediment and metals." (Mercola, The Most Dangerous Types of Water You Can Drink 2010)

Comparison Table of Water Filters – Advantages vs. Disadvantages

Type of Filter	Advantages	Disadvantages
Jug	– Convenient – Inexpensive – Easy to change the filters	– Least cost-effective in the long-term – Small storage ability – Shorter filter lives (must change often) – Only filters 5 or less contaminants
Reverse Osmosis	– Removes the largest amount of contaminants	– Expensive outlay – Filters essential minerals (which need to be replaced) – Uses a lot of energy – Wastes up to 85% of water in the filtration process
Deionisation	– Balances the minerals in the water – Removes dissolved inorganics effectively – Regenerable – Relatively inexpensive initial investment outlay	– Doesn't effectively remove particles, pyrogens or bacteria – Can generate resin particles that culture bacteria – High operating costs long-term

Type of Filter	Advantages	Disadvantages
Distillation	– Removes a broad range of contaminants – Reusable	– Some contaminants can be carried into the condensate – Requires careful maintenance to ensure purity – Consumes large amounts of energy – Takes a large amount of space
Carbon Block A. Tap Fitted B. Counter Top C. Under Sink	– Very effective at removing contaminants	
- Tap Fitted	– Convenient – Small and easy to use – Easy to replace the filters	– Slows the flow of the water – Can't be used on all taps
- Counter Top	– Filters large amounts of water without plumbing modifications – Less likely to clog up than jug or tap-mounted – Quick to install	– Clutters the counter top – Can't be used on all taps
- Under Sink	– Filters large amounts of water without taking up precious bench space – Doesn't have to be attached to an existing tap – Unlikely that the tap will clog up	– Requires plumbing modifications – Takes up space under the sink – More expensive outlay

*UV Treatment is another useful advantage of a water filter, as the ultraviolet light is used to disinfect the water. Please note that UV light only works on relatively clear water; otherwise, the light can't penetrate sufficiently. (Mercola, The Most Dangerous Types of Water You Can Drink 2010)

NUTRITION AND FUELLING YOUR BODY

The "Healthy" Food Pyramid

According to the Nutrition Australia website, The Australian Healthy Living Pyramid was created to *"encourage food variety and a diet of minimum fat, adequate fibre, limited salt and sufficient water that is balanced with physical activity. The 'Move More' base of the Pyramid shows moving legs to remind us that physical activity is an essential part of the energy balance equation that should be combined with healthy eating."* This food pyramid has evolved over time, but it still encourages a high carbohydrate intake, reduced fat spreads and even margarine, which I don't consider healthy!

Reprinted with permission from Nutrition Australia

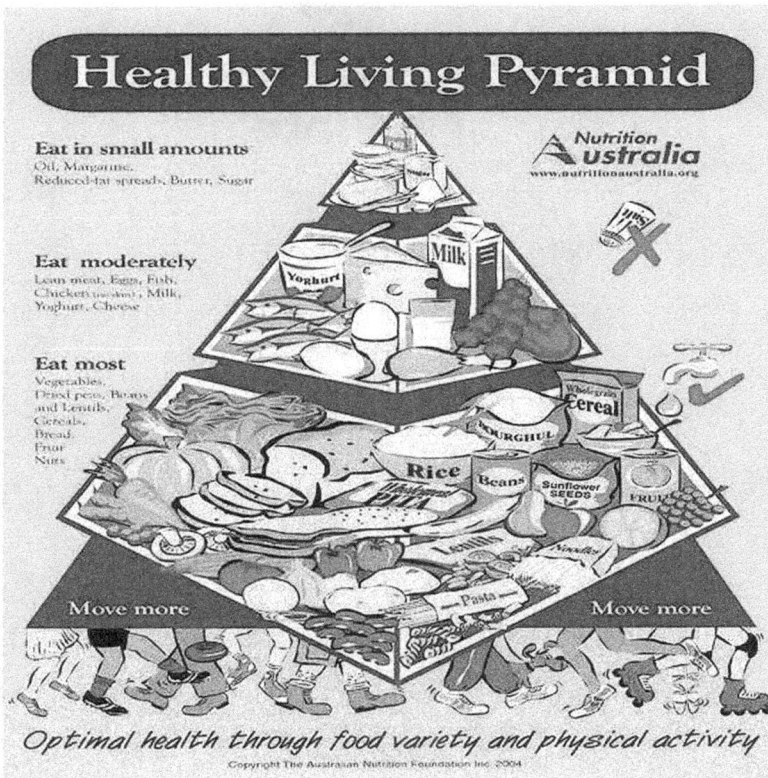

I believe there are better and healthier recommendations than Nutrition Australia's Healthy Living Pyramid. For example, there is a group of scientists who compare the US Governments "Food Plate" health recommendations with their improved version, the PHD Food Plate (reprinted with permission), on their website Perfect Health Diet. (Jaminet 2011) *I really like the idea behind the PHD Food Plate, but don't necessarily agree with everything. I think some people can tolerate properly prepared grains and legumes; however, when you are sick, this may not be the case.*

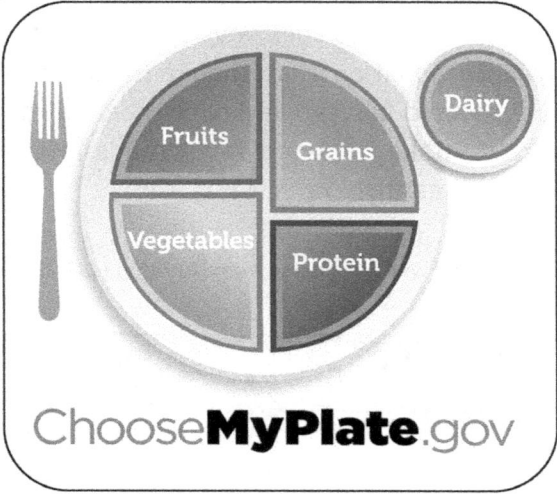

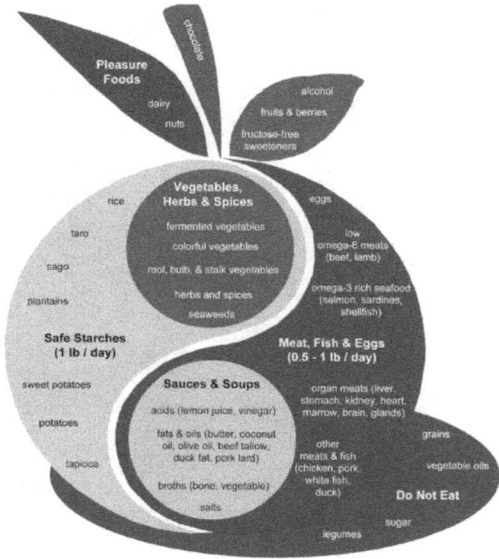

US Government Food Plate and PHD Food Plate (reprinted with permission)

I also love Ben Greenfield's very detailed Super Human Pyramid, which I have included in Appendix E:13. You can check it out at http:// superhumancoach.com/what-is-the-superhuman-food-pyramid/

Getting Back to Basics with Nutrition

Hippocrates said, "Let food be thy medicine." Sometimes I think we forget that food has healing and life-saving properties. Unfortunately, our food is not what it used to be, due to a whole host of factors including over-farming (which causes nutrient-poor soil as well as cross-contamination of foods), the use of pesticides, hormones and synthetic chemicals, advances in refrigeration, plastics used for storing food, pasteurisation, homogenisation, and GMO, just to name a few! I hear many people ask, "Well, how do I know what is best? This person says butter is bad and this person says butter is good. How am I supposed to know?" There are a few rules of thumb when you want to eat healthy. These rules should apply to everyone, but if you are sick, then it is even more imperative that you stick as closely as possible to them. Although the internet makes information easily accessible to us, we sometimes forget that anyone can write something on the internet; however, that does NOT make it a fact! Stick to these common sense rules and you can't go wrong:

❖ If it comes from a packet, it's not real food (if your great-great grandparents wouldn't recognise it, then don't eat it!)

❖ Don't eat it if it has more than five ingredients.

❖ If you can't pronounce the name of an ingredient, it's best not to eat it.

❖ Fresh, whole foods are best.

❖ Buy straight from the farmer at farmers' markets to have the best chance of getting fresh produce (or even better, grow it yourself!)

❖ Limit your sugar and, by the way, anything ending in "-ose" *is* sugar.

❖ Avoid reheating food (especially in a microwave, as it depletes the food's nutrients).

❖ Don't fall for marketing ploys like *lite* (lite in colour and nutrients, most likely), *low-fat* (code for high sugar and often extra chemicals due to the process used to remove the fat), *natural* (could literally be anything found in nature—edible or not), *no added sugar* (this doesn't mean that it doesn't have any sugar, just that it's not added, like in fruit-based products. So check the label to see how much sugar the product really contains).

❖ If a product doesn't go bad or mouldy quickly, then it's probably preserved and, therefore, not good for you (there are exceptions, like honey, and pickled and fermented foods).

❖ It's not food if it's called the same name in different languages, (e.g., McDonalds).

❖ Eat animals that have eaten well (how many cows in nature do you see eating grains?) So grass-fed and finished meat, and ideally raised in good conditions to avoid increased stress hormones.

❖ Just because it says organic on the label doesn't mean it is organic. Learn the symbols that indicate true organic produce (some companies have their brand name as organic!)

❖ Don't eat breakfast cereals that change the colour of the milk.

❖ The whiter the bread, the sooner you will be dead!

❖ Sweeten and salt your food yourself.

❖ Pay more, eat less.

❖ Eat when you are hungry (not bored).

❖ Sit down to eat so you can digest effectively.

❖ Stay hydrated to avoid overeating.

❖ Stop eating BEFORE you are full.

❖ Serve the proper portions and don't go back for seconds.

❖ Avoid the rule: "You have to eat everything on your plate or you can't leave the table."

❖ Have your own vegetable and herb garden, and grow your own fruit trees.

❖ Eat slowly and chew your food properly.

If you want more information about common sense eating, read Michael Pollan's *Food Rules: An Eater's Manual*.
(Pollan 2009)

The 80/20 Rule

I have always been a big believer in the 80/20 rule. If 80% of the time you are healthy and looking after yourself, then 20% of the time you can afford to indulge. Unfortunately, if you are not experiencing optimal health, then this rule is a luxury that you can no longer afford. The closer to 100% you are, the better you are going to support the healing process and the quicker your healing should be. Having said that, some people struggle to make healthy changes and are constantly unhappy. If this is the case for you, then take a step back and ask yourself: "What can I add to my diet or lifestyle that can enhance my health but is enjoyable as well?" It may be to drink more water or get a water filter, or to have a healthy snack before a sugary snack so you aren't as hungry, or even to eat basmati rice instead of white rice. I find that this philosophy of *add* rather than *take away* works better for many people. Making changes gradually is the key. As you start to feel better, you will naturally lean towards healthier options. For example, I love bread and pasta but I very rarely eat it. It wasn't a conscious decision, like a diet or detox, where I said, "I'm not eating bread and pasta anymore." It was because I had learnt how to prepare yummy vegetables, bone broths and meals using different herbs and spices that were both filling and appetising. Naturally, over time, I left the bread and pasta behind. I haven't bought or had bread or pasta (excluding rice noodles) in my house for over 10 years. However, if I am out or at someone's house, then I can eat it as a treat as part of my 20% indulgence!

Is Organic Produce a Healthier Option or Is It All Just Hype?

I think organic is better because the farming practices are more sustainable and it's well-governed. The key is not just to consume the most nutrients possible, but to also avoid harmful toxins in your food. Of course, caring for your environment so your kids and grandchildren have good soil to farm with later on is another added benefit. The more naturally the product is grown and farmed (i.e., how long since it was picked / harvested / slaughtered / etc.), and the fresher it is has a huge impact on your health. The only way to eat fresh and in season and really know everything about what you eat is to grow it yourself. Many people are doing this and making it a hobby for themselves and their families. The next best option is to go to local farms and pick fruit yourself, or you can buy from local growers' markets. If these are not viable options for you, then buying certified organic meat, fruit and vegetables ensures that they will be free of chemical fertilisers, synthetic pesticides, GMOs, antibiotics, growth hormones, sludge, waxes and irradiation. Be careful when shopping for certified organic because many companies have sneaky marketing tricks like using the word organic in their name or saying they use organic ingredients (which might be one organic ingredient whilst the rest are full of rubbish!).

Look for these certified organic labels (reprinted with permission):

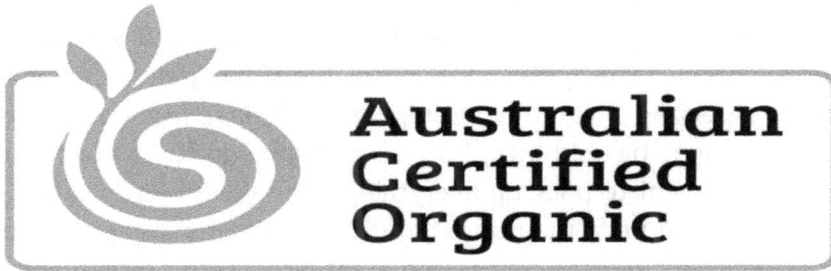

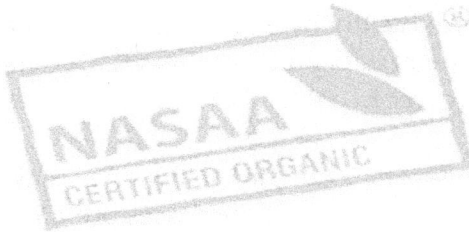

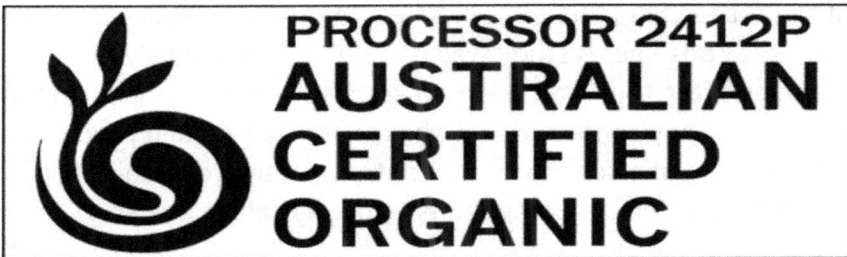

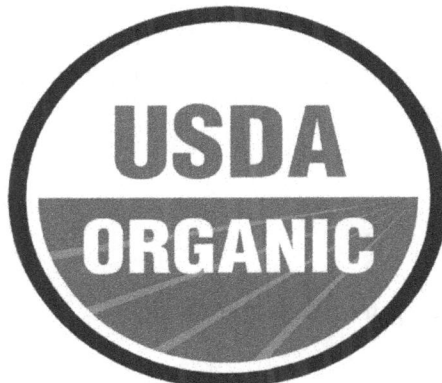

What If I Can't Afford Organic?

Being smart about how and when you shop can save you money (see some of my tips in How to Eat Healthy and Save). If you go to the farmers' market at the end of the day, you can get some amazing bargains, especially if you buy in bulk. You will have less choice (as the popular stuff may be sold out), but you can save up to 50% because the farmers don't want to pack up everything and take it home. Eating 100% organic might not be in the budget, but eating mostly organic can be no more expensive if you are smart! Red meat, fish, eggs, chicken and dairy are best sourced fresh and ideally organic if you are serious about your health. Eat better quality and less quantity is my rule of thumb! Eating organic is a long-term health investment and should never be seen as a quick fix, as often the results and benefits are not immediately evident. Not only is eating organic healthier, but it usually tastes better, too!

For fruits and vegetables, you can follow the Dirty Dozen and Clean Fifteen guidelines to decide which purchases are a must for organic and which ones are less essential. These lists were compiled by a group of scientists, researchers and policy makers in order to reduce the amount of toxins we consume. A study was done on conventionally grown fruits and veggies after they had been washed to see how many chemicals and pesticides they contained. It makes sense that certain produce, such as those with thicker or more resistant skin that we usually don't eat, would be better for us. Some fruits and vegetables are sprayed more than others, too, depending on what pests are attracted to them. Please know that washing produce does NOT get rid of the pesticides and chemicals. It merely reduces them! The Dirty Dozen and the Clean Fifteen are regularly updated, but here are the most up-to-date lists at the time of writing:

The Dirty Dozen

Produce that should be purchased organically:

❖ *celery*

- ❖ peaches

- ❖ strawberries

- ❖ apples

- ❖ blueberries

- ❖ nectarines

- ❖ capsicum

- ❖ spinach, kale and collard greens

- ❖ cherries

- ❖ potatoes

- ❖ grapes

- ❖ lettuce

The Clean Fifteen

Produce that is safest to purchase conventionally:

- ❖ avocado

- ❖ onions

- ❖ sweet corn

- ❖ pineapples

- ❖ mango

- ❖ sweet peas

- ❖ *asparagus*

- ❖ *kiwi fruit*

- ❖ *cabbage*

- ❖ *eggplant*

- ❖ *rockmelon*

- ❖ *watermelon*

- ❖ *grapefruit*

- ❖ *sweet potato*

- ❖ *sweet onions*

How to Eat Healthy AND Save Money!

Many people think that the quality of the products we eat and use doesn't make a big difference to our health in the long run, or they say they can't afford it! But I pose these questions: Does the extra money you spend on good quality items mean you spend less on health care (or more likely sick care)? Does it mean that you get to actually enjoy this life more, now that you are healthier? For me, it is a resounding, "Yes!" As I explained with the 80/20 rule, it doesn't have to be all doom and gloom. Think about this: most of the modern day diseases didn't exist in our ancestors' day, so is it possible our diet and lifestyle are big contributors to our ill health? You do your own research and make your own decisions. In the meantime, here are some handy tips to have your cake and eat it, too! (i.e., have quality food without the necessarily high price tag!)

- ❖ Grow your own fruits and veggies (or at least some of them!)

❖ Make your own sauces, condiments, yoghurt and bread (all the staples anyway, as they will be healthier and cheaper that way)

❖ Buy in bulk (this can be shared amongst a group if you are organised!)

❖ Shop online to get the best prices (you don't even have to leave your home)

❖ Pick your own fruit if you have local growers (it's a fun family activity and saves you a fortune, not to mention you are guaranteed freshness!)

❖ Shop at the local farmers' markets

❖ Order a weekly fruit and veggie box for home delivery (this varies depending on the season)

❖ Take advantage of sales, especially for things like herbs and non-perishable goods

❖ Get as many samples as you can. Not only are they free, but you can try things before you buy them, so you won't buy a whole lot if no one likes it!

Fat Does Not Necessarily Make You Fat!

Contrary to popular belief, not all fats make us fat! In fact, eating good fats is essential to optimal health. The first three fats listed (LCSF, MCT, MFA) should form the bulk of your fat intake and are important for balancing cholesterol (and essentially hormones), increasing muscle mass, supplying adequate energy and balancing mood. Check out Chris Kresser's 9 *steps to Perfect Health* PDF (Kresser 2015) for a full report, but I have summarised some of the information:

❖ **Long Chain Saturated Fats (LCSF):** Early research showed that eating LCSF contributed to high cholesterol, obesity and heart disease, and we have been brainwashed to think that it's true. Now I hear you saying, "Hang on! I still think that!!" Check out the research and decide for yourself, but understand that the research done over the past 50 years or so was all done on grain-fed meat! What do we know about grain-fed meat now? It causes inflammation! Inflammation is a contributor to many diseases including heart disease, obesity and high cholesterol. LCSF are found mostly in milk and the meat of animals, like sheep and cows. As long as the animals are raised in a stress-free environment and are grass-fed as nature intended, the fats consumed in meat are healthy for us in moderation.

❖ **Medium Chain Triglycerides (MCT):** MCTs are found in coconuts and mothers' milk. They are easily digestible because they don't require bile to break them down, so you can consume as much as you want.

❖ **Monounsaturated Fat (aka oleic acid – MFA):** MFA is found primarily in beef, non-refined olive oil, avocados, lard and certain nuts. These fats are healthy to consume in large amounts, but beware: some of the MFAs contain omega-6 polyunsaturated fats which are NOT healthy in large amounts.

❖ **Polyunsaturated Fatty Acids (PUFA):** PUFA is divided into omega-3 and -6. They are fragile and vulnerable to oxidative stress, which causes free radicals that predispose us to many diseases. PUFAs should account for no more than 4% of the total calories in your diet and be consumed at a ratio of 1:1 (omega-6: omega-3).

1. OMEGA-6 PUFA: (AKA LINOLEIC ACID – LA): LA, an essential fatty acid (EFA), is found in small amounts in fruits, vegetables, cereal grains, some nuts, poultry and meat. LA is also found in larger quantities in industrial-processed and refined oils. Our EFA intake is supplied by simply consuming small amounts of the natural foods described in this chapter. Excess omega-6 from processed foods can contribute to inflammation and many modern diseases (especially if not balanced 1:1 with omega-3).

2. OMEGA-3 PUFA: Omega-3 PUFA are further broken down into alpha-linolenic acid (ALA), a short chain fatty acid and long chain

fatty acids. Most people know of ALA if they supplement with flaxseed or EPA and DHA, and most people have heard of long chain fatty acids if they use supplements such as fish oil. Sources of omega-3 are seafood and meat. ALA is considered an EFA, but it's very hard to convert ALA to EPA and DHA, so supplementing or eating foods high in EPA and DHA is usually your best bet!

Trans Fats: are covered in the Foods section.

Grass-fed Meat

Many people have strong opinions about cruelty to animals and consuming meat. Some find the thought of eating animal meat emotionally overwhelming. Having said that, research shows that it takes at least 10 generations to change a food chain, and there are very few cultures who historically did not eat meat (with the exception of Hindu Indians, for example). I rarely see a long-term vegan or a vegetarian who I consider to be optimally healthy, but that opinion can vary depending on your definition of optimal health. However, if you are going to eat meat, then I recommend grass or pasture-fed and finished meat (and there is plenty of research to support it as a better nutritional choice). Anyone who eats meat knows that grass-fed and finished meat also tastes far superior.

Organ Meat or Organ Supplements

Organ meat has almost come full circle. Yes. I said organ meat!! Do I recommend you eat it? Absolutely! When our ancestors killed an animal, they would use and eat the whole thing, not just because it was good for them, but because they could die from starvation if times were tough. Many farmers still have this mentality: use the whole animal to avoid waste and get the most for their money. The truth of the matter is that organ meats are packed full of just about every nutrient, mineral, healthy fat and essential amino acid you can think of. I remember eating liver, kidneys and brains as a child before I had the awareness to think it was gross. No wonder I was so healthy back then!

What Organ Is The Best To Eat?

I learned from my TBM study that eating a certain organ meat supports the healthy function of the corresponding organ. So, if you have liver trouble, you should eat liver. If you have a heart condition, you should eat heart. If you are adrenally fatigued, you should eat adrenal and medulla glandular, and if you have fertility issues, then you eat ovaries or testes! I know this might sound terrible, but the main reason we think this is so awful is because we are socially trained to think eating organ meat is disgusting.

Does the Source of the Organ Meat Matter?

Just like sourcing free-range, grass-fed meat is important, it is also important to eat organ meat from animals raised in a healthy way. Would you want to eat the heart or adrenals of a stressed cow? Imagine how many extra stress hormones it would contain, not to mention how tough it would be! So be smart and only eat good quality organ meats.

What If I Just Can't Stomach Organ Meat? Is There an Alternative?

Start slowly by hiding it in foods or curries, or just having one tiny bite. I have seen long-term vegetarians over time convert to eating organ meats. However, if you are just unable or unwilling to stomach it, then you can buy organ meat in freeze dried capsules. Once again, the quality of the organ meat is essential, and the process to freeze-dry it is, too.

Where Do I Buy Organ Capsules?

In my opinion (and I am supported by many other health care profession-als), Dr. Ron's Ultra-Pure™ are the best capsules on the market. They are made from grass-fed, New Zealand animals and freeze-dried. The website is www.drrons.com/organ-and-glandular-supplements/index.html.

What Sort of Organ and Glandular Capsules Are Available?

There is organ delight (a mixture of nine different organs), adrenal (with adrenal cortex and liver), brain, heart (with liver), kidney, liver, ovary (with liver), pancreas, prostate, spleen, testicle, thymus, and thyroid (with liver). (Dr. Ron's Ultra-Pure: the additive free company 2015)

The Brilliance of Bone Broth

What Is the Difference Between Broth, Stock and Bone Broth?

BROTH is made with meat and a small number of bones. It is cooked for a short period of time (1–2 hours) and is high in protein

STOCK is made with bones (ideally bones are roasted and may contain a small amount of meat), cooked for a medium period of time (2–4 hours) and is high in gelatin

BONE BROTH is made with bones (ideally bones are roasted and may contain a small amount of meat), cooked for a long period of time (24 hours plus) and is high in protein, gelatin and minerals

What Are the Health Benefits of Bone Broth?
RICH IN PROTEINS

A) Gelatin

❖ supports good skin health (may even prevent / eliminate cellulite)

❖ supports digestive health and heals the gut (plays a critical role in the Gut and Psychology Syndrome [GAPS] diet)

❖ slows / prevents degenerative joint disease

❖ supports the connective tissue in your body that helps fingernails, skin and hair to grow and be strong

B) Glycosaminoglycans (GAGs) which are part of collagen
E.G. glucosamine and chondroitin

❖ protects joints

❖ slows / prevents degenerative joint disease

❖ decreases joint pain and arthritis

❖ improves connective tissue health

❖ improves gum health

RICH IN AMINO ACIDS

A) Glutamine assists in the treatment of leaky gut

B) Glycine supports the body's detoxification process

❖ boosts the production of endogenous (produced in the body) antioxidants such as glutathione and uric acid

❖ clears out excess methionine (naturally preventing increased levels of homocysteine, which in the process of its breakdown, increases the need for B vitamins)

❖ stimulates the secretion of stomach acids to assist digestion, which is great for people with acid reflux, IBS and FODMAPS intolerance (where short-chain carbs, or sugars, cause symptoms of IBS such as gas, pain and diarrhoea)

❖ a component of bile acid necessary for fat digestion and the maintenance of healthy cholesterol levels

❖ vital for healthy connective tissue (ligaments, joints, cartilage, blood vessels, around organs, etc.)

❖ decreases inflammation

❖ supports immune system function

❖ assists healing of SIBO (Small Intestine Bacterial Overgrowth)

❖ involved in the synthesis of DNA, RNA and many proteins

❖ assists in the optimal functioning of the nervous system

❖ improves wound healing

❖ regulates blood sugar levels

❖ enhances muscle repair / growth

❖ inhibits excitatory neurotransmitters which has a calming effect on the body and mind

❖ converted into serine which improves mental alertness, memory and mood

C) Proline

❖ supports good skin health (especially when taken with vitamin C)

❖ vital for healthy connective tissue (ligaments, joints, cartilage, blood vessels, around organs, etc.)

❖ reverses atherosclerotic deposits by enabling blood vessel walls to release cholesterol buildups into your blood stream, decreasing the size of potential blockages in your heart and the surrounding blood vessels

❖ helps your body break down proteins for use in creating new, healthy muscle cells.

RICH IN MINERALS

❖ calcium, magnesium, phosphorus, potassium and other trace minerals that are more easily absorbed by the body due to the extra fat content of the broth

ENHANCES IMMUNE SYSTEM FUNCTION

❖ especially chicken broth, as it stops the migration of neutrophils to help minimise colds, flus and upper respiratory infections

❖ enhances brain health due to the link between the gut and the brain

CONTAINS BONE MARROW

❖ creates healthy blood production

❖ repairs cellular damage

❖ contains high concentrations of stem cells that influence genetic material

NOURISHES THE KIDNEYS (traditional Chinese medicine perspective)

SUPPORTS ADRENAL FUNCTION

SUPPORTS ORAL HEALTH

❖ remineralises and strengthens teeth (via saliva)

❖ prevents / treats tooth decay

❖ prevents tooth loss via strengthening connective tissue

Tips for Making Bone Broth

1. Purchase bones from grass-fed animals (many butchers will just give them to you).

2. Roast bones first for 20–30 minutes.

3. Place bones in a pot or slow-cooker and cover with filtered water.

4. Use apple cider vinegar to make the water slightly acidic. This increases the leaching of minerals and nutrients from the bones into the bone broth.

5. Add onion, garlic and ginger for extra nutrients.

6. Keep all your off-cuts from vegetables to throw in.

7. Cook for at least 24 hours.

8. Freeze some broth in ice cube trays to use for braising.

9. Use a slow cooker if you have one. It's easier to cook for 24-48 hours without the fire danger of doing it on the stove for such long periods.

What Can I Use Bone Broth for?

❖ Drink as is, seasoned with salt and pepper

❖ Use it to braise vegetables and meat

❖ Make soups, stews and sauces

Who Should Drink Bone Broth?

Everyone! However, conditions that would particularly benefit include:

- ❖ osteoarthritis

- ❖ GIT issues – leaky gut, IBS, SIBO

- ❖ chronic inflammatory conditions

- ❖ autoimmune diseases

- ❖ poor immune function

- ❖ sports injuries

- ❖ skin conditions

- ❖ mineral deficiencies

- ❖ adrenal issues

- ❖ tooth decay / gum disease

(Health Benefits of Bone Broth 2012), (Bone Broth, Broths and Stocks 2015), (What's In a Bone? 2015)

Fermented Foods and Beverages

Fermentation involves the conversion of carbohydrates to alcohols and carbon dioxide or organic acids, using yeasts and bacteria or a combination of both under anaerobic conditions (in the absence of oxygen). This is how alcohols, like beer, wine and cider, are made. In our ancestors' days, fermented foods were a way to preserve food for up to six months. These days, we have come full circle as more people realise that eating fermented foods improves the beneficial bacteria in the GIT and, therefore, improves our immune function and overall health.

Purpose of Fermented Foods and Beverages

❖ Enriches the diet by creating a diversity of flavours, aromas and textures

❖ Preserves substantial amounts of food through lactic acid, alcohol, acetic acid and alkaline fermentation

❖ Biologically enriches food and beverages

❖ Eliminates anti-nutrients

❖ Decreases cooking time and fuel requirements

Benefits of Fermented Foods and Beverages

❖ Produces natural probiotics

❖ Reduces cancer of the colon and bowel

❖ Increases the natural levels of B12 and folic acid

❖ Destroys certain anti-nutrients, such as phalates and oxalates, that can interfere with the absorption of important minerals such as iron, magnesium and calcium

❖ Improves absorption of calcium and magnesium

❖ Lactobacilli strains assist in maintaining optimal concentrations of Helicobacter pylori to prevent peptic ulcers

❖ Assists in treating food allergies by balancing and enhancing the gut flora

❖ Enhances beneficial bacteria in the gut which in turn supports a healthy appetite, aids digestion, strengthens the intestines and improves the absorption of nutrients consumed

❖ Stimulates peristalsis in the gut which assists digestion and assimilation

❖ Strengthens metabolism

❖ Improves intestinal tract health

❖ Enhances immune system function

❖ Enhances the bioavailability of nutrients

❖ May reduce symptoms of lactose intolerance in susceptible individuals

❖ Some probiotic bacteria break down the milk protein casein into smaller and more digestible units to decrease the chance of, or provide relief from, intestinal inflammation that can cause allergic manifestations

❖ Increases immunoglobulins and, therefore, the ability to fight infection

❖ Fermented milk is believed to create certain peptides (chains of amino acids) which inhibit certain enzyme activity that contributes to increased blood pressure

❖ Naturally reduces high cholesterol levels

Types of Fermented Foods and Beverages

BEAN-BASED: miso, natto, soy sauce, stinky tofu, tempeh, soybean paste, Beijing mung bean milk, kinama, iru

GRAIN-BASED: amazake, beer, bread, choujiu, gamju, injera, makgeolli, murri, ogi, sake, sikhye, sourdough, sowans, rice wine, malt whisky, idli, dosa, vodka

VEGETABLE-BASED: kimchi, sauerkraut, mixed pickle, Indian pickle, gundruk

FRUIT-BASED: wine, vinegar, cider, perry, brandy, atchara, nata de coco, asinan, pickling

HONEY-BASED: mead, metheglin

DAIRY-BASED: cheese, kefir, kumis (mare milk), shubat (camel milk), cultured milk products such as quark, filmjölk, créme fraiche, smetana, skyr, yoghurt

FISH-BASED: fish sauce, bagoong, faseekh, garum, shrimp paste, shidal

MEAT-BASED: jamon iberico, chorizo, salami, pepperoni

TEA-BASED: pu-erh, kombucha, jun

WATER-BASED: Mexican kefir (can be made with coconut or any variation of flavoured water)

You can make your own fermented foods very easily, especially fermented veggies, kombucha, and both water and milk kefir. To get started, I recommend Sally Fallon's book Nourishing Traditions. *There are many companies now who make and sell fermented products, and they are becoming much more readily available in health food stores and even some supermarkets.*

Foods and Other Substances to Avoid

As we learn more about our health, you would think that we'd get smarter and implement healthier strategies when it comes to what we consume. However, the multibillion dollar industries that recommend diets consisting of low-fat, high carbohydrate, processed, preservative-filled and genetically modified organisms (GMO) are not only **not** making us healthier, but they are likely contributing to the steep decline in health and the explosion of modern diseases. It would be ignorant to think that our lifestyle is not contributing to this epidemic of disease and that our nutrition (or lack of) is a big part of it! Following are some foods and beverages to avoid if you want to improve your health (these apply to healthy people and even more so to those who are already sick).

REFINED OLIVE OILS – Olive oil is only good for you in its purest form. Cold-pressed, extra virgin olive oil means it comes from the FIRST press of the olives, heat has not been used (heat changes the chemistry of olive oil) and no chemical processes have been used to extract the oil. Please note that oils labelled as pure olive oil, olive oil, 100% olive oil or light olive oil are all REFINED oils that are no longer good for you, so read the labels carefully.

INDUSTRIAL SEED / VEGETABLE OILS – Historically, industrial oils, such as sunflower, safflower, cottonseed, corn, canola and soybean, have not been part of our diet, but they have been promoted as "healthy" to many unsuspecting consumers. NIH researcher Joseph Hibbeln has published a few research papers saying that the increased consumption of industrial oils is one big human experiment. He believes, without a doubt, that its consumption has directly contributed to the increase in violence, depression, cardiovascular mortality and inflammatory disease.

MARGARINE – You probably know that margarine is made from vegetable oils, which are oils extracted from seeds like rapeseed (canola oil), soy-bean, corn, sunflower, safflower, etc. What many people don't know is that these oils (unlike butter and coconut oil) can't be extracted natural-ly or cold–pressed; the oil must be removed using heat and many toxic chemicals. To make margarine, these oils are extracted under high heat and pressure, hydrogenated (so margarine can harden), steam-cleaned (extracting vitamins and antioxidants, but leaving the pesticides there!), emulsified (smoothing the lumps), steamed and deodorised (removing the smell), and then bleached (removing the charming grey colour).

SUGAR – Not all sugar is created equal. Sucrose (white table sugar) is made up of fructose and glucose. Glucose is a required nutrient for health. It is absorbed very quickly into the bloodstream for uptake in the cells in order for them to function optimally. Fructose, on the other hand, has no satiety (which means it will never make you full), and is directed straight to the liver (like any toxin) in order to be detoxified so it doesn't cause damage to the body (unlike glucose which is absorbed via the bloodstream). Not only does fructose make the liver work overtime, but any excess is converted to fat. Fructose in fruit is offset with the high fibre content, which is why juicing fruit is not actually considered healthy, despite popular belief.

Sugar also increases inflammation and suppresses immune system function. Sugar stimulates the pancreas to release insulin, which continues long after the sugar has been metabolised. This, in turn, decreases growth hormone release, which not only affects our growth and repair, but impacts immune system function. Many studies show that just one teaspoon of sugar can suppress the immune system for up to 16 hours! Sugar feeds yeast, and for anyone with Candida issues (which, let's face it, is most of us), it doesn't matter what treatments or diets you do for Candida, they WILL NOT WORK as long as you are consuming sugar in any form (yes, even sugar from fruit!).

Sugar is hidden almost everywhere and still affects your body in the same way whether it's natural or artificial. There are many names for sugar: sugar, invert sugar, brown sugar, sugar in the raw, sucrose, glucose, maltose, fructose, stevia, honey, syrups (maple, rice, corn, high-fructose corn), concentrated fruit juice, agave (90%+ fructose!!), sugar alcohols (xylitol, mannitol, sorbitol, malitol), aspartame (Nutrasweet®, Equal®), saccharin (Sweet'N Low®), acesulfame potassium (ACK, Sweet One®, Sunnet®), neotame, and cyclamate. A must-read (especially if you are finding it hard to avoid sugar) is the book *Sweet Poison*, by David Gillespie. He also wrote *Sweet Poison Quit Plan*. Hot tip: if you are struggling with sugar cravings, try taking a chromium supplement or eating more cinnamon as they help decrease sugar cravings! Being hydrated also helps!

SWEETENERS – At the end of the day, artificial sweeteners still impact the pancreas and insulin production in a similar way to regular sugar. The main reason most people use sweeteners is to decrease their caloric consumption in order to lose weight. They also use them because they are marketed as a "healthy" alternative. Historically, honey was the natural sweetener used, although many people believe it should be used medicinally more so than nutritionally (excluding Manuka honey).

My advice is to avoid sweeteners altogether (especially processed ones), but if you must use them, research supports the minimal use of honey or stevia, which have benefits due to their antibacterial and antioxidant properties. Natural sweeteners, such as maple syrup, molasses or coconut sugar, are composed mostly of sucrose. They do contain some minerals, so using small amounts when cooking is also a good option. A commonly used sweetener that is a known carcinogen is aspartame, which can also trigger neurological symptoms, so please avoid this one.

PROCESSED SOY – Soy is often consumed as a health food due to the false belief that it has kept Asian cultures healthy for centuries. On the contrary, it is *fermented* soy that they eat. It's the fermentation process that partially neutralises toxins found in soybeans and increases its natural probiotic content. It also makes it healthy to consume. Fermented soy includes miso, natto, tamari and tempeh. Soy that is not fermented is used in many foods in the form of soy lecithin, soybean oil, soy milk, soy flour and soy protein isolate. Soy contains phytoestrogens, which are endocrine disrupters (normal speak for "screws up your hormones" in both females and males), contributes to estrogen-based tumours and exacerbates or even causes thyroid problems. According to Chris Kresser (in one of his podcasts), soy also affects protein digestion, decreases the absorption of many essential minerals (like calcium, iron and magnesium), often contains MSG and glutamic acid (either due to the way it is processed or because it is simply added to make food taste better) and decreases sperm count. It only takes small amounts of soy (about a glass of soy milk per day) to create these sorts of health concerns. So yes, that one soy latte is negatively affecting your health. And don't get me started on the use of soy-based baby formulas!

CEREAL GRAINS (ESPECIALLY IF NOT PROPERLY PREPARED) – Cereal grains, such as wheat, oats, rye, corn, rice, barley and sorghum, are often considered healthy by many unsuspecting people. Once again, if you look at the evolutionary process, you can understand why some plant foods and grains are not fit for consumption in their raw state. Unlike animals, plants can't protect themselves by running away, so they developed mechanisms to protect themselves, such as coatings that are toxic or indigestible to humans and animals. That's why grains often have to be soaked or lightly heated to overcome this toxic factor and make them more digestible.

GLUTEN - Is found in wheat, oats (excluding organic oats), rye and barley (and any foods made from these grains such as cereals, muesli bars, flour, bread and pasta) and is often added to many foods under a variety of names. Many people find it hard to digest gluten (about 35% of people depending on what research you read). It is extremely inflammatory and causes damage to the intestines, which contributes to leaky gut and has the potential to affect almost any tissue or organ in our body, including the brain. For those with Lyme disease or a chronic disease, it's likely that you already have inflammatory or auto-immune symptoms, so you would do best to eliminate gluten for good (even after you beat your illness)! Chris Kresser blogs about the research that shows many more people are likely to be gluten intolerant, even if they have tested negative with the conventional testing. Lastly, gluten has a molecular structure similar to many other foods, so it's common that people who have issues digesting gluten also have problems with foods like dairy (alpha and beta casein, casomorphin, milk butyrophilin, cow's milk, cheese), chocolate, all cereal grains, corn, sesame and other grains such as quinoa (gluten-free seed of a leafy plant distantly related to spinach), amaranth, buckwheat (which is actually a fruit in the rhubarb family), tapioca and rice. Read Chris Kresser's 9 *Steps to Perfect Health* PDF for more info (Kresser 2015).

DAIRY - Almost everyone has a difficult time digesting dairy products, especially from cows, as the proteins in cow's milk are very different from those in human milk. So, from an evolutionary standpoint, we do not have the correct enzymes to properly break lactose and casein down. Many people understand that they shouldn't eat dairy when they are sick or phlegmy, because dairy causes inflammation that triggers mucous in the body; however this is constantly happening when you eat dairy, you just notice it a lot more when you are already sick and mucousy! Yoghurt is fermented, so it is generally easier to digest, and goat milk proteins are more similar to human milk proteins, so they are usually easier to digest as well. Anyone with chronic inflammation (hands up Lymies!) should limit or avoid dairy altogether, especially if they have respiratory conditions (such as sinusitis, asthma, wheezing and/or a productive cough).

TRANS FATS - There are two types of trans fats. Firstly, there are naturally occurring trans fats (NTF) that can be safely consumed and are found in small amounts in the meat, fat and dairy products of animals that digest their food via the natural ruminating process. Secondly, there are artificial / synthetic / industrial / manufactured trans fatty acids (ATF), which are fats and oils that have been chemically altered during processing. ATFs are found in products such as sweets, fast foods, fried foods, battered foods, pastries, shortening, packet food (cake mixes, icing, pancake mix, biscuits), flavours (used in some ice-creams), non-dairy creamers, microwave popcorn, frozen or creamy products (such as soft serve ice cream), frozen dinners and margarine. Trans fats are added to foods to enhance the flavour and texture and make them last longer. Even if the nutrition label on a product says no trans fat, it doesn't mean that there are no trans fats. You need to check, because trans fats can be labelled as hydrogenated oil or partially hydrogenated oil. Learn to read labels, as even products with the National Heart Foundation of Australia's "tick" of approval can still have up to 1% trans fats included. Trans fats increase cholesterol and inflammation in the body and are bad for your heart health. For those who are ill, you already have enough toxins and inflammation in your system without adding more from the trans fats!

MSG (monosodium glutamate) - Is a flavour-enhancing additive for food. While there is no substantial research to support the negative effects of MSG on our health, short-term studies by Metcalfe (Metcalfe 1998) show side effects such as headaches, body temperature fluctuations, heart palpitations, nausea, chest pain, weakness, hyperactivity and dry mouth, just to name a few. This is also supported in other studies (Izikson 2006) (Gladstein 2006). So, it seems obvious that in the long-term, MSG is not a safe or healthy additive to consume! Unfortunately, many people believe that because glutamate is a naturally forming amino acid that the body both uses and needs, it is safe to consume it in its synthetically manipulated form. However, MSG has been labelled an excitotoxin and can have detrimental effects even in healthy people. So do yourself a favour and avoid it.

Manufacturers have to state if there is MSG in their product. However, it may be labelled under any variety of names including the names of other substances that contain factory created, free glutamate (the form that is harmful and found in MSG) such as: monopotassium, glutamate (E620), glutamic acid (E620), calcium caseinate, vegetable protein extract, soy protein, soy protein concentrate, soy protein isolate, ajinomoto, gelatin, hydrolysed vegetable protein (HVP), hydrolysed plant protein (HPP), sodium caseinate, senomyx, magnesium glutamate (625), vestin, calcium glutamate (E632), textured protein, yeast extract, yeast food or nutrient, autolysed yeast, any hydrolysed protein, monoammonium glutamate (E624), natrium glutamate or anything autolysed or hydrolysed. (Anglesey 2014)

GMOs - Genetically modified organisms do not have to be displayed on labels in the United States or Australia, unlike Europe and South America. (Lynch and Vogel 2001) So there is really no way of knowing if a GMO is contained in a product unless the company makes a conscious choice to label their products certified non-GMO (which, like certified organic, has a strict and regulated system in order to earn that label). While there is not enough long-term research yet, I feel it's best to avoid making ourselves part of this unregulated research by steering clear of GMOs altogether! The Institute for Responsible Technology (IRT) has created a brochure about the health risks of GMO food that states, "*In 2009, the American Academy of Environmental Medicine (AAEM) stated that, 'Several animal studies indicate serious health risks associated with genetically modified (GM) food,' including infertility, immune problems, accelerated ageing, faulty insulin regulation, and changes in major organs and the gastrointestinal system.* (Health Risks 2010) *The AAEM has asked physicians to advise all patients to avoid GM foods.* (American Academy of Environmental Medicine 2015) You can check out the website and see what you think!

Chris Kresser, in his GMO research, suggests other potential side effects of GMO consumption. He says that our gut bacteria are capable of acquiring DNA sequences from GM plants, which could lead to antibiotic-resistant microbes (if you are someone who is completely affected by an increased microbial load already, then you don't want this, right?), liver and kidney damage as well as negative effects on the heart, spleen and adrenals (these have all been seen in GMO corn-fed rats!). Not to mention there have been links with low sperm count and infertility. The list goes on. (Kresser 2015) My advice: go GMO-free by sticking to a whole food and paleo-style menu as much as possible!

ANYTHING PROCESSED - As mentioned in the section Getting Back to Basics with Nutrition, if you can't pronounce the name of a food or it comes in a packet, it's likely to be processed! Not all things that come in a packet are necessarily harmful, but they may not always be the best source of nutrition (there are always exceptions to the rule, and of course for convenience, there are certified organic foods that come in a package and are a better choice than many other processed foods!). Just remember: the more refined the food is, the more likely it is to have harmful toxins like chemical additives and preservatives. Another great rule of thumb is to avoid anything white where possible (flour, sugar, bread, etc.) as well as anything that contains processed sugars (such as high fructose corn syrup [HFCS], seed oils and processed soy, as previously discussed). If you want a head start on decreasing your toxic load, then avoid processed foods!

FLUORIDE - Fluoride was first introduced to drinking water in Australia in 1953 at Beaconsfield in Tasmania. Currently, over 80% of Australian water supplies are now fluoridated. Organisations such as the World Health Organisation (WHO) and Australia's National Health and Medical Research Council (NHMRC) endorse water fluoridation as a safe and effective public health measure.

For years, the question as to whether fluoride is safe for consumption has been hotly debated. Despite the research describing fluoride as a dangerous and toxic poison that can accumulate in the body over years, the Australian government and many dentists and health professionals still advocate the use of fluoride to prevent dental decay. In the documentary *An Inconvenient Tooth* (Wagner 2012), Dr. Paul Connett, Professor of Chemistry at St. Lawrence University in New York, states that there are many things that the public doesn't know about fluoride when the research is scrutinised. I have summarised some of his major points and added extra information so that you can scrutinise the "facts" that you have been fed (and believed for a long time) about the safety of fluoride. Then you can make an educated decision for yourself.

Dr. Mercola's fluoride facts (Mercola 2014)

➤ Many developed countries do NOT fluoridate their water supply.

➤ Fluoridated countries do NOT have less tooth decay than non-fluoridated countries (according to WHO, there has been a decline in dental health across the board, despite some countries having fluoridated water while others don't).

➤ Fluoride does not just affect the teeth, but is an endocrine disrupter that affects hormones, bone, brain and blood sugar levels. (National Research Council, 2006 n.d.)

➤ There is not a single process in your body that requires fluoride.

➤ Fluoridation is NOT a natural process, and the fluoride that is added is usually fluorosilicic acid as opposed to the naturally occurring substance.

➤ Formula-fed babies (formula mixed with tap water) consume 100–250 times the levels of fluoride than breastfed babies, and studies show they not only have more likelihood of developing dental fluorosis, but overexposure to fluoride has been linked to lower IQ scores as well. (Table 1: Characteristics of epidemiological studies of fluoride exposure and children's cognitive outcomes 2012) This is apparently supported by 25 other studies!

➢ Fluoridated water is the only "drug" to be added to public water, meaning mass medication of the public without informed consent.

➢ Fluoride toxicity is exacerbated by conditions that occur frequently in low socio-economic areas such as nutrient deficiencies, infant formula consumption, kidney disease and diabetes.

➢ Scientists from the EPA's National Health and Environmental Effects Research Laboratory have classified fluoride as a "chemical having substantial evidence of developmental neurotoxicity."

➢ According to the Centers for Disease Control and Prevention (CDC), 41% of American adolescents now have dental fluorosis (unattractive discolouration and mottling of the teeth) that indicate overexposure to fluoride.

➢ A study done with mice showed that fluoride damages sperm chemotaxis (the process by which sperm are attracted toward an egg), which plays a critical role in allowing fertilisation to occur. This is believed to significantly affect male fertility in humans. (Lu, et al. 2014)

➢ Over 100 animal studies have also linked fluoride to brain damage. (Brain n.d.)

➢ Regular daily monitoring of fluoride levels in Australia drinking water shows as much as 2.8mg of fluoride per litre when the recommended safe guidelines are only 1.5mg/L! It's ridiculous that you need to call Poison Control if someone swallows 0.25mg of fluoride from their toothpaste, yet a glass of tap water could potentially contain this same amount, if not more!

With the addition of processed foods and drinks, it is most likely our modern Western lifestyle that has increased the incidence of dental decay. Since Western food was introduced, there has been a shift away from natural, unprocessed, organic foods. People used to eat what grew in their native environment including unpasteurised dairy products and fermented foods. Not only that, but a significant portion of their food was eaten raw, and the whole animal was eaten including animal products, organ meat and full fat butter! It is hard to believe that this shift has not impacted our dental health (especially the increased consumption of sugar) as well as myriad other lifestyle diseases.

Combating fluoridated water

The best way to avoid fluoridated water is to get a water filter. The activated carbon filters found in water bottles and jug-type filters, such as Brita and Pur, do NOT remove fluoride (or much else for that matter). The three types of filters that can remove fluoride are reverse osmosis, deionisers (which use ion-exchange resins) and activated alumina. Each of these filters should be able to remove about 90% of the fluoride.

Unfortunately, you can't always avoid drinking tap water, so taking lycopene (which is a carotenoid antioxidant) has been found to counteract and protect against the toxic effects of fluoride. (Mansour and Tawfik 2012)

Beverages to Avoid

Alcohol

The first and most important thing to avoid is alcohol. As everyone knows, alcohol overloads the liver, so give your poor liver a break and leave it some energy to perform its already overburdened role! If you are taking medications (especially antibiotics), be aware that alcohol can impact the effectiveness of the drugs, as it adversely reacts with many medications. Generally people who are sick cannot tolerate alcohol well, and the mega hangover from even small amounts of alcohol can be enough to turn you off drinking anyway! If you are super sensitive, you may even react to the alcohol base of many herbal remedies and homeopathics. In this case, you can put the homeopathic remedy into warm water to allow most of the alcohol to burn off.

Caffeine

First and foremost, the liver has to process caffeine, so similar to alcohol, we want to minimise the stress on your liver so it can get rid of the bugs and detox more efficiently and effectively. Caffeine also stimulates the adrenal glands, so if you are drinking coffee to function or stay awake, you are going to worsen your fatigue problems over time. Caffeine affects the absorption and production of many essential vitamins and minerals as well, such as iron, B6, B12 and folate. It is best to avoid it until you are well again, and then your body can often tolerate and enjoy it in small doses (depending on your genetics!).

Soft Drinks

I believe that no one should ever drink soft drinks, as they are full of sugar, preservatives, artificial flavours, colours and all things nasty. Whether or not you feel the ill effects, DON'T give in to the craving. You could try substituting a healthier option to fulfill the craving like sparkling water or kombucha. Kombucha is an amazing tasting and healthy probiotic drink that comes in several flavours, such as ginger (tastes similar to ginger beer), lemon, passion fruit and berry, and the fizz and flavours provide a great and HEALTHY substitute for you and your family, regardless of your health issues. Water kefir provides similar properties to kombucha and is very satisfying for those who are sick of drinking water.

Energy Drinks

Don't get me started on energy drinks. They should be banned. If you drink things like V, Monster or Red Bull, then you can never expect to be healthy, especially if you are chronically ill already. Some of these energy drinks have up to four times the amount of caffeine as compared to a cup of coffee, not to mention the sugar or the sweeteners (don't be fooled by the no sugar label; sweeteners are just as bad, if not worse for you). They are also very addictive so they can be hard to stop drinking. Do your liver, pancreas and adrenals a favour and don't start drinking them, and if you regularly drink them, STOP immediately!

Fruit Juices

I would not recommend drinking packaged fruit juices, regardless of the No Added Sugar or All Natural Ingredients claims. Fruit contains fructose, and no matter how you look at it, fructose is BAD for us. Now, fruit itself has beneficial vitamins and minerals and, of course, fibre, so it is best to eat the whole fruit rather than juicing it. If you are going to juice, then stick to low fructose options such as greens. Carrots and beetroots are juicing favourites but are higher in sugar then some fruits. Your best option is to buy a good blender, throw the whole fruit or vegetable in with some ice and make a frappé! Then, at least you are getting all the nutrients! Once again, organic and fresh is best. The longer it has been away from its natural source, the less nutrient dense it is.

Reading Food Labels

You must familiarise yourself with food labels. Terms like *organic, all natural, no added sugar, fresh,* and *made with whole grains* are all clever marketing ploys. Unfortunately, regulations are minimal, so people can plaster their labels with claims that use a play on words to trick our minds into thinking something is healthy or good for us. Here are some handy tips when reading labels:

Servings per Container: Always look at how many servings are in a product. The container may seem small, but don't assume it is only one serving. Manufacturers will often make products more than one serving so the calories (or other ingredients) seem lower in comparison to other products.

% Daily Value: This value is based on a daily diet of 2000 calories, so take this into consideration because not all of us require 2000 calories (weight, age, gender and exercise level all need to be considered).

Ingredient List: Manufacturers must list ALL the ingredients contained in their product. The ingredients are labelled in order of weight from highest to lowest. For example, if you buy a product that has sugar listed as one of the first ingredients, you know that it is VERY high in sugar.

Total Fat: This is broken down into saturated and trans fats. Trans fats may be listed as hydrogenated vegetable oil or partially hydrogenated vegetable oil, which can trick you into thinking there is minimal or no trans fats. Please note that companies are allowed to list 0g of trans fats if one serving contains less than .5g of trans fats, so never assume it is trans fat-free just because it says 0g.

The Chemical Maze is a handy, pocket-size book that helps you identify food additives (and cosmetic ingredients), as there is no possible way to remember them all. MSG has a multitude of names that even I can't always remember! This is a must-buy book if you are serious about arming yourself with up-to-date information about additives and chemicals in our food and cosmetics!

ADDRESSING INFLAMMATION AND PAIN

Inflammation and its causes are outlined in the Collateral and Concurrent Conditions section. However, knowing what inflammation is and trying to address it effectively are two very different things!

General Tips to Decrease Inflammation – Internal and Topical

❖ Hot and cold compresses.

❖ Diluted clove essential oil applied on joints.

❖ Hot Epsom salt bath.

❖ ½ tsp of turmeric powder with warm water 3x a day. Or, take 1 tsp of turmeric in hot coconut milk to cure all kinds of body pains.

❖ Rub aching joints with hot vinegar before going to bed.

❖ Drink 1 tsp of apple cider vinegar and ½ tsp of honey dissolved in a small glass of warm water up to 3x a day.

❖ Drink plenty of water to keep the body hydrated and assist the lymphatic system to remove inflammation.

❖ Exercise in water as it may reduce pain and improve flexibility.

❖ Earthing – For 20 minutes a day, walk or have your bare feet on land outdoors (not on cement). You may also buy gadgets to use indoors.

❖ Sun Gazing – Heals by filling the body with light energy; may help with eye disorders and appetite. Stand outdoors, bare feet preferably, and gaze in a relaxed way at the sun one hour after sunrise and one hour before sunset only. Start with 10 seconds and work up to a minute (or more).

❖ Fasting for a day – Drink only filtered water.

❖ Potato poultice – Place a grated or peeled potato on the skin of the affected area. Cover the potato with a tea towel and then wrap with plastic wrap. Remove after 30 minutes. Use daily or as necessary.

❖ Caster oil pack – See instructions in the Physical Healing section.

❖ Take 2 tbsp of rosemary with food.

❖ Use at least 4 tsp of dried ginger in boiling water for a brewed ginger tea.

❖ Horsetail heals tissues and reduces inflammation. The joints of this herb can be steeped in boiling water for a brewed tea or can be ground and applied on the inflamed area and covered with cloth to form a poultice.

Decreasing Chronic Inflammation – The Lyme Inflammation Diet (LID)

The Inflammation Diet was adapted by Dr. Kenneth Singleton, the first physician to publish a holistic Lyme-specific approach to treating Lyme disease. In his book *The Lyme Solution*, Chapter 5 highlights the crucial role that nutrition plays in healing. By eliminating foods and beverages that trigger or contribute to an inflammatory response, detoxification capacity improves and enzyme balance is enhanced. The multiphase program explains step-by-step which foods to eliminate, which foods to add and how to slowly reintroduce additional healthy foods. This diet is best supported using a holistic approach of regular exercise (where possible), stress management and quality sleep. (Singleton 2008)

Phase I – Induction Phase: Phase I is restrictive because it's designed to jump start the body's detoxification process and decrease inflammation-causing mechanisms within the body. It is the most challenging phase but only lasts a week, so in the scheme of things, it's really not that bad! Most people who are chronically ill will have already cut out many of the *nasties* and processed foods from their diet anyway just to survive! A list of allowed foods and beverages is included in the book to make it easier for you.

Phase II – Early Re-entry: Phase II allows you to slowly (one at a time) reintroduce certain foods that have a low risk of triggering inflammation to see how your body tolerates them. This process is usually done over a period of at least three weeks, gradually adding new groups of food every second day. Once again, a handy food list is supplied for you. If you react to any food upon reintroduction, then stop eating it until your body has had more time to heal, and then try it again later! Note: I would recommend introducing new foods every 3-7 days if you are sensitive.

Phase III – Late Re-entry: Once you have safely reintroduced Phase II foods, you may start Phase III. Foods (from a provided list) that are considered healthy (but may cause inflammation in predisposed or ill people) are reintroduced one at a time over at least four weeks. Add a new food no quicker than every second day, and if the first few foods exacerbate inflammatory symptoms, then revert back to phase II for a little longer.

Phase IV – Maintenance: If all goes well, you will enter Phase IV within about eight weeks after starting the LID. This phase allows you to further add healthy foods slowly back into your diet until you have a diet with lots of healthy options whilst still maintaining little to no chronic inflammatory symptoms. During maintenance, you need to follow the usual rules in terms of food consumption if you want to stay inflammation-free (or low inflammation) while you are healing. These are outlined in Getting Back to Basics with Nutrition if you need a reminder!

Laura Piazza (a Lyme sufferer) and her mother, Gail, took the Lyme Inflammation Diet one step further by working with Dr. Singleton (and his wife) to create an amazing companion recipe book called *Recipes for Repair: A Lyme Disease Cookbook*. It combines the Lyme Inflammation Diet information with yummy recipes, easy-to-read codes and shopping lists!

Can I Use More Objective Testing to Know If I'm Inflamed?

The best way is to get a C-reactive protein (CRP) blood test done in order to assess inflammation or infection in the body. The *Recipes for Repair: A Lyme Disease Cookbook* has a chronic inflammation self-assessment tool on page 30–31 that is very handy, too.

Anti-inflammatory Topicals

❖ Homeopathic arnica gel or cream applied topically relieves inflammation

❖ Lyprinol

Anti-inflammatory Herbs

❖ Anise essential oil

❖ Boswellia (Boswellia serrata)

❖ Magnesium, cod liver oil, omega-3 oils, ginger, turmeric, rosemary

❖ Boswellia liquorice root

❖ Bromelain – assists the body to repair our cells, and when taken on an empty stomach, this enzyme can break down the by-products of inflammation, thus clearing the way for cellular repair

❖ Cat's claw (Uncaria Tomentosa)

❖ Celery apigenin

❖ Cetyl myristoleate

❖ Curcumin

❖ Devil's claw

❖ Extract of tumeric and ginger combined

❖ Ginger (Zingiber officinalis)

❖ Goldenseal

❖ Grape seed extract

❖ Green tea (Camellia sinensis) – four cups daily for effectiveness

❖ Horsetail heals tissues and reduces inflammation

❖ Japanese honeysuckle vine (anti-inflammatory)

❖ Jojoba oil

❖ L-glutathione

❖ Meriva curcumin

❖ MSM (Methylsulfonylmenthane)

❖ Olive leaf extract (OLE) decreases inflammation from viral infections

❖ Papain

❖ Pycnogenol

❖ Quercetin

❖ Rosemary

❖ Rutin

❖ Slippery elm

❖ St. John's wort

❖ Turmeric (Curcuma longa)

❖ White willow bark liquorice

Anti-inflammatory Tips for Decreasing Edema or Fluid Retention Associated with Inflammation

❖ Herbal tea made from horsetail

* Celery seed capsules

* Celery seed and dandelion capsules

* Dandelion and celery

* Alfalfa – it is a diuretic and also contains amino acids that will reduce inflammation

* Rife 775.30

General Pain Tips and Tricks

The following herbs and Rife setting may help relieve pain. They do this by decreasing the excitability of the nerves and nerve centres. Antispasmodic (antiparalysis) herbs are quite similar in function.

* Ecklonia cava

* Quercetin

* Curcumin

* Chamomile

* D-Flame™

* Echinacea

* Ginger

* Gravel root

* Mistletoe

* Nervines

❖ White willow

❖ Wood betony

❖ Epsom salt baths

❖ CuraMed® (750mg)

❖ Rife 376

TREATING COGNITIVE DYSFUNCTION THAT HAS A ZOONOTIC ORIGIN OR CAUSE

Chronic diseases, like Lyme disease, may not only affect cognitive function, but may also mimic many psychiatric disorders. The most common disorders of the brain besides the cognitive disorders and brain dysfunction are anxiety disorders, mood disorders (depression), psychotic disorders and eating disorders.

Improving Cognitive Function

❖ Camu-Camu (Myrciaria dubia)

❖ Lithium Orotate 5mg – Improves thinking, protects the brain from toxins, elevates mood, and decreases anxiety and nervous system irritability

❖ Fish oil capsules for depression (high dose DHA)

❖ DL-phenylalanine (DLPA) – for depression

❖ Balance all vitamins and minerals (most especially the B vitamins)

❖ Aim to reduce the brain inflammation with heavy-duty daily detoxification and by eradicating bacteria (or whatever the offending microbe is)

Lifting the Layers of Brain Fog

❖ Stop putting toxins and poisons on / in the body

❖ Stop smoking cigarettes – nicotine is not just the toxic part, it is what has been added to the cigarette that is truly toxic (try hypnotherapy to quit)

❖ Remove the metal, vaccination, radiation, chemical, and drug poisons stored in the body with zeolite or other metal detox products

❖ Remove all parasites, amoebas, flukes and tapeworms

❖ Remove all types of fungus

❖ Remove oneself from a mouldy environment that is releasing mould spores

❖ Open sluggish lymphatic and liver pathways with pathway cleansers to allow toxins out of the body

❖ Move, move, move to pump the immune and lymphatic system

❖ Promote detoxification through foods, hydration and a balance of vitamins and minerals

❖ As soon as possible, eradicate any unfavourable bacteria, viruses, rickettsias and protozoans

Natural Anxiety Treatment Tips

❖ Breathing exercises (see Supportive Treatments in Chapter 6 for tips on breathing)

❖ 30 minutes of walking per day, or as often as necessary or able

❖ Benzoin essential oil – dab on the base of the skull once daily

❖ Hypericum Perforatum – used both externally and internally and is similar to St. John's wort

❖ Bach Rescue Sleep – a fast-acting spray that naturally calms the restless mind

❖ Valerian root extract - also known as amantilla, phu, garden valerian, setwall

❖ Passionflower

❖ Lady's slipper

❖ Skullcap

❖ Lime (linden) blossom

❖ Mistletoe

TREATING THE BIOFILM

As explained earlier, the biofilm is one major block to healing the body from chronic illness. The treatment and break down of the biofilm is tricky, and no one can confidently tell you exactly what to do. Enzymes, such as lumbrokinase, nattokinase or serrapeptase, and even mucolytic enzymes can break down fibrin and possible strep in the biofilm so that the medications and antimicrobials you are taking can actually get to the pathogenic microbes and do their job to eliminate them. The Byron White Formula A-BIO™ is believed to be quite effective as well. Dr. Peta Cohen, M.S., R.D., who specialises in working with autistic children using a biomedical approach and is the founder of Total Life Center in Northern New Jersey, rotates a variety of antimicrobials such as berberine, artemisinin, citrus seed extract, black walnut hulls, artemisia herb, echinacea, goldenseal, gentian, tea tree oil, fumitory, gentian, galbanum oil, oregano oil and neem. She also uses pharmaceuticals, such as Vancomycin, Diflucan and Gentamycin, when necessary. Dr. Sapi has done lab experiments and believes a combination of Cat's claw and Otoba bark extract (called Samento and Banderol in the Cowden Protocol's NutraMedix® program) is effective for the removal of nearly all biofilms.

Using binders to help mop up debris and microbial die-off is really important. There is once again debate as to which binders should be used (if at all). However, if your primary practitioner prescribes them, then they may choose from binders such as chitosan, citrus pectin, organic germanium, chlorella and activated charcoal (the Cowden Protocol uses zeolite as a binder). Sometimes the breakdown of bacteria can cause the body to become acidic, so using buffering supplements such as buffered vitamin C or any product that helps alkalise your body can also help speed up the healing process.

Be sure to have your minerals assessed when doing this sort of treatment and replace / supplement as necessary. This testing could be blood, stool, hair and/or urine testing, so ask your doctor for more information.

GIT SUPPORT

As mentioned earlier, optimal GIT function is the foundation for a healthy functioning immune system. Keys to improving gut health include supporting and protecting the natural gut flora, addressing the microbial load, decreasing inflammation and supporting overall digestion.

Supporting Natural Gut Flora: According to Chris Kresser, "The human gut contains 10 times more bacteria than all the human cells in the entire body, with over 400 different strains." (Kresser 2015) It is essential to supplement with probiotics, and there many great products on the market. I tend to use and prescribe both Metagenics and Bioceuticals® products, which have a great range of probiotics to suit different GIT dysfunctions. It's best to rotate different ones. Even better, do some functional stool testing to find out exactly which strains of bacteria YOU need so you can supplement accordingly.

Eliminating Pathogenic Microbes: Ideally, this is done using antimicrobials, and sometimes your doctor will suggest antibiotics if results are not forthcoming. Some of the herbs used might include grapefruit seed extract, olive leaf extract, TOA cat's claw, Japanese knotweed and barberry.

Decreasing Inflammation: Most common causes of gut inflammation include infections, autoimmune reactions / disease, poor diet, environmental toxins and dysbiosis. Supplements that contain glutamine or specifically Intestamine® from the Bioceuticals range are great for decreasing inflammation in the gut and intestines, respectively. You can also add any of the anti-inflammatory supplements from the table included earlier and drink bone broth.

Restoring Stomach Acid Production: Stomach acid (HCL) is essential for digestion and the absorption of fats, carbohydrates and proteins. HCL stimulates the release of pancreatic enzymes for carbohydrate digestion and triggers the production of pepsin for protein breakdown. If stomach acid is too low, then undigested proteins and carbohydrates can sit in the GIT and cause symptoms such as bloating, gas, reflux and other digestive symptoms. Undigested proteins can escape into the bloodstream and set off an allergic response. The main factors that cause low stomach acid include infections (such as H.pylori), certain drugs, chronic stress, poor diet and ageing, so supplementing with HCL, decreasing stress, avoiding drugs and improving your diet are all going to help! If you work out how to slow the ageing process, then let me know! Supplementing with HCL (e.g. Metagenics Metagest® or Professional Botanicals Di-Aide Enzymes) may take 3–6 months to restore optimal stomach acid, so be patient and work with a practitioner who knows how to test and administer it safely.

Optimising Enzyme Production: Enzymes are essential for breaking down larger molecules from food into absorbable proteins (carried out by protease), fats (carried out by lipase) and/or carbohydrates (carried out by carbohydrases). The main causes of lowered enzyme activity are low HCL, chronic stress, poor diet, ageing and the lack of coenzymes (vitamins and minerals), which help them work. A natural way of increasing stomach acid is by supplementing with bitters such as goldenseal root, dandelion, fennel, ginger and beetroot.

Addressing Acidity: Certain parts of the body are meant to be acidic (like the stomach), which is essential for killing microbes and breaking down food, whereas the blood (best tested via urine but can be tested using saliva), ideally, should be alkaline (7.2–7.4). If your stomach is not acidic, you may not be producing hydrochloric acid, so supplementing with Metagenics Metagest® or Professional Botanicals Di-Aide Enzymes™, which both contain HCL and digestive enzymes to aid digestion in the stomach and intestines, may be necessary. See the Creating an Alkaline Environment section for information on how to address this more thoroughly.

Avoiding Sugar: especially processed sugar, but also limit fruit, which is full of fructose (even though fruit is also packed with nutrients and soluble fibre, it's best to keep to a minimum due to the fructose content).

Eating Fermented Foods: like kimchi, sauerkraut, kefir, kombucha

Eating More Fermentable Fibres: such as yucca, yams and sweet potato

Allergy Testing and Eliminating Inflammatory Foods: The biggest culprits are usually dairy, gluten, anything *white* (flour, bread, etc.) and processed foods. Try eliminating these if you are getting any adverse GIT symptoms and then reintroduce them one at a time (or just leave them out!). You can also cut out some of the guess work and have allergy testing done to see what triggers an IgG response. Often allergies / intolerances will ease off or even be eliminated once the body is functioning optimally again.

Moving the Bowels: It's so important to move your bowels daily (ideally 2–3 times a day). If you are constipated, then some natural remedies include:

❖ drink more water

❖ add more fibre such as apple pectin, ground flax seeds, slippery elm and psyllium husks to your meal or smoothie

❖ increase your magnesium and vitamin C doses to increase bowel motility

❖ increase insoluble fibre by eating lots of fresh vegetables

HORMONAL SUPPORT

Adrenal Support

It is very important to address the adrenals in any chronic illness and Lyme disease treatment plan.

Lifestyle Factors: must be addressed first. With that in mind, for most sick people exercise will need to be adjusted. Although it's important to keep moving, any extra stress on the body can slow the healing process. Exercise like yoga is great to get the body moving while still keeping the body in a predominantly parasympathetic rest-and-digest state. In this way, you can still heal and not over-stress your adrenals. Most people with Lyme disease will be advised against aerobic exercise, and some won't be able to do it anyway. However, on those days when you can, make sure you get plenty of rest before and after, drink plenty of water and supplement. Lifestyle changes, like scheduling naps or down time and decreasing your exposure to stressful situations including work, are very important. In fact, decreasing stress in all forms is very important. Although it's not possible to eliminate all stress (and let's be honest, in a healthy person, a little stress can be helpful), the better you can do this, the quicker your adrenals will heal and the better you will feel!

Nutritional Factors: As with anything, the better you eat and the fewer toxins you consume, the better your body is going to heal. Your adrenal nutrition is no different (please see the Nutrition and Fuelling Your Body section for complete nutritional information), but the general rules of thumb are to avoid caffeine and sugar (especially processed sugar), keep your diet low GI and high in protein to regulate your blood sugar, and stay hydrated. Nothing is a substitute for water (ideally filtered) but bone broths and soups can be great, especially if you have lost your appetite.

Adrenal Autonomic Recovery Meal: In TBM land (kinesiology), if you find it hard to get to sleep, if you wake up regularly in the night for no known reason or because you are hungry, or if you wake up tired despite being in bed for a sufficient amount of time, it often indicates your adrenals are overactive or fatigued. To support the adrenals while you sleep and recover, drink the following shake just before bedtime: *half a banana, ⅛ cup full fat cream, ¼ cup natural full fat yoghurt and one raw egg blended.* Ideally these ingredients should be organic. Yes, I know it sounds disgusting (it took me two weeks to get up the guts to try it, especially because I don't really like yoghurt and I despise cream!), but it is actually really nice (if you like banana smoothies, it tastes exactly the same), and in the summer, I throw in some ice cubes as well. I actually looked forward to it each night for dessert because of the sweetness of the banana. If you don't like banana, you can substitute with berries, but I can't guarantee it will have the same effect because I haven't tried it. The blend of fat, protein and sugar feeds the adrenals so they can rest instead of wake you up in the night. Most people report sleeping like a baby almost immediately after starting the shake. If you have lactose issues, I suggest working with a TBM practitioner to harmonise these first (or you may feel a little sick, like I did initially).

Adrenal Glandulars: Dr. Ron's Ultra-Pure™ brand sells adrenal (plus cortex and liver) capsules or you can get the Organ Delight, which has a combination of nine organs (including adrenal). For more information on supplementing with organ meat (or equivalent freeze-dried capsules), see the Nutrition and Fuelling Your Body section in Chapter 7.

regulate exhausted adrenals when cortisol production is low and serum levels fall short, and reduce your cortisol levels when adrenals are overactive. Adaptogenic herbs are also helpful for those who have adrenal imbalances, which cause a mixture of adrenalin and cortisol bursts that can leave you feeling anxious and wired, yet also drained and exhausted. These are best used in the early stages of adrenal fatigue and shouldn't be relied upon as a crutch; it's absolutely essential that dietary and lifestyle changes are made in conjunction with adpatogen herbal supplementation. Adaptogens include ginseng (Siberian and Korean), ashwagandra and Rhodiola rosea.

Other Adrenal Supportive Herbs: liquorice root

Adrenal Supplements: Metagenics makes a great herbal product for adrenal support called Adrenatone. It can be prescribed by any health care professional trained in the distribution of Metagenics' products. Professional Botanicals has a great product called ADR that you can buy from their website (I recommend working with a TBM practitioner when taking ADR). Bioceuticals® also does an adrenal support called Adrenoplex, which you can pick up in most health food stores if you don't have access to Metagenics' products. Vitamin C supplementation is also helpful for the adrenals.

Adrenal Precursors: Some practitioners may use DHEA and/or pregnenolone, as they are the hormones that help create the adrenal hormones

Isocort: When cortisol levels are extremely low or high, you may want to supplement with Isocort, a plant-based cortisol that actually contains small doses of cortisol. At the time of writing this book, this supplement was no longer available, but I added it with the hope that either Isocort or something equivalent would be available again in the near future. Please remember that this is NOT fixing the cause of the adrenal issues. Instead, it's giving your body cortisol so that the adrenals can rest and recuperate. Short-term use is recommended only.

Thyroid Support

Natural support for the thyroid includes the following:

❖ Iodine, which is a precursor for the production of thyroid hormones T3 and T4 (except if you have Hashimoto's thyroiditis in which it is contraindicated)

❖ Tyrosine is also a precursor for thyroid hormone production

❖ Supplementation with zinc and selenium (if low) is essential for T4–T3 conversion

Herbs such as kelp (very high in iodine) and bladderwrack are also good for thyroid support.

Some doctors may recommend taking a thyroid hormone supplement, but this is beyond the scope of this book and, in my opinion, more of a last resort if lifestyle, dietary changes and natural supplementation have not worked.

Reproductive Support

Chaste Tree: If your menstrual cycle is affected, then it's more than likely that your progesterone is the cause of your hormonal imbalance, so chaste tree (Vitex) as a spray or a homeopathic can be useful. This really helped me to regulate my cycle and decrease the pain and emotional symptoms associated with PMS (in fact, I don't get PMS anymore, and even my husband agrees!).

Fertility Herbs: Shataran and false unicorn root from MediHerb.

Menopausal Herbs: Liquorice root, red clover and black cohosh

Chinese Herbs: In my opinion, the best way to get your reproductive hormones back on track is with regular acupuncture in combination with Chinese herbs. These herbs will be prescribed on an individual basis depending on your symptoms, history, pulse and what your tongue looks like (this is how traditional Chinese medicine practitioners diagnose and treat you).

LOW DOSE NALTREXONE (LDN) FOR IMMUNE MODULATION

History and Use of LDN

LDN is used in many illnesses and is known for its use with cancer and autoimmune diseases, but not so much for its use in Lyme disease until recently (especially in Australia). LDN is often particularly useful in the treatment of Lyme disease where it is used as an immune modulator to balance the immune response without overstimulating it. Since 1984, naltrexone has been used to wean heroin or opium addicts from their drugs by binding to opiate sites in the brain and blocking their effect. In 1985, LDN use was found to improve HIV sufferers' immune response to the infection. In the mid-1990s, a doctor started prescribing LDN to his cancer patients and reported prompt control over many of his autoimmune patients' symptoms (mostly lupus).

So How Does LDN Help Immune Modulation?

Research by Makman shows that opioid receptors are located on immune cells and, therefore, have a direct effect on immune system functioning. (Makman 1994) Low doses of naltrexone taken just before bedtime (between 9pm and 2am) cause a brief blockage of these opioid receptors between 2–4am, which creates increased endorphin and enkephalin levels. This, in turn, may up-regulate parts of the immune system, decrease the deterioration of helper T-cells (CD4+), induce tumour and cancer cell death, and increase natural killer cells. (Roy and Loh 1996) It's also believed that the restoration of the body's normal endorphin production is a huge part of the therapeutic action of LDN.

Are There Other Benefits to LDN Besides Immune Modulation?

Chronic diseases such as Lyme disease (and its co-infections) can have a huge impact on the immune system, which is why LDN can be so effective. It helps strengthen the immune system and gets it to work more effectively and efficiently (as it's meant to do!). When the immune system is working better, then people often also notice improvements in sleep, energy and pain levels.

What Dose Is Considered Low in LDN and What Dose Is Usually Prescribed?

Naltrexone doses were initially 50–300mg doses whereas LDN is much smaller doses of 1.5–4.5mg (doses lower than 1.5mg are likely to have no effect, while doses above 4.5mg are likely to decrease its effectiveness by blocking opioid receptors and endorphins for too long). Many doctors will start you on 1.5mg and build up to 4.5mg over a week or two. I initially started on 4.5mg (in one capsule) and had no sleep disturbance, which is sometimes reported when you first start. If you are quite sensitive or sick, then I recommend starting with lower doses and building up, but consult your doctor who will know what's best for you. Please see the Cautions and Contraindications following for exceptions to these doses.

Are There Side Effects or Contraindications, or Can Anyone Take LDN?

There are no known side effects to LDN except that you may experience some sleep difficulty that will usually resolve itself within the first week. Like any medication or treatment, not everyone has amazing results with LDN, but it's rare that it will make you worse so, in my opinion, it's worth a try.

Cautions and Contraindications

❖ Anyone taking narcotic pain medications such as morphine, tremadol or any medications containing codeine

❖ Anyone taking immunosuppressive medications such as transplant patients, as LDN may counter the effect of the those medications

❖ Anyone with Hashimoto's thyroiditis (low thyroid) must begin at the lowest dose of 1.5mg and monitor their thyroid function closely, because as the immune system responds, they will often need to decrease or even stop taking their thyroid medications

❖ People with MS who get muscle spasms are recommended to build up to 3mg and stay at that dosage

How Much Does LDN Cost and Where Do I Buy It?

You will need a script from your doctor, and then you'll need to find a good compounding chemist. In Sydney, I use Kingsway Compounding Chemist at Brookvale, but there are plenty others available. It costs about $50 for a month's supply depending where you purchase it. Most compounding chemists will compound LDN in whatever capsule strength you are prescribed (from 1.5–4.5mg).

When Do I Take LDN?

Take at bedtime, ideally after 9pm but before 2am.

TREATING FUNGAL INFECTIONS AND CANDIDIASIS

There is no definitive way to test for yeast overgrowth; however, there are blood tests or stool tests for yeast overgrowth that may be helpful. Skilled practitioners may use Live Blood Analysis (Dark-field therapy), and some may blood test for antibodies to intestinal yeast or conduct stool tests, but none of these methods are an exact science. The best way to diagnose yeast infections is clinically with history and symptoms. The Healing Arts Partnership uses a screening questionnaire (Appendix E:10) which is a great tool to evaluate the likelihood of a yeast infection based on risk factors, and symptom type and intensity. A score of 140 or higher is considered significant and treatment is recommended. Yeast infections may have similar symptoms to Lyme disease and Herx reactions, so it is important to get rid of fungal infections, not just to improve healing capacity, but so you can eliminate some of the symptoms that may be overlapping or exacerbating one another. For those with vaginitis or genital thrush, douche with Loalsan (purchase here: www.tbmseminars. com), and for those with fungal nail infections, soaking the feet and hands in Loalsan works a treat.

Douche or Soak with Loalsan: 3x a day for 3 days, once a day for 4 days and once a week for a few weeks. Afterwards, you will need to replace the beneficial flora using yoghurt or even a probiotic douche. Using TBM and kinesiology can also fast track your treatment.

Yeast and a Sugar-free Diet: Yeast feeds on sugar, so eliminating it from the diet for somewhere between 2–8 weeks will help facilitate your body to address yeast overgrowth / infection. I adapted my yeast-free diet from the TBM manual and Adele Reising (see Appendix E:11 for a copy).

Replenishing the Good Bacteria in the Vagina: Sometimes taking a multi-strain probiotic will be enough. For women, you will often notice a white coating or thrush in your vagina if you have thrush. In my experience, you will need to address the colonies of good bacteria vaginally as well as get the gut bacteria sorted out. My remedy is to douche to kill any bacteria and fungi, and then use organic apple cider vinegar to douche twice a day for three days to optimise the vaginal pH. At bedtime, cover a tampon with organic natural yoghurt and sleep with it in. Other options include putting yoghurt directly inside your vagina (the tampon tends to hold it in better) or inserting a probiotic capsule into your vagina. Do this every night for 1 to 2 weeks whilst you continue to take probiotics orally as well. You can also try Fem-Dophilus, an oral probiotic that is designed to restore optimal vaginal flora.

Garlic Tampon: Garlic is antibacterial and antifungal, so another trick you can use (if you don't find it too gross and can tolerate garlic) is to peel a piece of garlic and put it inside your vagina before going to bed. You will know it has absorbed because you will be able to taste garlic in your mouth in the morning.

Antifungal Supplements, Oils and Herbs: The best supplement I have found for Candida is Canicid Forte from Molecular Products. Other oils and herbs that have great antifungal properties are olive leaf extract, grapefruit seed extract, cinnamon, clove, peppermint, oil of oregano, neem leaf, tea tree and Nutrimedix products' Banderol and Cumanda. Stephen Buhner (Forsgren 2010) believes that the use of equal parts of desert willow and chapparo amargosa tinctures blended together can have an anti-Candida effect (½ tsp 3x daily for 30 days, supported by an anti-Candida diet). Cinnamomum verum (Sri Lankan) is believed to not just kill fungus such as Candida, but also spirochetes, viruses, protozoans and rickettsiae.

Fasting: If you still can't beat Candida, you may want to read Stephen Buhner's book *The Fasting Path.* He believes that sometimes, the only way to beat tough Candida is to fast. (Buhner 2003) I am skeptical of fasting when you are sick, but as a last resort, it may be worth a try!

TREATING RECURRENT UTIs

Due to suppressed immune system function and often an overuse of antibiotics, urinary tract infections, which include the bladder and kidneys, are unfortunately quite common in Lyme disease patients. Please note that they may be asymptomatic, mild or severe. Over 90% of UTIs are believed to be caused by E.coli entering the urinary tract, whilst a small percentage are believed to be from other causes such as biofilms forming in the urogenital tract (There are those nasty biofilms again. They're like bullet-proof vests for cheeky bacteria.). Often doctors will prescribe antibiotics to treat UTIs, but in my opinion, this is a short-term fix which can create even more challenges long-term, as antibiotics may wipe out the overgrowth of E.coli, but they also deplete the beneficial bacteria. Even worse, they can create antibiotic-resistant strains of E.coli. Antibiotics are a last choice option here.

The main treatment for UTIs caused by E.coli is D-Mannose, a naturally forming sugar found in large quantities in cranberries and cranberry juice (100% cranberry juice you buy from health food stores and some grocers, not that sugary stuff you buy in the local supermarket).

I recommend eating organic cranberries or drinking a shot of 100% cranberry juice each day to maintain good urinary tract health. You can also dilute 100% cranberry juice with water, as it is very sour!

There is also an array of cranberry capsules on the market. By far the BEST brand in my opinion is Professional Botanicals Cranberry Complex (and I had tried probably 20 brands before I tried this one). It has vitamin C and immune-boosting herbs such as echinacea root, reishi, cordyceps and goldenseal as well as enzymes! Even though you need to order it from America, it is still cheaper and probably twice as effective in comparison with anything else on the market, in my opinion.

The KEY to getting long-term results is to take one cranberry capsule daily for a year after the initial regimen – start with 3 capsules 3x a day for 3 weeks and repeat if acute. Most people take them for a few months, forget (yep, that was me!) and then have to start all over again! Do yourself a favour and make a note or reminder in your diary, and take it for a year! I also douched with Loalsan. If you have a yeast infection and UTI issues, then douching with Loalsan or the equivalent will kill two birds with one stone. After you have douched, you can use Fem-Dophilus, an oral probiotic that is specially designed to restore optimal vaginal flora, or you can just put yoghurt or any other brand of probiotic straight inside your vagina!

If you are one of the 10% who has a UTI caused by something other than E.coli, then the cranberry treatment just isn't going to work for you. You will also need to address the biofilm that is protecting the bacteria. Chris Kresser (Kresser 2015) suggests using Lauricidin®, nattokinase or apolactoferrin (lactoferrin) and has some supportive research on his website if you are interested. Any of the biofilm treatments that you are already doing for Borrelia should also help this problem.

ADDRESSING AND TREATING MOULD TOXICITY

I am no expert in mould toxicity, but I have learned quite a lot along my journey that I would like to share with you. However, I suggest that you enlist the help of a mould specialist if you think that this is a major concurrent issue creating your symptoms.

Did you know that not all moulds are toxic to humans and that some are only toxic at very high levels? Well, now you do!

Mould, Mould Spores and Mycotoxins Explained

Mould refers to different types of fungi that grow in filaments and reproduce by forming spores (often these spores are invisible to the naked eye!). Mould can grow indoors or outdoors and thrives in damp, humid, warm environments but can be found in any environment in any season, so don't be complacent!

Spores refer to the tiny (often microscopic) particles that allow mould to reproduce. They survive extreme conditions (often where mould cannot) and travel through air. Once the spores land on a moist surface, mould can then reproduce and grow.

Mycotoxins refer to the toxic chemicals that are present in mould spores and small fragments of mould and fungus, and are dispersed in air.

Symptoms of Mould Toxicity

Take note that there is a huge crossover with Lyme and mould symptoms. It's sometimes hard to know if adverse symptoms are being caused by moulds or Borrelia, or both (or even Candida!). The main symptoms of mould toxicity include, but are not limited to: fatigue, muscle pain, joint and nerve issues (cramps, weakness, aches, stiffness, numbness, tingling, tremors), ice pick pain headaches, eye and visual disturbances (light sensitivity, red eyes, blurry, floaters), respiratory symptoms (cough, shortness of breath, sinus issues), brain issues (poor memory, decreased

293

focus / concentration, word recollection issues, decreased ability to learn new information, confusion, brain fog, disorientation), mood swings, appetite swings, night sweats, temperature dysregulation, excessive thirst, increased urination, vertigo and a metallic taste in the mouth.

Diagnosing Mould Toxicity

Many people often look fine when they are being afflicted by mycotoxins. For those with Lyme disease, does this sound familiar?! People continually say to you, "You look fine to me!" and you want to scream or even worse, punch them in the face as you might look well but you certainly don't feel well! Why do some people get really sick and toxic with exposure to mould while others who have been exposed to the same environment remain healthy? The answer is in your genes. Some people have a faulty or mutated HLA-DR gene and are, therefore, genetically more susceptible to mould toxicity. In terms of genetics, everyone is coded differently, and how the body deals with inflammation (and therefore mould) is no different. About 25% of people have an affected HLA-DR gene, so instead of creating an antigen to fight mould after the first-time exposure, that antigen not only doesn't fight to disable the mycotoxins, but it stays in the body, which causes the body to keep increasing inflammation in response. Eventually the body starts to attack itself in what is known as an autoimmune response.

Online VCS Screening Test – go to http://www.survivingmold.com/store1/online-screening-test and take the Visual Contrast Sensitivity Aptitude test and accompanying survey as a starting point to see if it's likely that you might have mould toxicity.

Treating Mould Toxicity

Address the Environment First

KNOW WHERE MOULD CAN BE FOUND. Mould and its mycotoxins are not just found in damp places that smell musty. They are also found in places such as contaminated foods (especially leftovers, even if they are refrigerated), foods packaged in plastic, nuts, dust, concrete slabs and cars (especially if you live in a wet or humid area).

AVOID EATING LEFTOVERS. Foods grow mould very quickly; just because you can't see mould doesn't mean it isn't there. If you do eat a lot of leftovers or nuts, a great idea is to lightly heat and sauté them in an attempt to kill the mould before ingesting.

AVOID KNOWN MOULDY PLACES. This is not always possible, but keeping your car, workplace and home clean and dry can really help. If you live in an old, damp place, then it would be wise to consider moving, or at the very least, get a good air filter.

HAVE YOUR HOME AND WORKPLACE ASSESSED FOR MOULD. There are companies that specialise in this. If your environment doesn't smell musty or feel damp, then sometimes there are still things you can do to eliminate the mould that is there (assuming it's not going to build up again!). There are many ways buildings become home to a toxic mix of microbes (including mould) such as construction defects, ineffective ventilation, basements that are below water level (and leak), flat roofs and water leaks that haven't been cleaned up or fixed. If you Google *mould remediation* or *mould removal Australia* (or your country), you will get plenty of information.

> Here's a helpful PDF: http://inspectapedia.com/sickhouse/Australian_Mold_Guideline-2005.pdf. It gives an overview of the different assessment (and treatment) options and includes questionnaires, visual inspections, surface sampling, air sampling and dust sampling.

Treating (or Preventing) Mould in the Environment

Remember, when you "kill" mould, it will release toxins. While you are addressing mould issues in your environment, you should stay out of that environment for at least a few days, but ideally a week.

CLEAN UP SPILLS IMMEDIATELY. If something is leaking, there is water in the bathroom after everyone has showered, or something gets spilt (even just a tiny bit), make sure you clean it up before it has time to seep into the cracks.

USE A DEHUMIDIFIER. This will help pull water out of the air in humid areas and prevent mould from growing. It will also make your environment more comfortable so it's likely you will sleep better and help decrease populations of pests.

USE HEPA FILTERS. The best vacuums and air filters are ones with a HEPA filter. They are expensive but worth the investment for your health. Most air filters only purify particles larger than 0.3 microns in size, but up to 90% of fine particles are smaller than this. So, buying a cheap air filter will only help filter about 10% of the particles, leaving pollen, pet hair and mould spores untouched! In my opinion, if you have a mould problem (or allergies or multiple chemical sensitivities), then the best thing you can do is to buy a good quality air filter that filters particles as small as 0.003 microns. Then you can filter out allergens (mould, dust mite, pollen or animal hair), VOCs (volatile molecular compounds) and air pollution (from chemicals, tobacco or wood fire smoke) as well as odours (pets, musty or cooking). If you want more information about good quality air filters as well as EMR and radiation shielding, go to http://www.breathing-easy.net. (Room Air Purifiers n.d.)

USE MOISTURE POTS AND HANGING BAGS. You can buy various brands of pots and hanging bags (for your wardrobe) from local supermarkets such as Coles and Woolworths, and also at Bunnings Warehouse. They work by absorbing excess moisture from the air when the special pellets inside them are exposed to air, and then they convert that moisture into brine (salt solution). Just place them strategically around the house—in cupboards and damp areas—to draw moisture into them. The ones I use in my home are called DampRid (www.damprid.com). They are a non-toxic, septic-safe and environmentally friendly way to deal with humidity and dampness in the environment (home, work, car). They have a very strong smell though, so I tend to put them in my cupboards and shut the doors!

GET FRESH AIR AND SUNLIGHT. Open windows, hang portable things like clothes outside and give your place as much air and sunlight as possible, as mould doesn't survive well in these elements. Using a fan (especially in the bathroom) and opening the windows helps to circulate the air and prevent mould buildup.

USE VINEGAR AND ESSENTIAL OILS. White vinegar is a safe, cheap and effective cleaner for the whole house, and is particularly effective against mould and bacteria. You can use it on a sponge or have it in a spray bottle. Soak the affected area for a few hours. Then, scrub it off and ensure the area is fully dried. If you don't like the smell of vinegar, try adding some essential oils such as tea tree oil or grapefruit seed extract (tea tree has a strong but pleasant aroma, and grapefruit seed oil has no smell at all! Plus, both have additional antifungal properties). Tea tree and grapefruit seed oil are a lot more expensive than vinegar, and tea tree oil has the strongest antifungal properties of the three.

CLEAN WITH BAKING SODA. Baking soda is another great cleaning product. Because it is mildly abrasive, it is good for areas that need scrubbing like bathrooms, grout and cracks. Rinse with white vinegar to prevent leaving any white residue on the surface.

GET RID OF THE CARPET. Many allergens, including mould, are very hard to remove from carpet, even if it is vacuumed and cleaned regularly. Use a HEPA filter vacuum as suggested, but if you own your home, then your best bet is to pull up and replace your carpet, as it will be much better for you health without any carpet!

I still think the best way to eliminate mould from your environment is to call in the experts.

Dealing with Mould in the Body

The approach to mould in the body is three-pronged.

1. PREVENT MOULD BY ADDRESSING YOUR DIET. The best approach is to follow the yeast-free diet and eat fresh and unpackaged

items as often as you can. Remember: just because you can't see mould doesn't mean that it isn't there! Rules of thumb include the following: avoid eating leftovers (especially anything that has been stored for more than 24 hours), fruit (especially high glycaemic fruits), grains, alcohol, aged cheeses, vinegar (and vinegar-based products), alcohol, nuts and cured meats. If you are going to eat fruit, make sure that it is thoroughly washed and, ideally, organic. Soaking nuts (especially in lemon juice) can help remove the mould unless you are eating them fresh from where they are grown (with the exception of cashews which you should never eat raw) or you are storing them in the fridge in an airtight glass container.

2. KILL THE MOULD THAT EXISTS. This is done with antifungals such as olive leaf extract, grapefruit seed extract, cinnamon, clove, peppermint, oil of oregano, the product TriGuard Plus and Nutramedix® products Banderol and Cumanda.

3. BIND THE DIE-OFF. This process is not unlike the "mop-up" process from the die-off from Borrelia to minimise or prevent Herxing. Many of the same binders can be used. If mould is really bad, some doctors, including James Schaller and the doctors who treat Lyme in Germany, recommend using a drug called cholestyramine. This drug was created to lower cholesterol, so if your cholesterol is already low, this drug may not be an option for you. Speak to your GP first. Another option may be activated carbon, but that is beyond the scope of this book.

The Shoemaker Protocol

Shoemaker regards treatment like a trip up a pyramid. If eliminating mould exposure at the bottom of the pyramid eliminates the symptoms, then the job is done. If not, then you must continue up the pyramid. Next steps include a thorough history combined with lab testing (MMP9, VEGF, C4a and TGF beta-1) and a VSC test. These results are used to monitor and implement the appropriate treatment strategy until full health and recovery is achieved. (What Do I Do? n.d.)

Log onto http://www.survivingmold.com/treatment for an overview of this method and http://www.survivingmold.com/treatment/step-by-step for the step-by-step process you can work through with your primary health care practitioner.

HOMEOPATHY

The German physician Samuel Hahnemann, who found the conventional medicine techniques in Germany at the time to be less than sufficient and felt that the "state-of-the art" treatments were causing more harm than good, discovered homeopathy. Whilst working as a medicinal translator, he translated an article about a particular Peruvian bark that, due to its bitter nature, was successfully used to treat febrile states. He thought it was utterly absurd and decided to experiment with it by taking it himself. Low and behold, the ingestion of a small amount of the bark made him sick with the exact symptoms that the bark was supposed to cure!

Over the next 10 years, Dr. Hahnemann turned himself, willing colleagues and even his family into human experiments by administering medicines and herbs and studying their symptoms (both physical and emotional). He found that the symptoms were reproducible in all healthy individuals. He then departed from accepted scientific research and applied the information he had learned to sick people instead of healthy ones! What he discovered was that when administering a substance capable of producing similar symptoms to the actual symptoms of their disease, resolution of the symptoms and illness often occurred. This effect is known as the Law of Similars (i.e. like cures like). He also found that by diluting the substances more and more and shaking the bottle (known as succusion), the substances not only became less toxic, but became more potent as well. This is known as the Law of the Minimum Dose. To make a long story short, homeopathy works by administering a very diluted substance (generally from a plant or herb) that would typically cause symptoms in a healthy person, but in a sick person causes the body to intensify its own healing response towards that particular illness and often resolve the symptoms! Despite people's scepticism, homeopathy has still managed to spread to every continent on Earth. I *know that I personally respond amazingly well using homeopathy, especially for emotional symptoms.*

Because homeopathy focuses on the whole body rather than a medical diagnosis to determine where the imbalance is occurring to cause adverse symptoms and ultimately disease, it is helpful then in treating chronic diseases. For Lyme disease, homeopathy is also believed to help activate dormant layers of the spirochete infection (and cyst form), which makes unfavourable microbes more vulnerable to other adjunct therapies such as antibiotics, Rife therapy, acupuncture and medicinal herbs. Homeopathy, of course, works best in combination with optimal lifestyle strategies such as a healthy diet, adequate hydration and stress reduction techniques.

Dr. Cindee Gardner uses homeopathic remedies such as "Sepia, Sulphur, Tellurium, Ledum, Syphilinum, Carcinocin, Kalmia, Arnica, Rhododendron, Bryonia, Gelsemium, Rhus Toxicodendron, Arsenicum Album, Apis, Hyper-icum, Ruta, Symphytum, Silica, Cimicifuga, Argentum Nitricum, Mercury, Colchicine, Pulsatilla, Lac Caninium, Glycyrrhiza, Lyssinum, Spilanthes, Ixo-des, Trombidium, Arbuts, Myristica, Carboneum Sulphuricum, Cimex, China, Psorinum, Toxoplasm, Viscum, Tuberculinum, Natrum Sulphuricum, Candida Albicans, AIDS nosode, Mezurium, and Thuja, and several different Lyme no-sodes, among other remedies."(Gardner Revised 2012)

From his research, presented in "Homeopathy and Lyme Disease," Dr. Ronald Whitmont (Whitmont 2012) concludes that homeopathic treatment is effective in the worldwide treatment of infectious diseases because it supports rather than suppresses immune system function. More research is needed in this area to convince the medical world, but personal success is enough for me, so try it for yourself!

ESSENTIAL OILS

Essential oils are often considered the life force of the plant and are stored in special cells, ducts, glands, roots, seeds, flowers, bark or leaves of the plant. The plant uses these oils to protect itself from animals, insects and other microorganisms. This is why essential oils can have the same healing and protective effects when used as medicines for healing. They are obtained from the plant in various ways: by compression, distillation with steam, dissolving the oils out (extraction) or absorbing them, and by pressure and maceration.

I am not an expert in essential oils, but in order to give you some other treatment options, I'd like to share which oils have helped me. To be effective, make sure you take the oil(s) for long enough. If you have not experienced improvements or a Herx within three months, then I suggest you change the dose or try another oil. No symptom changes may indicate the oil is either ineffective or not specific for your needs.

Essential oils generally work by impacting / killing / eradicating infections so the body can take charge and heal itself. They are best used as an alternative or at different times than antibiotics, as they often counteract each other.

Grades of Oils

Be sure to buy good quality, pure, undiluted, organic and therapeutic grade essential oils for best results. Some oils are safe to ingest, but synthetic oils should NOT be consumed. Talk to your herbalist before taking an essential oil orally.

How Are Essential Oils Sold?

Single One oil within one bottle – sometimes pure or sometimes mixed with a carrier oil.

Blend More than one essential oil in one bottle along with a carrier oil that is not an essential oil.

A Patch Test for Allergies

It is very rare for anyone to have a skin reaction or allergy to essential oils but better to be safe than sorry! Put a drop on the underside of your arm and leave for 10 minutes. If there is no reaction, then you can safely apply it to your skin.

Essential Oils Useful in the Treatment of Lyme Disease and Its Co-infections

The following list includes essential oils that target Rickettsia, Bartonella bacteria, Babesia protozoa, spirochetes of Lyme, STARI, Borrelia myamotoi, TBRF (Tick-borne Relapsing Fever) and encysted form, Babesia, Bartonella, mycoplasmas, viruses, other zoonotic bacteria and fungi, including all types of Candida.

- ❖ Cannabis sativa

- ❖ Cinnamon verum leaf from Sri Lanka – works without upsetting the gut flora

- ❖ Citrus reticulata (Mandarin)

- ❖ CHUM-FLUOX-AVIVA – okay with drugs and herbs; also targets the cysts of Lyme and Morgellons fungus

- ❖ Origanum marjorana (France) or Thymus mastichina (Spain)

Other Oils That Target Spirochetes and Cysts

Cinnamon Bark, Marjoram, Myrrh, Orange, Pine, Rosemary, Rosewood, Tangerine, and Wintergreen (not all of these can be ingested)

The Lyme Bullet

This is a natural treatment method to use when you are bitten by a tick (and to prevent zoonotic infection). I have not used this personally but it was shared with me by a fellow Lymie. Put 20 drops of the following in a capsule and take every 4 hours for 3 days, then every 8 hours for 4 days.

❖ 2 drops of frankincense

❖ 6 drops of oregano

❖ 12 drops of thieves

Taking Oral Essential Oils

Oils are generally not added to liquid as they don't mix or absorb well. Do not put under the tongue like homeopathic remedies.

1. Drop the required dose on a cracker or a slice of bread (or other foods) and have with a meal. Be careful with capsules if you have low stomach acid.

2. Slowly increase the drops every day or every other day.

3. If a Herx is reached, then decrease the dose or stop for as long as it takes for the body to safely detoxify. Then resume at a lower dose and continue to slowly increase.

4. Repeat until you have done for 65 days straight without a Herx.

5. Continue for another 35 days if fungus is present (including Candida and/or mould).

Other Methods to Use Essential Oils

❖ Rub on your skin (usually combined with a base oil like olive or almond oil)

❖ Old-fashioned inhalation – drop a few drops in a bowl of boiling water and drape a towel over your head and shoulders as you lean over the steam with your eyes closed

❖ Use a facial steamer (similar to inhalation)

❖ Diffuser / atomiser / nebuliser – less potent because its dispersed throughout the whole room, but it continually exposes you to the oils and can be helpful for sensitive people

DETOXIFICATION

If the liver or any of the detoxification organs are under stress, you can use treatments and strategies that supercharge and support the detoxification process, minimise the toxic load by decreasing your toxin intake (internally, externally, in your environment and in your mind) and prevent detoxifications issues in the first place (or at least lessen them).

Toxins and Toxicity

A toxin is something that has the ability to create disease in the body in high doses. It is something that causes the body to expel it in order to maintain or move towards optimal health. Many people think that the word toxin solely refers to things like pesticides, preservatives and pollution, but even seemingly natural and beneficial nutrients, like vitamin C or water, can be toxic in high doses. Toxic levels will be different for each person depending on their genetics, immune function, detoxification capacity and amount of exposure or consumption. If your immune system and detoxification capacity are good, then you may be able to tolerate small amounts of toxins, such as a sugary treat or a swim in a chlorinated pool, but the more of each toxin you are exposed to or consume, the more toxic it becomes due to buildup.

Toxicity is unavoidable. Over an extended period of time, small daily doses of multiple contaminants have a cumulative detrimental effect on physiologic pathways, which can eventually impair homeostasis and cause disease. Every year, it is believed that thousands of new chemicals are invented and released in to the environment from advances in manufacturing, farming, medicine, and science, to name a few. Check out the video on YouTube about toxins in our environment (https://www.youtube.com/watch?v=Hgbv3Bz6zTY). It is American, but I'm sure many industrialised countries are similar.

How Do Toxins Get in?

Ingestion, breathing, olfaction, skin absorption and vertical transmission (mother / father to foetus)

Total Toxin Load = Total Toxin Exposure minus Ability to Detoxify and Ability to Eliminate Toxins

Generational Toxicity

It is now known that the burden of toxicity is passed from one generation to the next. Babies are being born *pre-polluted* and have disturbing levels of toxicity in their cord blood. If they are breastfed, it is believed that as much as 20–70% of a woman's pesticide burden is released into her milk supply over a six-month period (due to the fat soluble nature of toxins), as the mother releases fat stores to produce milk. So detoxing BEFORE a pregnancy is extremely important. (Nickerson 2006)

Factors Affecting Toxin Resistance

Individual resistance to a certain toxin exposure varies greatly between individuals due to a variety of factors:

❖ Current health status

❖ Genetic susceptibility

❖ Blood type

❖ Age – the older you are, the higher the chance of exposure and accumulative burden

❖ Exposures – timing, pattern, duration

❖ Nutrition and lifestyle – diet, hydration, exercise, etc.

❖ GIT function and integrity – digestion, absorption, microbiome

❖ Genetic detoxification capacity – Phase I, II, III liver enzymes and function

❖ Immune function and status

❖ Environment – air quality, pesticides

❖ Water quality and quantity

❖ Movement – engaging lymphatic and circulatory systems

❖ Mood, emotions and perceptions

❖ Drugs and supplements – past and present

❖ Breathing

Supercharging the Detoxification Process

Two key factors in detoxification are to 1) reduce the toxic burden and 2) improve toxin resistance. First, let's focus on what you can do to supercharge your body's natural detoxification and, thereby, increase toxic resilience.

Supporting the Body's Natural Detoxification Pathways

❖ It is essential that you have daily bowel movements (ideally 2–3 times a day). If you aren't, then you need to drink more water, add more ground flax seeds, slippery elm and psyllium husks or fibre (such as apple pectin) to your meals or smoothies. You can also try vitamins that have a natural laxative effect when taken in excess, such as magnesium or vitamin C, as they increase bowel motility in higher doses (not to mention, Lymies are often low in magnesium anyway, and extra vitamin C has many other benefits including immune support!).

❖ Drink filtered water to flush the kidneys and support liver function. The general rule is 43ml per kg per day.

❖ The Indian spice turmeric is not just effective for natural inflammation reduction, but also assists detoxification by increasing the expression of glutathione S-transferase, which assists in methylation.

❖ Vitamin C aids in overall detoxification and when combined with B3 helps tissues expel toxins.

❖ Garlic is antimicrobial and has detoxification capacities, so add it to your food whenever possible. Make sure you let it rest for 10 minutes after you peel and chop / crush it so you benefit from the active healing component of allicin (if you are freezing it, leave it for 10 minutes and then put it in the freezer so you will get the most allicin possible).

❖ Exercise, infrared saunas, steam rooms, drinking water and deep breathing also move the lymphatic system and support lung excretion.

❖ Avoid putting things on your skin that will affect the way it breathes and expels toxins, especially chemical-based products that can seep into the skin and cause extra toxicity (see more specific tips in Detox Your Body from the Outside).

❖ Avoid medications where possible because they put extra strain on the liver due to the processing required to metabolise them, not to mention the extra toxic burden on the entire detoxification system.

Improving Detoxification

Supporting the body's natural detoxification pathways, decreasing the amount of toxins dumped into the body and using binding agents to speed up elimination, will all help improve detoxification capacity, but the key is to ensure all three phases of liver detoxification are working optimally.

Detox programs are great, but only if done properly. Most commercial detox programs focus on mobilising the toxins without supporting Phase II and III liver function. This is very dangerous because for every toxin that is mobilised in Phase I, there is a free radical created which can cause damage to the cells. So if Phase II liver detoxification is not working optimally, then you are essentially making yourself more toxic! So it's super important that Phase II detoxification is supported in order to neutralise those free radicals. Then you can eliminate the toxins and avoid making a bad situation worse! Boosting the body's ability to naturally create glutathione (or supplementing, which is not as powerful) and improving methylation is the best way to support and improve detoxification. This way, you are looking to the cause of the detoxification issue rather than trying to fix the symptoms it's creating.

BOOSTING NATURAL GLUTATHIONE

The best approach to boost natural glutathione is to eat certain foods and take supplements whilst minimising foods and habits that deplete natural sources. It's best to create a holistic approach rather than just picking one category from the table, or one supplement or one food. A combination approach usually works best! Please note that certain genetic mutations may affect the way your body methylates (especially CBS, a gene that converts homocysteine into cystathionine and eventually into glutathione), so if glutathione supplementation makes you sick or doesn't seem to help, you will need to consult your doctor for further testing and help. (Kresser 2015)

Things that deplete glutathione levels	Things that boost natural glutathione levels	Nutrients required for natural glutathione synthesis/levels	Botanicals
Toxins (e.g., environmental, endotoxins, medications) Stress (physical, chemical and emotional) Exposure to infectious agents Nutrient deficiencies	Exercise Raw dairy Raw eggs Fresh unprocessed meats Sulphur-rich foods (onions, garlic) Cruciferous vegetables (kale, horseradish, collard greens, cabbage, broccoli, spinach, cauliflower, bok choy, radish) Avocado	B6 B12 N-acetyl-cysteine (NAC) ALA Selenium Glycine	Milk thistle Cordyceps Broccoli seed

For more information, see Chris Kresser's website
www.chriskresser.com (Kresser 2015)

IMPROVING METHYLATION

A healthy body makes plenty of methyl groups whilst an unhealthy body does not, and health declines if the body is not methylating optimally. Improving natural methylation includes eating foods that naturally contain methyl groups such as good quality red meat. The less cooked the red meat, the more methionine and the better you will methylate, so steak tartare, or rare steak, is a good choice (but only if the meat is organic or grass-fed and finished, of course).

Foods supporting natural methylation	Supplements that support methylation
Red meat Chicken Beetroot Quinoa Dark green, steamed leafy vegetables	Active B12 Folate B6 Betaine

Improving Elimination Pathways

PRIMARY ROUTES OF ELIMINATION – bowels, bladder, skin, breathing, voice and menses which are all outlined as follows. The primary routes of elimination all have direct access to the outside of the body and occur as the "normal" daily bodily toxins and wastes are excreted. Some toxins are able to be directly excreted through the primary routes of elimination, whilst others must first be transformed by the liver. Through a series of reactions, the liver is able to convert some toxins to a more water-soluble form, which will aid excretion in the urine, breath or sweat. Other toxins are combined with bile into a fat soluble form to aid excretion via the bowels. Therefore, the liver plays a large role in the conversion and detoxification of toxins and is a vital organ in the eliminatory process.

1. Bowels – The bowels are the major route of elimination of toxins from the body. Food is ingested and passes through the digestive tract. Nutrients are absorbed during this process and the waste is eliminated via the stool, which protects the body from toxic accumulation. So, ensuring your bowels are working properly is essential for detoxification. If the stools are not passed efficiently and effectively, not only is it completely uncomfortable (bordering on torture), but it does not allow toxic release and may even allow toxins to be reabsorbed back into the body.

The first time I was ever constipated was in 2012 in Italy. I didn't go for eight days, despite having a whole tub of vitamin C powder in two days, overdosing on magnesium powder and having several coffees a day! I was in so much pain that I finally went to a chemist and asked for an herbal laxative (very funny trying to explain what I wanted when the pharmacist didn't speak much English! You get the picture!). Even the laxatives he gave me took 48 hours and three doses to work! That was the first time I understood what my clients felt when they told me they were constipated. That's also what babies feel like when they don't move their bowels regularly (despite many health professionals saying it's "normal" to not poo for up to three weeks sometimes).You try not pooing for even a few days and tell me that it's normal!!! I feel awful if I don't poo multiple times a day! After six months of antibiotic use, I also had really bad constipation and it took me 10 months to get my bowels back on track post-antibiotic treatment. Poo is important and there are varying classifications of what constipation means. To keep it simple, if you are not going daily, have to strain to go or are a 1, 2 or 3 on the Bristol Stool Chart, YOU ARE CONSTIPATED and need to act immediately. The Bristol Stool Chart is also a great way to alleviate embarrassment when talking about poo with your health professional.

The Bristol Stool Chart

Bristol Stool Form Scale		
Type	Description	Image
Type 1	Separate hard lumps, like nuts	
Type 2	Sausage-shaped but lumpy	
Type 3	Like a sausage or snake but with cracks on its surface	
Type 4	Like a sausage or snake, smooth and soft	
Type 5	Soft blobs with clear-cut edges	
Type 6	Fluffy pieces with ragged edges, a mushy stool	
Type 7	Watery, no solid pieces	

Type 1: Separate hard lumps, like nuts

Typical in acute dysbiosis (aka disbacteriosis) post-antibiotic use, in de-hydration or when people have low fibre diets causing a microbial imbalance in the GIT. Balance of benign and beneficial microbial colonies in the GIT are necessary for functions such as digestion, absorption of nutrients and protecting the body from penetration of pathogenic microbes. Type 1 stools are missing bacteria and fibre. Therefore, they have nothing to retain the water with, which creates hard and abrasive lumps usually about 1–2cm in diameter that may be painful to pass (with the likelihood of anorectal bleeding). Flatulence is unlikely because the fermentation of fibre isn't taking place.

Type 2: Sausage-like but lumpy

Type 2 is similar to Type 1 except that the hard lumps are joined together by some bacteria and fibre components to make a single mass with a diameter of about 3–4cm. This form occurs due to prolonged transit time where the stool can remain in the colon for up to several weeks instead of the usual 24–72 hours. These are the most destructive and painful stools to pass due to the size and hardness (almost certainly causing anal canal damage and bleeding of varying degrees). Anorectal pain, dehydration, withholding or delaying defecation (which I call "over baking") and a history of chronic constipation are the most likely causes. Extreme straining can cause haemorrhoids, anal fissures, anal canal laceration and diverticulitis. These stools are indicative of IBS and minor flatulence is probable. Be careful with adding extra fibre to your diet as the fibre will expand the stool and may cause damage in the small or large bowel.

Type 3: Like a sausage but with cracks in the surface

This form is similar to Type 2 but has a quicker transit time (1–2 weeks) and, therefore, a slightly smaller diameter of 2–3.5cm. Type 3 is typical of latent constipation where IBS is likely, flatulence is minor and straining is required. It has similar adverse effects to Type 2 (especially exacerbation of haemorrhoidal disease).

Type 4: Like a sausage or snake, smooth and soft

This form is 1–2cm in diameter and normal for someone defecating once daily.

Type 5: Soft blobs with clear-cut edges

This form is ideal and has a diameter of 1–1.5cm. It is typical for a person who has stools two to three times daily after major meals.

Type 6: Fluffy pieces with ragged edges, a mushy stool

With Type 6, it may be difficult to control the urge, so it can be a messy affair! The looseness of the stool suggests a slightly hyperactive colon (faster motility), which can be caused by excess dietary potassium, sudden dehydration, a spike in blood pressure related to stress, the consumption of too many spices, drinking water with a high mineral content or the use of laxatives.

Type 7: Watery, no solid pieces

This is known as classic diarrhoea.

2. Bladder – The bladder stores and excretes urine after the urinary system filters blood, and it breaks down metabolic waste into byproducts such as uric acid and nitrogen.

3. Skin – The skin removes toxins stored in fat tissues through sweating. Sweating may be stimulated via exercise, fever or a hot environment (weather, sauna, steam room, heater, etc.)

4. Breathing – The lungs expel carbon dioxide (a naturally occurring toxin) via the breath in order to maintain pH balance and homeostasis within the body.

5. Voice – The voice is an important way for the body to express true feelings and emotions (whether positive or negative) and is an important part of detoxification in the body.

6. Menses– Menstruation is a primary route of elimination for women each month as blood and uterine lining are shed, which eliminates unwanted waste. Dark, heavy, painful periods are often a sign of toxicity. The further away from "normal" the period is in terms of pain, length, clotting, etc., the more likely you are toxic.

SECONDARY ROUTES OF ELIMINATION are nasal discharge, ear wax, tears, hair, leucorrhea (excess vaginal secretions), phlegm, mucus or blood in the stool and sneezing.

Secondary routes of elimination kick in when the primary routes are overburdened with toxins. The body attempts to shed unwanted toxins from the system by utilising the secondary routes.

Improving Gut Integrity

The gut is the foundation for detoxification and health. The gut is the interface for many vital functions and communicates a significant amount of information about immune function, inflammation, and toxic and nutritional status. The delicate microbiome and the gut wall play important roles and have the potential to be both barriers and sources of inflammation. As such, the gut wall can be considered the gatekeeper to inflammation, which in turn is believed to be a key driver of chronic disease. The "leakier" the gut is, the more inflammatory triggers the body has to deal with, and this can be exacerbated again by dysbiosis. Toxins that come through the mouth (food, drink, drugs) go through the gut, which is the first line of defence. Should the gut fail to eliminate the toxin(s) completely, then the toxin(s) move through to the liver and kidneys, which is how these organs become overburdened. Should the liver and kidneys fail to remove the toxic load, then cellular function is impaired. So an intact gut barrier keeps food, bacteria and gut-generated toxins from entering systemic circulation in large quantities. It also has its own detoxification capacity with Phase I, II and III enzymes, just like the liver! Even your blood type can affect your gut function. For example, Type O blood types are genetically better equipped for optimal gut function! The gut function and treatment could be a whole book on its own, but I just wanted to point out the importance of getting the gut right as a priority.

Genetic and Genomic Testing

Genetic testing is available to determine what genes you've inherited. You could technically test all 25,000 genes, but it would be very expensive, and not enough is known about all the genes and their functions yet. Because all genes have not been mapped for specific characteristics, the information would be useless (until scientists unlock the meaning to more of the genes anyway). In order to have a more cost-effective option in which more meaningful information can be gleaned, there are tests that target a narrower range of genes. Through this testing, you can identify which genes have specific mutations, or single nucleotide polymorphisms (SNPs). Most genetic testing will test between 20–35 SNPs, which can cost anywhere from $100–$1600, so it is important that you test with reputable labs that will provide consistent and accurate results. The information can then be used to target treatment and/or preventative strategies. Some people may find the knowledge of such mutations scary. In my opinion, there is no point testing something that you either don't have the ability or knowledge to change, or don't plan to change even if that information is available to you. Most tests are done with either a saliva swab or pin prick blood test so are not particularly invasive.

Dr. Amy Yasko uses an interesting and easy-to-understand analogy to describe the difference between addressing mutated genes as done in nutrigenomics as opposed to just trying to supercharge the detoxification process alone. She explains that detoxification is like a revolving door. When working properly, people can come and go just as toxins do. However, if the door is not working well and it lets in more people than it lets out, then at some point there will be congestion. This is what happens when you have a genetic mutation that affects your methylation; it allows the accumulation of toxins. Supercharging the detoxification pathway using chelation and/or binding agents is said to be like letting people (accumulated toxins) out the side door; it allows detoxification but doesn't actually fix the main issue—the broken front door. So as soon as the side door is shut or becomes impaired or broken, then the accumulation of toxins builds up all over again. Nutrigenomics addresses the primary concern (the broken front door) by using targeted nutrition to bypass the mutation and get the door working again. This allows the natural exit (which is much more efficient) to be used again. (Yasko 2008)

Dr. Amy Yasko will test about 30 methylation SNPs (single nucleotide polymorphisms). You may need a doctor's prescription. It is considered to be a highly accurate test and gives you information about what foods and supplements are best for your genetics.

A cheaper test can be found at www.23andme.com. It is less expensive than Amy Yasko's test but not as comprehensive. You will need to Google their genetic genie to upload the raw data you receive in order to make sense of the information.

I used genetic testing by FitGenes, which tests a whole panel of genetics and also includes the MTHFR panel.

I've also heard that smartDNA (smartdna.com.au) is a good company.

Treating MTHFR Defects

The goal would never to be to change a defective gene (well it's not possible yet anyway), but you can help it do its job better to optimise your health. *I have MTHFR mutations, so I know more than the average person and have done my research. Changing to activated B vitamins and folate has changed my life! B vitamin supplements always made me feel so sick! Then when I learned about MTHFR and started taking activated B supplements, I finally understood why!*

The MTHFR gene assists the conversion of folate and B12 to a more useable form, so if you have MTHFR mutations, you may have high folate and B12 on blood-testing panels because your body is not fully converting them or absorbing them. If this is the case, it is recommended that you avoid any fortified or processed foods with folic acid and limit whole foods that contain natural folic acid. Also steer clear of any supplements that have folic acid or B12 (cyanocobalamin) and instead opt for activated forms of folate (methylfolate) and B12 (methylcobalamin / methylB12). Start with low doses (especially methylcobalamin), because once your body has a usable form, it may cause a detox effect as it goes to work (you definitely don't need side effects, such as aching body and fatigue, especially if you are already unwell!).

Another good B vitamin is the methyl version of B6 called P-5-P.

Dr. Ben Lynch, an expert in MTHFR, has a great website www.mthfr. net. His advice is to repair the digestive system and optimise gut flora as the first steps in correcting methylation deficiencies. That especially includes treating Candida due to the toxins it releases that inhibit proper methylation. (B. Lynch n.d.)

I agree with experts to eat clean, such as organic and Paleo. Avoiding exposure to toxins is also important (see the Detoxification section in Chapter 7).

If taking methyl B vitamins causes you to over methylate, taking time-released Niacin 50 mg can slow it down. Symptoms of over methylation can include muscle pain or headaches, fatigue, insomnia, irritability or anxiety.

Minerals play a key role in several enzymatic functions. Vitamin C, E and bioflavinoids are antioxidants that can assist on a small scale to clear free radicals. Molybdenum 500 mcg helps break down excess sulfates and sulfites and is also recommended to assist the detox pathway of endotoxins to prevent Herxing.

Treating Histadelia (Under-methylation)

Histadelia is characterised by high histamine levels due to "under" methylation. The treatment of histadelia requires great patience, because it takes time to get the combination of the supplement right and then, of course, for the body to uptake and use the appropriate nutrients to make internal healing changes. It usually takes 4–10 weeks to feel significant changes and another 6–12 months to complete the treatment. Some people will be able to ease off or decrease their supplementation as long as significant lifestyle changes have been made, and others will need to continue on some sort of ongoing treatment plan to maintain these changes. The prognosis is good if the histadelic patient cooperates with treatment and works to give up detrimental addictions and improve their overall lifestyle choices that impact their diet (healthy fats and oils, 50%+ diet of fresh vegetables, high quality proteins with each meal, mineral dense sea or Himalayan salt, minimal caffeine, minimal alcohol) and quality of sleep. They should also quit smoking and decrease toxins and stress. I recommend that you read *Mental Illness: The Nutrition Connection* by Carl Pfeiffer, a pioneer in orthomolecular psychiatry.

Biochemically, treatment revolves around calcium and methionine. Vitamin C in the form of ascorbic acid, activated B6 (P-5-P), TMG (tri-methyl-glycine), magnesium, manganese, zinc, B2 and SAM-e (as long as you don't have an MTHFR defect) are also helpful. Copper may be supplemented if low because copper is part of the enzyme histaminase that is involved in the metabolism of histamine (which in excess can cause things like hay fever, allergy-type reactions, vascular headaches and may be a component of mental disorders such as depression, obsessive compulsive tendencies and oppositional-defiant disorder).

METHIONINE – Methionine is mostly found in red meat. However, if the meat is cooked too much, then the amino acid is destroyed. Therefore, maximise your methionine naturally by eating rare or raw meat such as steak tartare (which is surprisingly tasty!). Some argue that animal pro-teins should not be consumed due to the high content of histidine that is then converted into histamine. This is judged on a case-by-case basis.

Methionine supplements are hard to find. A great product that contains methionine is P2 Detox. However, it is a practitioner-only brand, so you would need to have it dispensed from a health professional like a naturopath, nutritionist or even some chiropractors (we stock it at our Health Space Clinics). I believe that there is no substitute for good quality, grass-fed and finished (ideally organic) red meat, and you should be eating it at least once a week to aid methylation. If you have a red meat allergy, then it may be a sign that your body is not detoxing or methylating optimally, so it's even more important to address these issues immediately.

A good compounded supplement is usually the best to get the right balance and form of nutrients, so speak to your doctor about testing and treatment options. If you are also diagnosed as pyrrole, the Kingsway Compounding chemist does a great pyrrole mixture for under-methylators called Primer Pyrrole Undermethylating Capsules. I noticed a huge boost in energy after about four weeks of taking these capsules. You will need a script from your doctor. Working with your doctor or herbalist and good compounding chemist is essential.

Oil Pulling

<u>WHAT IS OIL PULLING AND WHERE DID IT START?</u>

Oil pulling (also known as oil swishing) is an ancient Ayurvedic remedy to improve oral health, detoxification and overall systemic healing. It is mentioned in old Ayurvedic texts and was used long before it was comprehensible to Western medicine. It claims with long term-use to cure about 30 systemic diseases and restore and maintain optimal health. It is a simple process where pure cold-pressed oil is swished in the mouth for 10–20 minutes. These pure oils act as natural agents to pull harmful bacteria, fungi and other organisms out of the teeth, mouth, gums and throat but without affecting the natural micro flora.

WHAT ARE SOME BENEFITS OF OIL PULLING FOR ORAL HEALTH?

❖ Strengthening of the teeth, gums and jaws

❖ Prevention of mouth ulcers

❖ Prevention of diseases of the gums and mouth, such as cavities and gingivitis

❖ Prevention for bad breath

❖ Remedy for bleeding gums

❖ Prevention of dryness of the lips, mouth and throat

❖ Treatment for TMJ and general soreness in the jaw area

HOW DOES OIL PULLING HELP SYSTEMIC HEALTH AND DETOXIFICATION?

The benefits of oil pulling are believed to extend from dental health to systemic health due to the elimination of the development of dental foci. Teeth and their roots extend into the jaw bone, and if there is poor dental hygiene, microbes that enter the mouth find cavities in the damp and poorly vascularised environment. Microbes wait until the immune system is compromised before releasing into the systemic blood stream to affect the organs (it is believed that each tooth is specifically assigned to an organ). Root canals are believed to enhance this toxic effect as harmful microbes are trapped in the space where the root has been removed, slowly drip feeding into the body. Regular oil pulling can eliminate toxicity, heal cells, tissues and organs, and restore natural balance to the body. When your immune system is strong, you might not notice any ill signs or symptoms, but when you are immunocompromised, it can be enough to tip you over the edge! Many people have experienced significant health improvements immediately after having their root canals removed. I am one of those people. The minute my root canal tooth was out of my gum, I literally felt some of my brain fog lift and my energy increase about 20–30% immediately!

WHAT ARE THE SYSTEMIC BENEFITS OF OIL PULLING?

Research shows that oil pulling helps the lymphatic system by decreasing its load. As harmful microbes are removed, beneficial microfloras have a healthier environment in which to naturally flourish. Symptoms and diseases that may be decreased, eliminated and even prevented include:

❖ *Headaches and migraines*

❖ *Bronchitis*

❖ *Tooth pain*

❖ *Thrombosis*

❖ *Eczema and allergies*

❖ *Ulcers*

❖ *Asthma*

❖ *Nerves, paralysis and encephalitis*

❖ *Growth of malignant tumours*

❖ *Hormone imbalances*

❖ *Inflammation of arthritis*

❖ *Gastroenteritis*

❖ *Kidney function*

❖ *Sinus congestion*

❖ *Vision*

❖ *Insomnia*

❖ *Hangovers*

❖ *Pain*

❖ *Heavy metal toxicity*

HOW DO I PERFORM OIL PULLING?

❖ The best time to do oil pulling is in the morning on an empty stomach.

❖ Put 1 tsp of cold-pressed, extra virgin sesame oil (or coconut, sunflower or olive oil) in your mouth and swish it around for 10–20 minutes (this is ideal, but even 5 minutes is helpful!)

❖ This process mixes the saliva with the oil causing it to get thinner and whiter, enzymes are activated, and this along with the lipids draws out toxins and absorbs them into the oil.

❖ You ideally keep swishing it around until the oil reaches a thick, viscous white consistency, which indicates that the toxins have been maximally absorbed. Then, spit it out. DO NOT SWALLOW or you will reabsorb all the toxins you just released.

❖ Thoroughly rinse out your mouth to ensure no toxins are left to reabsorb.

❖ Be sure to clean your sink properly to remove any toxins.

❖ This process can be repeated 3x a day if necessary, but always before a meal on an empty stomach.

❖ If you are time poor, then even five minutes can be helpful, so give it a go!

IS THERE RESEARCH THAT SUPPORTS OIL PULLING?

According to an Indian research study in 2008, oil pulling significantly reduced counts of the Streptococcus mutans' bacteria in the oral cavity. (Asokan, Rathan, et al. 2008)

Another Indian study in 2009 showed that oil pulling significantly reduced plaque and improved gum health in a group of adolescent boys. (Asokan, Emmadi and Chamundeswari 2009)

2011 research supports oil pulling as a natural and effective substitute to mouthwash, as it improves halitosis (bad breath) by decreasing the microbes that may potentially contribute to it. (Asokan, Kumar, et al. 2011)

The benefits of oil pulling include a mechanical cleaning action in the mouth. (Kumar, Emmadi and Raghuraman 2011)

DETOXING AND DECREASING THE TOXIC LOAD

When people hear the word detox, they often think of those 1 day to 3 month programs that people do every now and again when they want to have a *"clean out"* or start a health kick. The problem with detox programs is that there is very little scientific evidence for their efficacy, and to be honest, many of them are downright dangerous. If you are not addressing all three phases of detoxification, you run the risk of just moving toxins around and making yourself quite sick! What you should be aiming for with detoxification is to create lifestyle changes to support and enhance detoxification for life. I'm a big believer in the 80/20 rule—80% healthy and 20% indulgence, but this rule changes when you have an unhealthy body. The sicker you are, the closer to 100% you will need to be with your detoxification in order to swing the scales back towards optimal health. It's all about being smart and choosing lifestyle and nutritional choices that you enjoy first and foremost, and working out what you will and won't give up. As you feel better, you will naturally make and implement healthier choices without the fuss and stress. For example, when using organic or chemical-free body products, I rarely can tell the difference, but it does mean a less toxic load, so I can enjoy an organic glass of red wine! See where I'm going with this! Let's breakdown detoxing into categories and give you some hints for some easy changes you can implement!

Detoxing Your Body from the Inside

Know the contents / toxins / reactants in foods and beverages *and try to avoid the nasties!*

❖ Basic contents – protein, carbohydrate, lectins, food pollen homology

❖ Natural processes – ageing, insects, worms, fungi, fermentation

❖ Protectant pesticides – pesticides, fungicides, antibiotics, etc.

❖ Spoilage – bacterial, fungal (mould), toxins, histamine, pathogens, heavy metals, etc.

❖ Genetic engineering – soy, coffee, squash, tomato, corn, beetroot, salmon, etc.

❖ Treatments – canning, freezing, heating, salting, smoking, marinating, microwaving

❖ Additives – preservatives, antibiotics, hormones, enzymes, colourings, flavourings

General Detoxification Tips and Tricks

❖ *Eat organic fruit and vegetables as much as possible (limiting fruit and root vegetables that are higher in starch to 1–2 pieces a day maximum).*

❖ *Eat free-range poultry and grass-fed and finished meats (ideally organic).*

❖ *Eat fish with the lowest mercury contamination and locally caught seafood.*

❖ *Eat healthy fats – e.g., nuts, seeds, avocado, good quality meats, oils, fish, flax, coconut, macadamia.*

❖ *Drink your minimum water intake daily (43ml per kg per day). Ideally, it should be filtered to remove toxins like fluoride, heavy metals and bacteria.*

❖ *Keep your body alkalised.*

❖ *Lemon in warm water every morning is alkalising, is a natural detoxifier and also stimulates healthy digestion.*

❖ *Avoid alcohol (this is usually pretty easy considering you feel hungover most of the time anyway when you are sick).*

❖ *Avoid all processed foods, especially ones with GMO, colours, flavours and preservatives.*

❖ *Avoid all food toxins including processed foods, vegetables oils, processed sugar and unprepared grains.*

❖ *Make sure you are moving your bowels daily (ideally three times a day).*

❖ *Infrared sauna (ideally daily)*

❖ *Exercise daily for at least 20 minutes (doesn't need to be strenuous).*

❖ *Epsom salt baths or float tanks*

❖ *Eat fermented foods / probiotics to balance gut flora and improve immune system function.*

❖ *Brush your skin daily to assist the lymphatic system and detoxification process.*

❖ *Don't overheat empty, non-stick pans (even better, don't use non stick or tephlon pans). Ideally use cast iron pans.*

❖ *Store all your food in glass containers.*

❖ *Transfer any food bought in plastic packages to glass as soon as possible (including meat on plastic trays).*

Foods that promote detoxification are: broccoli, artichokes, coriander, flaxseeds, garlic, apples, turmeric, beetroot, spinach, cabbage and asparagus.

Blood Purification Herbs

For centuries, traditional Chinese medicine practitioners have advocated the use of blood-purifying herbs to improve the detoxification of toxins from the spleen, kidneys, liver and bowels in order to improve health! Blood-purifying herbs include: barberry, cayenne, chaparral, chickweed, cleavers, dandelion, echinacea sassafras, garlic (kyolic), ginseng, goldenseal, gotu kola, liquorice root, poke root, prickly ash, red clover tops and yellow dock.

Supporting the Liver, Gallbladder and the Kidneys

The liver and kidneys are the body's natural detox system. Optimal liver function is important for everyone, but especially if you are sick. The liver, when working optimally, is designed to prevent pathogens from passing into the bloodstream and break down toxic chemicals from our lifestyle and environment. The kidneys are important for filtering waste from the blood and removing extra water waste via urine. There is plenty of information throughout this book about supporting them, but general rules of thumb are:

LIVER: Avoid omega-6 polyunsaturated oils, limit polyunsaturated and trans fats, eat fats from fish, eggs, animals and nuts, avoid refined sugar and minimise alcohol intake (or even worse, eating saturated fat with alcohol). Unfortunately, what we don't do these days is eat good quality, grass-fed liver! Liver contains all the nutrients we need for a healthy functioning liver. Alternatively, you could purchase freeze-dried capsules (I recommend Dr. Ron's Ultra-Pure™ brand, as you probably know by now!). Beetroots, carrots and cucumbers support liver function. Most Lymies or anyone with liver pathology from confirmed blood tests will need a liver support formula.

GALLBLADDER: Often people forget about the gallbladder. If the gallbladder is burdened, then so is your liver (it's even worse if you have had your gallbladder removed!). There is a great TBM kinesiology protocol you can do to dump gallstones from your gallbladder (and, essentially, your liver), but I recommend using this protocol under the supervision of your TBM health care practitioner (they will muscle test to see if this process is appropriate for you).

Gallbladder Dump – for Excreting Gallstones

TO SOFTEN:

Drink 235ml of apple juice night and morning for 7–9 days only. The malic acid clears the Kupffer cells of the liver and tends to reduce and soften gallstones.

TO DUMP:

Before Bed: Mix 150ml of classic regular canned Coke with 175ml of virgin olive oil and 15ml of lemon juice. Drink quickly at bedtime (much easier to drink if it's cold).

Next Morning: As soon as you wake up, drink a full 295ml bottle of Kruises Fluid Magnesia (buy online or at Chemist Warehouse)

This protocol should be done on a day when you can stay home and close to the bathroom. The more you rest, the better you will feel the next day! For maximum benefit, remove fried and junk foods from the diet at least a week before doing this protocol (although I hope that those foods were removed from your diet long ago!). This protocol is repeated every 3–7 days until no more gallstones come out.

Be warned: Green balls that float in the toilet bowl will come out! People won't believe you, and as gross as it is, you will want to show someone! Many of my clients have brought pictures to me!!! It's gross, but the process is VERY effective! For me, it took five rounds to dump my gallstones. The first time nothing happened, and then four more attempts until I could see nothing more in my stool. The drink is disgusting and I gagged trying to swallow it. It is not an easy protocol, but it is worth it.

KIDNEYS: First and foremost, drink your minimum water requirement, avoid fructose, and once again, eat organ meat (kidneys). Natural herbs and foods that support kidney detoxification are pineapple, parsley, celery, marshmallow root and burbur. Teas that support kidney function are celery seed, corn silk and watermelon teas.

Binding Agents in Detoxification

Binding agents can also be used to speed up the elimination part of the detoxification process. Binding agents generally pass through the gut and intestinal tract without being absorbed, so they can bind to toxins and assist their efficient removal before they end up being reabsorbed (bile excretes the toxins to the gut to be eliminated, but if the bowels are sluggish, then the bile can be reabsorbed again before the toxins have been dumped) or clogging up the system. Binding agents include activated charcoal, chlorella, cilantro and chlorophyl. I don't advise self-administering these binders. Instead, work with your primary health care practitioner to implement the right binder and dose for you. Binders are not appropriate for all people or during certain times in your treatment, and there is still some controversy as to whether they are effective or even safe at all.

Chelation and Metal Detoxification

Metal detoxification is not something to be taken lightly. You need to work with a practitioner who has experience and knowledge in chelation protocols. Once you know what metals are affecting you, a chelation protocol specific for the metals in your body is utilised. Chelators work to immobilise and make metals more water-soluble in order to bond to the metal for safe excretion. Chelating agents include DMSA, DMPS, EDTA and cilantro. Binders, which will bind and mop up anything in the bloodstream, include activated charcoal, chlorella, ground flax seeds, psyllium husks and apple pectin. Other natural agents used to support metal detoxification are glutathione, high dose vitamin C, NAC and ALA. The two products that I found most helpful were: BioRay's NDF Plus® (a blend of cilantro and chlorella with Polyflor™ cell wall lysates, blazei mushroom, reishi mushroom, cordyceps mushroom, horsetail and milk thistle seeds) and Zeolite HP from NutraMedix® (a compound formed naturally from volcanic rock and made up primarily of hydrated aluminium and silicon compounds). Not only were these supplements helpful with metal detoxification, but also with supporting and improving bowel motility. As the excretion of metals occur, don't be surprised if you feel worse before you feel better or have exacerbated detox symptoms including skin rashes.

There is also a theory that microbes die-off using this process, hence, the importance of targeting metals in Lyme disease patients. A well-functioning methylation cycle is also important for safe and efficient excretion of metals. I haven't added too much specific information here, as I don't believe you should be dealing with this on your own, but the following table provides an overview of chelating agents and their side effects.

PHARMACEUTICAL CHELATION OVERVIEW

Drug	Role	Side Effects
CaNa2EDTA	Detoxes bones Primarily chelates lead as well as radioactive elements (plutonium, thorium, uranium, strontium) Decreases high levels of Ca Removes copper in Wilson's disease Give as IV – continuous infusion recommended	Nephrotoxic Anorexia, nausea/vomiting, fatigue, zinc depletion, bone marrow suppression, anaemia Thrombophlebitis, hypocalcaemia, congestive heart failure
DMSA	Binds tightly to mercury, arsenic, lead, cadmium Low molecular weight so easily filtered via the kidneys into urine	Chelates copper, chromium, zinc Skin reactions, neutropenia, GIT upset
DMPS	Binds tightly to inorganic mercury, arsenic, lead, cadmium Low molecular weight so easily filtered via kidneys into urine	Chelates copper, chromium, zinc Allergic reactions such as itching, nausea, dizziness, fever, weakness, rash, fever
Dimercaprol	Used for arsenic, mercury, gold, lead, antimony and other toxic metal poisoning Chelates intra and extracellular lead that is excreted in bile and urine	Administered via deep painful IM injections Fever, nausea/vomiting, headaches, a tight sensation in the trunk and limbs, tachycardia, hypertension, nephrotoxicity
Penicillamine	Used for arsenic poisoning Forms a soluble complex with metals that is then excreted in urine	May worsen neurological symptoms Diarrhoea, taste alteration, proteinuria, thrombocytopenia, leucopenia

Commercial Detoxes and Cleanses

As I have already mentioned, most commercial detoxes tend to be fads that are marketed well in order to sell products to the willing consumer in order to make a buck. I'm not against them all, but it's important to work with a primary health care practitioner to ensure all parts of the detoxification process are addressed. To be honest, the best way to keep the body healthy is to avoid *toxifying* it in the first place as well as ensuring that the natural detoxification organs and pathways are supported for the toxins that do make their way in. Cleaning your body is like cleaning your house. You can do a massive spring clean, but if you don't keep it up, the house gets messy again pretty quickly!

The best detox support supplements I have come across are Paleologix, designed by Robb Wolf (who has a background in microbiology) and Chris Kresser. (Kresser 2015) If you want more information, go to http://paleologix.com. Metagenics also trains coaches, naturopaths and other health professionals on the safe implementation of their well-researched detox program. They also have great support on their website with recipes and research www.metagenics.com.au.

Identifying Toxins and Detoxing Your Body from the Outside

Environmental Toxins

Environmental toxins are found everywhere, in every person and on every planet. They can be found in soil, food, water, building materials and our bodies (in blood, fluids, tissues and breast milk). These toxins and chronic disease go hand-in-hand, and there is a lot of research to support that. In the most recent WHO World Cancer Report that was released in Feb 2014, air pollution and radiation (both environmental toxins) were listed as major sources of *preventable* toxins that cause cancer. Knowing the types and sources of environmental toxins is the first step in minimising or eliminating them. Types of environmental toxins include:

POPs (PERSISTENT ORGANIC POLLUTANTS): DDT, PFCs, PCB, Dioxin, PBDE, PBB, HCB

POPs have the ability to affect gene expression, disrupt endocrine function, increase insulin resistance, drive fatty liver and VAT (visceral adipose tissue), and are directly linked to obesity. These are all directly or indirectly linked to impaired detoxification!

ENDOCRINE DISRUPTORS: phthalates, BPA, PFOA and PBDE can interfere with the production, release, metabolism and elimination of hormones, or mimic the occurrence of natural hormones.

NUCLEAR RADIATION: from mining, transport, weapons, waste, power

HEAVY METALS: mercury, arsenic, aluminium, copper, Pb, antimony, etc.

EMF: power lines, cordless appliances, mobile phones, lights, WiFi

Other toxins include drugs, medication, alcohol and tobacco.

Common Sources of Endocrine Disruptors

HOUSEHOLD PRODUCT INGREDIENTS: chemicals found in appliances, vehicles, building materials, electronics, crafts, textiles, furniture and household cleaning products

PERSONAL CARE PRODUCTS / COSMETIC INGREDIENTS: chemicals found in products such as cosmetics, hair care products, lotions, soaps, deodorants, fragrances and shaving products

FOOD ADDITIVES: antioxidants, dyes and compounds used in food processing and packaging (e.g., colours, flavours, preservatives)

FLAME RETARDANTS: chemicals used to prevent fires (e.g., fire extinguishers)

PLASTICS AND RUBBERS: components, reactants or additives in the manufacture of rubbers or plastics

PESTICIDE INGREDIENTS: insecticides / acarides (miticides), herbicides, fungicides, rodenticides and biocides

ANTIMICROBIALS: chemicals that prevent the growth of or destroy micro-organisms

Plastics with Known Endocrine-disrupting Activity vs. Plastics with No Known Health Effects

Number / Name	Plastics with Known Endocrine-Disrupting Activity	Number / Name	Plastics with No Known Health Effects
1 PET or PETE	Polyethylene terephthalate Water, drink and other bottles Polyester material Avoid heating	2 HDPE	High density polyethylene Milk, juice, water, ice cream containers, bins Outdoor furniture
3 V or PVC	Vinyl or polyvinyl chloride (PVC) Soft plastics – bottles, toys, wire insulation, shower curtains, food packaging, plumbing pipes, bags	4 LDPE	Low density polyethylene Bins, tubs, tubing, cling wrap
6 PS	Polystyrene or Styrofoam Disposable plates, cups, meat trays, egg cartons, produce boxes, packaging	5 PP	Polypropylene Microwave safe ovenware, food containers (such as tomato sauce bottles, margarine tubs and yoghurt containers), crates, plant pots, car parts

Number / Name	Plastics with Known Endocrine-Disrupting Activity	Number / Name	Plastics with No Known Health Effects
7 OTHER	Miscellaneous – including polycarbonate and sources of BPA, some baby bottles, eating utensils, plastic coating for metal cans		

Common Sources of Bisphenol A (BPA)

BPA is a carbon-based, synthetic organic compound used in the manufacture of epoxy resins and other polycarbonate plastics. The primary source of human exposure to BPA is through dietary and oral routes where the BPA leaches from the protective, internal epoxy resin coatings of items such as plastic containers and drink bottles, into the food or liquid. The degree to which the BPA leaches depends on factors such as the temperature of the plastic (or food / liquid inside the plastic) and the age of the container.

DIETARY / ORAL SOURCES: canned foods, baby bottles, water bottles, plastic food containers, plastic disposable take-away containers, plastic cling wrap, plastic food wrappers, drinking water, plastic cutlery and dishware, cigarette filters, dust and breast milk

DERMAL: bath water, thermal papers (e.g., receipts), eye glasses (lenses and frames), sports equipment, children's toys (children's toys can also be an oral source as kids often put toys in their mouth), household detergents, cosmetics, personal care products and paint (fumes can also be breathed in)

INHALATION: indoor and outdoor air, and dust

SUBCUTANEOUS: medical equipment and procedures (Vandenberg 2013)

Identifying Toxic Metal Exposure

Sources, Signs, Symptoms and Manifestations of Toxic Metal Exposure

Metal	Source	Clinical Signs, Symptoms & Manifestations
Lead	Exposure to lead smelters Drinking water through old plumbing Old paint Air/traffic pollution	Abdominal pain, headaches, seizures, irritability, anaemia, lethargy, joint pain, stained teeth, cognitive dysfunction (poor memory and concentration), autistic spectrum disorders (ASD)
Mercury	Amalgam fillings High seafood diet Pesticides, fungicides, insecticides Cosmetics	Tremors, anxiety, excitability, disturbed sleep, memory loss, ASD, hypothyroid, fatigue, depression
Aluminium	Aluminium cooking utensils Metal manufacturing plants Antiperspirants Antacids Canned foods Cosmetics	Memory loss, learning difficulty, loss of coordination, disorientation, mental confusion, headaches, reproductive dysfunction
Arsenic	Chemical processing plants Cigarette smoke Fungicides	Sore throat, abdominal pain, vomiting, diarrhoea, mucosal irritation, increased risk of skin cancer, arrhythmia and cardiac collapse, type 2 diabetes
Cadmium	Battery manufacturing plants Colour pigments in paints and plastics Cigarette smoke Air/traffic pollution	Nausea, vomiting, abdominal pain, chronic obstructive lung disease, renal disease, migraines, growth impairment, emphysema, loss of taste and smell, poor appetite, cardiovascular disease, cancer

Personal Care Products

I am lucky enough to have spent a lot of time with Therese Kerr (yes, the mother of the gorgeous Miranda Kerr—and yes, I have met her, too!). We've had some great chats, I've been to her seminars, and of course, I've kept up with the latest information and research via her wonderful website www.theresekerr.com. Did you know that your skin is your largest organ and has the capacity to absorb toxins up to 10 times faster than via ingestion? "The average woman puts over 200+ chemicals on her skin everyday," and 65–70% of those chemicals are being absorbed straight into the bloodstream through the skin! (Why Certified Organic n.d.)

TYPES OF PERSONAL CARE PRODUCTS

There are so many toxic products that we put on or in our body without even thinking about it including:

Skin and body care – sunscreen, moisturiser, lotion, oil, antibacterial hand wash / wipes / gel, shaving cream, after-shave, body scrub, tanning products, massage oil

Face care – cleanser, scrub, mask, toner, moisturiser, sunscreen, primer, eye cream, lip balm

Hair care – shampoo, conditioner, leave-in conditioner, serum, mousse, hairspray, wax, keratin hair straightening products

Nail care – nail polish, nail polish remover, glue for fake nails

Oral care – toothpaste, mouth wash, breath freshener

Baby care – nappy cream, nappy powder, wipes, antibacterial hand wash / wipes / gel

Cosmetics – foundation, bronzer, blush, lipstick, eye liner, eye shadow, mascara, lip liner, concealer, etc.

Bath and Shower – body wash, bubble bath, soap

Perfume

Deodorant

Did you know that the more personal care products you use on your skin, the higher your exposure and accumulation of toxins? A study done in 2011 showed that the levels of toxic phthalates in urine increased exponentially with every extra personal care product used! (Romero-Franco, et al. 2011) To determine this, they tested:

1. Shampoo only

2. Shampoo + one other product (e.g., perfume, anti-ageing cream, hair styling products, eye shadow)

3. Shampoo + two other products

4. Shampoo + three other products

DANGEROUS TOXINS FOUND IN OUR PERSONAL CARE PRODUCTS

You might assume that ingredients in personal care products are safe; if they weren't, we wouldn't be allowed to use them. However, the Environmental Working Group (EWG) states that the ingredients in cosmetics and personal care products are not regulated and that premarket safety testing is not necessarily carried out on those products. According to the FDAs website, "Cosmetic manufacturers may use any ingredient they choose, except for a few ingredients that are prohibited by regulation."([FDA] 2015)

However, you can check to see what chemicals the products you are using contain, (such as phthalates, parabens, and formaldehyde) by visiting the Environmental Working Group's Skin Deep® Cosmetic Safety Database. The online guide looks at the safety of more than 7,600 ingredients in nearly 62,000 products. You can use this database to narrow the cosmetics field and find potentially healthier products to use.

Some of the nasties that are used in personal care products include (Top tips for safer products n.d.):

❖ Phthalates – Fragrance almost always contains phthalates. Sometimes, ingredient names will have the suffix -phthalate, but you can't always rely on that. Acronyms of some phthalates used in cosmetics include DEP, DBP, and BzBP. Be wary of that phth because it shows up in the middle of words, too.

❖ Triclosan and Triclocarban – also labelled as Irgasan DP-300, Lexol 300, Ster-Zac, cloxifenolum.

❖ Nitro and polycyclic musks

❖ Parabens (specifically Propyl-, Isopropyl-, Butyl-, and Isobutyl-parabens)

❖ Fragrance – also labelled as parfum and aroma (sounds lovely, but it's not!)

❖ BHA

❖ Boric acid and sodium borate

❖ Coal tar ingredients (especially in hair dyes)

❖ Formaldehyde

❖ Formaldehyde releasers – Bronopol, DMDM hydantoin, Diazolidinyl urea, Imidazolidinyl, Quaternium-15

❖ Hydroquinone

❖ Lead

❖ Methylisothiazolinone, methylchloroisothiazolinone and benzisothi-azolinone

❖ Nanoparticles

❖ Oxybenzone

❖ PEGs / Ceteareth / Polyethylene compounds

❖ Petroleum distillates

❖ Resorcinol

❖ Toluene

❖ Vitamin A compounds (retinyl palmitate, retinyl acetate, retinol)

❖ Animal-based ingredients

❖ UV-filtering chemicals – May be labelled as any of the following: benzophenone, oxybenzone (benzophenone-3), octyl-methoxycin-namate, para-aminobenzoic acid (PABA), 3-benzylidene camphor (3-BC), 3-(4-methyl-benzylidene) camphor (4-MBC), 2-ethylhexyl 4-methoxy cinnamate (OMC), homosalate (HMS), 2-ethylhexyl 4-di-methylaminobenzoate (OD-PABA).

NATURAL PRODUCTS TO USE AS ALTERNATIVES ON YOUR BODY

❖ Almond oil – moisturiser

❖ Apricot kernel oil – moisturiser

❖ Cacao butter – moisturiser (also stabilises creams)

❖ Coconut oil – moisturiser, soap, antiseptic, put on infections (especial-ly fungal and bacterial), hair conditioner, massage oil

❖ Jojoba oil – moisturiser, antiseptic

❖ Walnut oil – moisturiser

❖ Rosehip oil – moisturiser (especially good for scars and wrinkles—or preventing them!)

So How Do I Know What Personal Care Products to Buy?

The truth is, you really don't know what is in the product unless the product you are buying is *certified organic* and contains the certified organic logo. As with food, a company can label or name their product *organic, pure, natural* or *safe*, but it may still contain thousands of harmful chemicals. Of the 10,500 main chemicals used in products, the EWG website says that only 13% to-date have actually been tested for safety! Not only that, but companies are only required to list some of the toxic ingredients because they can list the others as trade secrets!

Certified organic not only means that 95% or more of the ingredients are organic, but all processes from soil preparation, picking, packaging and dispatch are governed and require certification by an external body that has very strict regulations. There is an emphasis on environmental protection as well as consumer safety, and as consumers it is our responsibility to hold companies accountable if they are circumventing the law. The ACCC (Australian Competition and Consumer Commission) website states "consumers purchasing organic products should be able to feel confident that the ingredients are in fact organic. Misleading, false or deceptive organic claims are against the law."(Organic Claims n.d.) So make a difference and report companies and businesses that are not doing the right thing.

Where Can I Get Certified Organic Products?

Organic is not necessarily more expensive. Local farmers' markets cut out the middle man which can lower costs. In fact, I find that many of the personal care products and food I buy are a similar price, but organic products are much better quality and often last longer. The few products that are a bit more expensive are usually worth it. The more money you spend keeping your body healthy, the less you will have to spend fixing it. In my opinion, medications and operations are way more expensive in the scheme of things than buying organic! If you don't have the time or access to farmers' markets, online shops are another great resource. My personal favourite is The Organic Beauty Shop (http://theorganicbeautyshop.com.au). It's Australian, has a variety of brands and products, is well-priced and usually delivers within 24–48 hours! Other shops in Sydney include my very own Health Space Wholefoods, About Life, Egg of the Universe, Paleo Cafés, The Source Bulk Foods and local organic grocers.

SO WHY DOESN'T EVERYONE USE CERTIFIED ORGANIC PRODUCTS?

The world always works on supply and demand. If we continue to buy poor quality products, then this increases the demand for those products, and consequently, the supply is increased. To break this cycle, we need to increase the demand for certified organic products and force the bigger companies to comply or leave the market. This would bring the price down because companies would then be competing for a bigger share of the certified organic market. Every single person can make a difference by buying certified organic. It's better for you, your family and the environment.

10 Toxic Truths

I listened to Prof. Marc Cohen talk about the scientific basis of detoxification at the 2013 International Congress of Natural Medicine in Sydney. A big part of his talk focussed on the harm that environmental toxins are causing to our health. He talked about the 10 toxic truths, which really hit home and made sense to me. The take-away message was that each toxin or toxic exposure in isolation may seem insignificant, but the toxic soup combination has a major effect! Let me share the 10 toxic truths with you:

1. TOXINS ARE EVERYWHERE AND AFFECT EVERYONE: Toxins are often invisible and latent.

2. THE FULL EXTENT OF TOXINS IS UNKNOWN: Very few toxic chemicals are tested for toxicity.

3. TINY DOSES OF TOXINS CAN CAUSE BIG EFFECTS

4. CHEMICAL COCKTAILS ARE MUCH MORE DANGEROUS: "The dose, timing and mixture make the poison."

5. WINDOWS OF DEVELOPMENT ARE CRITICAL: Developing children, older people and people who are sick are more susceptible to toxins.

6. INDIVIDUAL RISK FACTORS AND GENETIC PREDISPOSITION MEAN CERTAIN PEOPLE ARE MORE AFFECTED OR AT RISK FROM CERTAIN TOXINS

7. THERE IS BIOMAGNIFICATION OF TOXINS OVER A LIFESPAN: Fat soluble toxins are usually not excreted and can accumulate over an individual's life span.

8. THERE IS BIOMAGNIFICATION OF TOXINS UP THE FOOD CHAINS: For example, some sea mammals are so toxic their carcasses have to be disposed of as toxic waste!

9. EFFECTS OF TOXINS ARE EPIGENETIC AND TRANSGENERATIONAL: Maternal exposure to toxins affects an unborn child, future grandchildren and great grandchildren.

10. INJUSTICE AND ACCIDENTS HAPPEN: Exposure to toxins varies with public policy, demographics, location, consumption and migration measures.

Lifestyle Measures to Decrease Environmental Toxins

❖ Take your shoes off inside.

❖ Eat fresh organic food. It decreases your chemical and pesticide load.

❖ Minimise food packaging (there are many toxins in these packages – glass is best!).

❖ Have indoor plants to absorb toxins and pollution in the air.

❖ Avoid plastic and BPA plastics (storage containers, take-away food containers, drink bottles, etc.) *and never re-use or heat them.*

❖ Avoid handling thermal receipts (did you know receipts from the cash register contain BPA?).

❖ The 10-second rule works for microbes but not for environmental toxins. Once your food contacts an environmental toxin, it will attach and you will consume it! Ideally, wash anything before you eat it (especially if it has been sitting in the fridge or a fruit basket, or been dropped on the ground!).

❖ Wash your hands with water not wipes – Studies show that people who use bacterial gels and wipes have a 3.3 times higher toxin load, as they tend to not wash their hands as much.

❖ Swim in the ocean rather than pools – There are many chemicals in pools.

❖ Monitor air quality (and, ideally, use a Hepa air filter).

❖ Use non-toxic building materials, paints, carpet and cleaning agents.

❖ Wash new clothing before wearing.

❖ Use natural cosmetics, body products and fragrances.

❖ Don't put anything on your skin that you wouldn't eat!

Detoxing your Home – Household Cleaning Products

Information and Statistics about Chemical Household Cleaning Products

Cleaning products are one of the biggest sources of toxins. These chemicals get on our skin and in our lungs, and afterwards, anyone who touches that area comes in contact with them. They might kill germs and make things look cleaner, but what else are they doing?

"Within 26 seconds after exposure to chemicals such as cleaning products, traces of these chemicals can be found in every organ in the body."

--CHEC's HealtheHouse

Many of the cleaners we use are labelled *do not swallow, if swallowed call the poison hotline immediately* or *do not allow contact with skin.* They smell awful, often give you breathing issues when you inhale them, are covered in poison labels and warnings, and need to be locked up and kept out of the reach of kids, yet we still continue to clean with them. I'm not sure about you, but this makes no sense to me! I feel the marketing industry has brainwashed us to think that we need all these fancy toxic cleaners so that our homes will be clean, but at what cost? Not only that, but many fancy cleaners are expensive!

"Of chemicals commonly found in homes, 150 have been linked to allergies, birth defects, cancer, and psychological disorders."

-- Consumer Protection Agency, United States

In my opinion, using these chemicals is way more harmful than a bit of dirt and a few germs! Not only that, but there are plenty of safer alternatives that do the job just as well, and they're a whole lot cheaper, safer and have much less of an impact on Earth's delicate ecosystem.

"Chemicals have replaced bacteria and viruses as the main threat to health. The diseases we are beginning to see as the major causes of death in the latter part of (the 1900's) and into the 21st century are diseases of chemical origin."

--Dr. Dick Irwin, Toxicologist, Texas A&M University

Now I, like many others, want my house to look clean, but there are alarming statistics when you read the research. For example, a kitchen sponge can harbour billions of species of bacteria at any one time. If ingested, our bodies are designed to deal with it. However, the sponge and the disinfectant used to clean the sink contain a harmful residue that your body can't break down. I think we need to reverse our thinking and look to strengthening the body so it can do its job of filtering out stray germs and creating antibodies to fight off these pathogenic microbes even quicker next time. It doesn't make sense to continue using all the chemicals that are not only harmful to us and the environment, but have now with their overuse created these superbugs that are actually becoming resistant to many of the chemicals we use anyway.

Unreliable Product Labeling for Household Cleaning Products

Just as we have learnt with food and body care products, labeling for household cleaners is also inconsistent and at times misleading, as their content lists may be incomplete or simply inaccurate. You need to learn to read labels and learn about ingredients, or even better, just make your own cleaning products!

Chemicals to Avoid in Household Cleaners (Rosa 2008)

❖ Alcohol

❖ Ammonia

❖ Bleach

- ❖ Butyl Cellosolve

- ❖ Cresol

- ❖ Dye

- ❖ Ethanol

- ❖ Formaldehyde

- ❖ Glycols

- ❖ Hydrochloric acid

- ❖ Hydrofluoric acid

- ❖ Lye

- ❖ Naphthalene

- ❖ Paradichlorobenzenes (PDCBs)

- ❖ Perchloroethylene

- ❖ Petroleum distillates

- ❖ Phenol

- ❖ Phosphoric acid

- ❖ Propellants

- ❖ Sulphuric acid

- ❖ Trichloroethylene (TCE)

If you want to know more about these toxins, read the book or e-book *The Awful Truth About Cleaning Products and Fertility Revealed* by the gorgeous Gabriela Rosa. With her permission, I have included information from her e-book and associated PDF (Rosa 2008) that outlines various chemicals, where they are found and their known health impacts.

Chemical Name	Health Impact	Commonly Contained In
2-Butoxyethanol	Liver and kidney damage Neurotoxin	All-purpose cleaners, window cleaners spray cleaners, scouring powders
Akanol amines	Carcinogen [precursors]	All-purpose cleaners
Alkyl phenoxy ethanols	Hormone disruptor	Laundry detergents, all-purpose cleaners
Amyl acetate	Neurotoxin	Furniture polishes
Cresol	Liver and kidney damage Neurotoxin	Disinfectants
Crystalline silica	Carcinogen	All-purpose cleaners, scouring powders
Dichloroisocyanurate	Reproductive and immune system development disruptor	Tub and tile cleaners, scouring powders, dishwasher powders
Diethanolamines	Carcinogenic [nitrosamines]	All-purpose cleaners, detergents, dishwashing liquids
Dioxane	Immunosuppressant Carcinogen	Window cleaners, laundry liquids, dishwashing liquids

Ethylene glycol	Neurotoxin	All-purpose cleaners
Formaldehyde	Carcinogen	Deodorisers, disinfectants, germicides

Tips for Switching to Natural Household Cleaning Methods and Products
(Rosa 2008)

❖ You can either replace your commercial cleaners with a homemade substitute as you run out of each one, or if you are like me and want those chemicals out of your house, you can get rid of them now. Make sure they are disposed of safely. Do NOT pour them down the sink or into the garden. Some of the products are considered hazardous, so it may not even be safe to dispose of in your council garbage bin. Contact your local waste management department for information and advice.

❖ Although non-toxic cleaning products do not pose the same health risks as traditional toxic cleaners, they can still be dangerous in high dosages, so don't be careless with them. Always keep your cleaners in a baby / childproofed area and store them in the area in which you use them (i.e., bathroom cleaners in the bathroom cabinet, kitchen cleaners in the kitchen, etc.)

❖ Store your cleaners in reusable airtight containers. Do not reuse bottles from commercial cleaners. Instead, purchase empty spray bottles or recycle milk jugs. Be sure to label each container with the ingredients, date made and purpose.

❖ Remember to replace your expensive scrubbers and cleaning tools with healthier homemade or recycled alternatives.

❖ Get an apron with lots of pockets to save you time when cleaning. Put all your homemade cleaning tools in the pockets for easy access.

❖ Try colour coding your cloths for different areas – e.g., bathroom, kitchen and toilet.

❖ Remember when cleaning that the actual chemicals are only one part of the danger, so be sure to wear protective clothing and a face mask when in areas of dust, mould, fumes, heavy metals, asbestos, etc.

Making / Recycling / Buying Your Own Cleaning Tools (Rosa 2008)

OLD SOCKS – great for cleaning textured areas like walls (little pieces break off the sponges when you try to scrub textured surfaces).

SCRUBBERS / SCOURERS – Cut up pieces of mesh potato bags and tie into a small ball.

SPONGES / CLOTHS – Throw your dirty sponges and cloths in the dishwasher or boil them with a bit of baking soda on the stove to make them look like new again. If you want to purchase a good cloth, the ENJO brand is the best and can be used over and over with great results! Any microfibre cloth is money well spent!

BROOM – Find a broom with bristles.

TOWELS – Cut up old towels instead of throwing them away and use them as rags and dish cloths.

TOOTHBRUSHES – An old toothbrush is very handy to scrub floors and tiles, stains on clothing, light switches and other nooks and crannies!

MOP – To make a new mop head, cut up strips of old towels, shirts or socks. Rubber band or tie the top ends of the strips together and then secure to the mop stick.

NEWSPAPER – works well to clean windows.

RAZOR BLADE – great for stubborn grime, soap scum or food blobs that can't be easily removed with a toothbrush.

PAINT SCRAPER / PUTTY KNIFE – also great for removing stubborn blobs if you don't have a razor blade.

DUSTER – Dusting moves dust from one place to another. Sometimes this is handy if you are trying to clean high and hard to reach areas that collect dust. Then you can vacuum or clean it up once it's moved to a lower place. It's best to buy a duster (ostrich feathers are supposed to be the best). I like the ENJO All purpose Flexi because it also has an extension handle. You can also try making a homemade one similar to the mop.

SPRAY CONTAINERS – Buy or save spray containers (not from those nasty chemical cleaners though) to use for your own homemade cleaners.

VACUUM CLEANER – A vacuum with a HEPA filter is the best.

Ingredients for Natural Cleaners (Rosa 2008)

BAKING SODA (AKA BICARBONATE SODA) – is a great all-purpose, non-toxic cleaner that cleans, deodorises, scours, polishes and removes stains (and has a very long shelf life).

BORAX – deodorises, removes stains, boosts the cleaning power of soap, prevents mould and odors and is a great alternative to bleach.

CORNSTARCH – cleans and deodorises carpets and rugs, and can be used in place of baby powder and under your arms to soak up sweat.

LEMON JUICE – is great for whitening items and removing grease and stains on aluminium and porcelain.

PURE SOAP – cleans almost anything and is mild.

SALT – Regular table salt makes an abrasive, but gentle, scouring powder.

SODIUM CARBONATE – cuts grease and disinfects.

WHITE VINEGAR – has a long shelf life and works by neutralising alkaline materials, so it's great for whitening, cleaning hard surfaces, windows and shiny metal surfaces, removing soap scum, alleviating odours and removing mildew, stains, grease and wax buildup (be sure not to use brown or apple cider vinegar as it may stain).

GRAPEFRUIT SEED EXTRACT – is a powerful antibacterial agent.

TEA TREE OIL – is a powerful antibacterial agent (smells nice, too!).

LIQUID CASTILE SOAP (VEGETABLE OR GLYCERINE-BASED) – is great for removing dirt.

COCONUT OIL – is great to use in soaps, as it lathers, stabilises mixtures, does not stain and is easy to wash off (great as a moisturiser for the skin, too).

LINSEED OIL – is great for polishing and finishing wood (be careful as it will harden when exposed to air).

Using Essential Oils in Household Cleaning

Essential oils are not just for aromatherapy massage, perfume and oil burners. They are fabulous for use as natural household cleaners, insect repellants and air fresheners. Quality is the key, so make sure you purchase 100% pure essential oils, or they won't work well or last as long as household cleaners. The other option is to make your own by purchasing a home distiller. Unless you have way too much time on your hands or an outlet to also sell them, I would personally stick to buying them! The following information is reprinted with permission from Gabriella Rosa's e-book. (Rosa 2008)

Essential Oil	Properties
Basil**	Antiseptic, antibacterial
Bay	Antibacterial
Bergamot*	Antibiotic
Camphor	Antibacterial
Cardamom	Antibacterial
Cedar wood**	Antiseptic, antifungal
Chamomile**	Antibiotic, antibacterial
Cinnamon	Antiviral
Citronella	Antibacterial
Clary sage**	Antiseptic, deodorant
Clove	Antibiotic, antiviral
Cypress	Antibacterial
Eucalyptus	Antibiotic, antifungal, antiviral, antibacterial
Frankincense	Antiseptic
Geranium**	Antiseptic, deodorant
Ginger	Antibacterial
Grapefruit*	Antiseptic, disinfectant
Hyssop	Antibiotic, antibacterial
Jasmine**	Antiseptic
Juniper**	Antifungal, antibacterial
Lavender	Antibiotic, antifungal, antiviral, antibacterial
Lemon*	Antibiotic, antifungal, antiviral, antibacterial
Lemongrass	Antibacterial
Lemon verbena	Antibacterial
Lime*	Antibiotic, antibacterial
Marjoram	Antibacterial

Myrtle	Antibiotic, antifungal
Neroli	Antiseptic, antibacterial, deodorant
Nutmeg	Antibiotic
Orange*	Antibacterial
Oregano	Antibiotic, antiviral
Palmarosa	Antiseptic, antiviral, antibacterial
Patchouli	Antibiotic, antifungal
Peppermint**	Antiseptic
Pine	Antibiotic, antibacterial
Rose**	Antiseptic
Rosemary**	Antibacterial
Rosewood	Antiseptic, antibacterial, deodorant
Sage**	Antifungal, antibacterial
Sandalwood	Antifungal, antiviral, antibacterial
Savory	Antifungal
Spearmint	Antibacterial
Tea-tree	Antibiotic, antifungal, antiviral, antibacterial
Thyme**	Antibacterial, antifungal, antiviral, antibacterial
Verbena (aka vervain)	Antibacterial
Wintergreen* **	Antibacterial
Ylang ylang	Antiseptic

*Exercise caution when handling these essential oils. Wearing protective gloves is recommended.

**Avoid using if you are pregnant.

Recipes for Homemade Household Cleaners

Michelle Shaeffer from Natural Frugal Cleaning has some great natural formulas and tips. I have summarised and converted them to metric. Check out her website for more details. (Shaeffer n.d.)

GENERAL AND MULTI-PURPOSE CLEANERS

❖ Mix 3 tbsp of baking soda with 4 cups of water and put in a spray bottle.

❖ Mix ¼ cup baking soda, 1 cup white vinegar and 3.7L warm water in a tightly sealed and labelled container for everyday use.

❖ Mix 3 parts water to 1 part white vinegar and use in a spray bottle.

❖ For stained areas, make a paste of baking soda and water and put it over the stain to soak in, and then scrub it off.

Glass and window cleaner

Mix 2 tbsp cornstarch, 1 cup white vinegar and 3.5L warm water in a bucket and use to scrub windows or glass. Using newspaper can help minimise streaking.

Add ½ cup white vinegar to 3.5L warm water. Just mix and scrub.

Use straight lemon juice and dry with a soft cloth.

Use plain club soda and scrub with old newspaper.

Tile and lino cleaner

Soak 5–7 green or black tea bags in a big bucket of scalding water overnight and use as a natural cleaner and sanitiser.

Laundry detergent

❖ First option – Use washing soda or soap in lieu of detergent.

❖ Second option – Mix equal quantities of detergent and baking soda (in this way, you'll only use half the amount of detergent that you usually do). Ideally, choose eco-friendly or decreased chemical versions of detergent to start with.

❖ Third option – If you don't have access to washing soda, then make your own: Preheat your oven to 200° C. Sprinkle some baking soda onto a shallow baking tray and put into the oven for about an hour or until the powder changes composition. Look for the baking soda which is powdery, crystalised like salt and clumped together to change its composition to a grainy, dull, opaque substance with separate grains. It will get easier to see the changes once you've done it a few times. (Sarah 2012)

Homemade powdered detergent – You can also make your own pow-dered detergent using a basic recipe of 5 cups of soap flakes and 7 cups of borax. Use ½ cup for each wash. If you have hard water, you can add 3.5 cups of washing soda to the recipe.

Homemade liquid detergent – For liquid detergent, shave a bar of vegetable gylcerin soap into a saucepan of boiling water (3–4 cups of water). Once it's dissolved, pour the liquid into a 3.5L bucket of pure water and add a cup of washing soda (you can also add ½ cup of borax if you want an added kick!)

Homemade stain remover

For stains or heavily soiled clothing, make a paste of washing soda and water and apply to the stains a few hours before washing with any of the three laundry detergent options previously mentioned.

Carpet Cleaners

For deodorising

❖ Sprinkle baking soda or cornstarch on carpet, using about 1 cup per medium-sized room. Leave for 30 minutes then vacuum.

❖ Mix 2 parts cornmeal with 1 part borax. Sprinkle liberally on carpet, leave for one hour and then vacuum.

To soak up big spills – Pour cornmeal on the spill and leave for 5–15 minutes before sweeping into a dustpan and then vacuuming.

For spills or stains – Put ¼ cup liquid soap or detergent in the blender with ¼ cup water and blend until foamy. Apply to spots on the carpet and then rinse with vinegar.

For general cleaning – Once every two months, steam your carpets. Hire a steamer and add a cup of white vinegar instead of the store's chemical concoction.

Spot or stain remover

Remove spots as soon as possible for best results.

Blood stain – Repeatedly gently sponge with cold water and pat dry with a towel until the stain is gone.

Red wine – Immediately dab moisture with an absorbent cloth and then cover the stain with salt. Let the salt sit for several hours and vacuum when dry.

Ink stains – Wet fabric with cold water and apply a paste of cream of tartar and lemon juice. Let it sit for 1 hour. Then soak in cold water and wash as usual.

Perspiration stains– Sponge stain with a weak solution of white vinegar and water, or lemon juice and water.

Grease stains– Squeeze some real orange, lemon or lime juice on the grease. You might have to let it soak a bit in some sudsy water, but the acid in citrus can degrease like you wouldn't believe. This is great for surfaces, plastic furniture and toys, dishes and the stovetop (Note: lemons work best for surfaces; oranges are great for dishes; and don't use citrus on anything that can be stained, like wood or fabric).

Upholstery and rug cleaner

Clean stains immediately with soda water.

Sink cleaner .

Combine baking soda and salt to scrub stainless steel.

Wall cleaner

Dissolve 3½ tbsp borax in 2L of water (Scrub a really dirty wall from the bottom up. If you scrub from the top down, the dirty water will run down over the dry, soiled wall leaving hard-to-remove streaks.).

Wood floor wax / cleaner

❖ Mix equal portions of oil and vinegar and apply a thin coat, making sure to rub it in well.

❖ Add ¼ cup of olive oil, which contains antimicrobial properties, to warm water.

❖ Wash painted wooden floors with 1 tsp of washing soda per 3.8L of hot water and rinse with plain water.

- ❖ To eliminate creaks, sprinkle a bit of baking powder in the cracks and wipe up with a damp towel.

Oven cleaner

- ❖ Sprinkle salt on spills when they are warm and scrub off.

- ❖ Mix 3 tbsp of washing soda with 1L of warm water.

- ❖ Use oven liners (trays) to catch spills and prevent a mess in the first place.

- ❖ Gently using steel wool for stubborn and burnt on spills can be useful.

Porcelain cleaner (sinks, tubs and toilets)

Mix borax and baking soda together in equal quantities and scrub away!

Coffee maker cleaner

Run a pot of half vinegar, half water through the machine followed by two consecutive pots of pure water (otherwise you're in for some terrible coffee).

Disinfectant

Mix 2 cups water, 3 tbsp liquid soap, 20-30 drops tea tree oil. This is best dispensed in a spray bottle. Spray on anything from benches to chopping boards to your baby's bottom!

Drain opener

Pour ½ cup washing soda into the drain followed immediately by 2 cups of boiling water.

For prevention, flush the drain weekly with boiling water.

Furniture Polish

❖ Mix 3 parts olive oil with 1 part vinegar. Use a soft cloth to apply.

❖ Mix 2 parts olive oil to 1 part lemon juice. Use a soft cloth to apply.

Metal cleaner or polish (brass, bronze, copper and pewter ONLY)

Mix 1 tbsp flour, 1 tbsp salt and 1 tbsp white vinegar.

Combine 1 tbsp of flour and 1 tbsp of salt in a small bowl and stir until blended. Add 1 tbsp of white vinegar and mix into a paste. Using a damp cloth or sponge, smear the paste onto the metal and rub gently. Let the polish dry for about an hour before rinsing well with warm water and buffing dry with a soft cloth.

For copper, you can also pour a mixture of vinegar and salt on it and rub.

Silver cleaner or polish

Place aluminium foil in the bottom of a clean sink with the plug inserted. Mix baking soda and salt in equal parts and then pour boiling water into the sink. Put tarnished silver or silver plated items into the sink and let them sit for 5-15 minutes. The tarnish will disappear from the silver and reappear on the foil. Alternatively, you could use the same method in a jar or container lined with aluminium foil. Buff with a sock or soft cloth.

Rub the silver item with toothpaste and a soft cloth. Rinse with warm water then dry.

Shoe polish

Polish leather with the inside of a banana peel. Then buff with a cloth.

Air freshener

❖ Leave an opened box of baking soda in the room.

❖ Add cloves and cinnamon to boiling water and let simmer.

❖ Use fresh flowers, essential oils and herbs in the room.

Insect repellant

Burn citronella in candles or an oil burner.

Plant sweet basil around the patio and house to repel insects, especially mosquitoes.

Smelly garbage disposal

Drop in a leftover lemon rind or two and grind away.

Detoxing Your Environment

Most environmental slogans include the words *reduce - reuse - recycle*, and I would like to add compost. First and foremost, we need to reduce the production of toxic waste, both in the form of manufacturing it in the first place and then having to dispose of it later. You might think that the job is too big for you, but waste and the toxic chemicals produced from its manufacture and disposal affects you directly. Waste we produce has to end up somewhere, and these chemicals, one way or another, end up in our environment and often make their way back into our bodies via recycled water or pollution. Waste that affects your health right now includes toxic chemicals from:

❖ Consumer products - e.g., cleaning products, garden chemicals, beauty products, plastics, toys

❖ Crops that have been sprayed with chemicals that can runoff into waterways and leach into the soil

❖ Industrial plants that are actually making toxic products and creating waste at the same time

❖ Incinerators and landfills that get burned into the air or leach into the soil

❖ E-waste (electronic waste) from companies who have no plan on how to safely dispose of it once it's broken or the consumer wants to upgrade

❖ Garbage dumped down drains

In the days of pre-industrial waste, most products were made from wood or metal and were often reused or recycled. People grew their own food and the food scraps and products that weren't used were either put into compost to put back into the soil, buried or burned (which was much safer due to the lack of chemicals contained in such products). During the Industrial Revolution, we transitioned to a disposable society that predominantly uses plastic and synthetic materials, which have caused a huge waste issue. Not only that, universities who teach chemistry do not teach toxicology, so students never learn what combinations of molecules make a molecule toxic, and the chemistry industry is completely unregulated (unlike the medical professions or engineers, for example), so they can essentially make whatever combination of toxic chemicals they like! If this sort of information interests you, read the book *Toxin Toxout* by Bruce Lourie and Rick Smith (who first wrote *Death by Rubber Duck*). Until then, here are some easy tips to get you started (Lourie and Smith 2013):

❖ Don't buy or use Teflon® or non stick pans.

❖ Use biodegradable cleaning products.

❖ Use cosmetics and body products that are, ideally, certified organic or at least chemical-free.

❖ Recycle at home and work.

❖ Dispose of e-waste in centres that dispose of it safely (safely as possible anyway).

❖ Compost your food scraps.

❖ Use glass instead of plastic.

❖ Avoid buying or using products that have a limited life span or will create waste once disposed of such as electronics, toys and plastic bags.

❖ When shopping, use reusable bags or boxes instead of the plastic bags provided.

❖ Have your own vegetable garden.

Detoxing Your Mind

Mind-made toxins include self-sabotaging thought patterns (such as guilt, fear, resentment, low self esteem), toxic relationships, toxic mindset, toxic attitude, toxic social influences and chronic negativity. Often we don't understand the importance of detoxing our mind, but our thoughts affect our chemistry and our ability to detoxify. I talk more about this in the Emotional and Spiritual Treatment section of this book!

"Everything is possible to the person who believes."

Jesus

CHAPTER 8 –
EMOTIONAL TREATMENT AND STRATEGIES

"It's not what happens to you, but how you react to it that matters."

Epictetus (Greek Philosopher)

FAMILY, FRIENDS AND PARTNERS

Telling Family and Friends

Everyone's health journey is different. If you have been really sick, then a diagnosis, even a serious one, may be a welcome relief. If you have had mild symptoms or only had symptoms off-and-on, then a serious diagnosis like Lyme disease may come as a surprise. If you are asymptomatic but were tested because a family member (partner or mother) may have passed it on, you could be in shock. Although it can be difficult for many reasons, you still need to let your family and friends know. I was lucky. Everyone in my life was very supportive, but I do know many people who have had family and friends literally turn their backs on them because they didn't believe Lyme disease was a real illness.

Your friends and family may ask a lot of questions, which you'll have to answer over and over, and it can be quite distressing. Although it is nice when people want to know because they really do care (and Lyme is such an interesting topic), I recommend that you write your story about how it happened so you don't have to tell it a million times.

The reactions of your friends and family can vary as well. Some people don't want to annoy you, so it may seem like they don't care. However, they may not know how to express their feelings at the time. Other people may smother you with attention and sympathy, which not everyone enjoys! I wrote this book to also help friends and family of someone diagnosed with Lyme or a chronic disease. It's hard for them, too.

Whether people care too much or not enough, it's still a challenge! As I became sicker, some of the people who I thought were my closest friends were nowhere to be seen. At first I was really upset. I told my husband that after all the years of helping people, I had no friends returning the favour. He wisely said to me that I didn't know what was going on in other peoples' lives. They may be busy, may find it hard to communicate or feel like they tried but received no response (because I was sick). He said that if I was upset about it, I should tell them or get over it. He was right. Only I have control over how I feel. I had a handful of amazing people doing amazing things for me, and so I started focussing what little energy I had on them. It's funny...when you are at the top of your game (like I was when I was the national champion and traveling the world), you have no shortage of people who want to be a part of that. But when you hit a bump in the road, it's your true friends who shine through, so see this as a positive thing. You can't be best friends with everyone (although if you are like me, you will give it a good dig!), but it's actually important to have a best friend and a group of close friends so you can share your time accordingly.

Challenging relationships also help us become better versions of ourselves because they force us to recognise our least desirable qualities and traits. I believe that the people in your life act as mirrors, reflecting back to you what you see or feel. If someone says something that hurts your feelings, then you also own that trait as you relate to it. So instead of being upset or hurt by what people say to you, look deep inside to see why it hurt you so much. Learn about yourself and how you can be a better person, and also let go of any emotions that you have no control over and clearly do not serve you. If you notice something positive about someone (like their generosity or their kind heart for example), then you, too, share this trait; otherwise, you would not be able to recognise it.

Besides my amazing husband and network of Health Space practitioners, I have had a few other people who were shining lights in my journey. Please read my dedication at the start if you haven't already, as these people are a very important part of my healing journey. They gave me inspiration when I felt alone.

"Just as rocks bumping into each other in a stream eventually polish each other smooth, life polishes us through the challenges of our relationships."

Miranda Kerr

How Family and Friends Can Help Someone Diagnosed with Lyme Disease

This section is especially for the family and friends of someone diagnosed with Lyme disease. As you can imagine, being diagnosed with any disease can be a stressful time, so please share this information with your loved ones so they can help you.

The Five Stages of Grief (and Healing)

The five stages of grief have evolved since their introduction, but they continue to be useful as a guide to deal with grief, even though everyone deals with it differently. Not everyone will go through every stage or in the exact order or even in the same amount of time. Some people might move through the process in a week, and some may never ever get through it. By being aware of the stages, you will be better equipped to deal with your grief or support a loved one through their grief process.

Although the stages of grief generally refer to the loss or pending loss of someone, the stages one experiences when they lose their health are quite similar. When I dealt with my illness, I went through all the stages of grief, and it was helpful to identify what I was feeling. Everyone at some time will experience grief, and awareness of these stages can really help one to cope, accept and move on with life after constructively dealing with the emotions associated with it.

Denial and Isolation – Your response to the loss is one of shock, and denial is the body's way of rationalising or blocking overwhelming emotions. Life no longer makes sense. You can't believe it has happened, and you try to go on as if nothing has. Denial helps you deal with grief as the world becomes overwhelming and at times meaningless. You might feel numb, which is nature's way of only letting in what you can handle at that time. This stage is characterised by "It'll be fine" or "I'm going to be okay" (re: health) or "The doctor must be wrong."

Anger – This is where reality and pain re-emerge, and the vulnerability is often expressed as anger, such as "Why me?" or "It's not fair." Anger has no limits and may be directed inward or at others. The more anger you feel, the more passionate or connected you are to the cause of the grief and the longer it may take to dissipate. Anger can also provide an anchor for you, giving you temporary support when you are feeling lost and vulnerable. Underneath anger, there is pain and other emotions, so the angrier you are, the more you can numb that pain and block yourself from feeling any other emotions. It's best to release your anger in constructive ways in order to move through the healing process.

Bargaining – When you experience a loss, even with your health or a possession, you will do anything to get it back. You want your life the way it used to be. During this stage, one believes that they can somehow change, postpone, extend or exchange the situation, and it usually starts with "If only I had..." or "I would do anything if I could..." You bargain—with God, the universe, yourself, etc., to negotiate your way out of your hurt. You will use phrases like "If only I had done / not done ..." "I will never do this again if..." "What if..." or "I will devote the rest of my life to helping others if..." and so on.

Depression – As you begin to acknowledge the reality of your loss, your attention will move into the present and grief will enter your life on a deeper level. The depression often feels unrelenting, as though it will last forever. Often you will withdraw, wondering if life is even worth living. Depression can be mild or severe and is often expressed as "Why bother?"

This type of depression is not a sign of mental illness but an appropriate response to the grief or loss you've experienced. Grief over the loss of something can be naturally depressing but is a necessary step in the healing process. It is both healthy and required, and should not be something you are told or feel you have to "snap out of." Mental illness may exacerbate the grief response, and in some cases, depression needs immediate help, so make sure you reach out for help if you need it (or provide help if you identify a friend / family member who is depressed).

Acceptance – Once the depressing feelings lift, you are able to come to peace with the grief. This can takes days, years or even forever depending on how you move through the stages. It does not necessarily mean that you understand it or are okay with what happened, but that you recognise there is a new reality. This stage is about accepting what you have lost and readjusting. At first, acceptance may just be having more good days than bad, and it is not until you have given grief its respect and time that you can begin to fully live again. It is characterised by the belief that "Everything is going to be okay."

As hard as it is to be the one going through it, it is equally hard but in a different way for close friends and family. Sometimes it's hard to know what to say or do, and every person will react differently and heal in different stages in their own time. I know that I personally tended to get sick of always talking about Lyme and how I was feeling, but I also felt disappointed when people who I thought were close friends weren't really there for me like I thought they would be. It's a hard balance! I think the key is to ask the person with the diagnosis what THEY want. Don't try and guess or treat them how you would want to be treated; that may not work for them. We all try to do our best and want to help our friends when they are in need, so ask them how you can help. For example, if someone asked me, "Can I do something to help you?" I would answer, "No thanks," because I wouldn't want to be a burden or put anyone out. So then that person feels like they can't help and might not ask again. A better question would be, "I would love to visit you. Is this something you would like?" Be specific with your questions and when possible, ask open-ended questions (i.e., questions they have to answer with more than just a yes or no). For example, "I am going to cook you some food on the weekend. What would you like me to cook for you, and is there anything you can't eat?"

Here are some other ways to help out your friend, especially if they are sick!

Visiting: Be flexible (we all have such busy schedules!). When your friend is sick, don't be offended if they cancel on you regularly or last minute; instead, tell them that you are glad they are putting themselves first. If they are not well, drop in for short visits, unless they ask otherwise. Sometimes when I was sick, I enjoyed having a friend over to watch movies with me. Other times, when I was really sick, I just needed to be alone. Once again, just ask them what they want, and you will be the best friend in the world. If they cancel on you or it takes awhile to organise a catch up, don't give up. It's not because they don't want to; it's just that when you are sick (especially if you have something like Lyme disease), you honestly don't know from hour to hour, let alone day to day, how you are going to feel!

Cooking: My beautiful friend, Kate Barbat, used to make me organic carrot soup. When I was sick and found it hard to eat, this was a lifesaver! Kate would also buy and deliver big fruit and veggie boxes so I could cook my own food (Well Nick would anyway!). The little things like this are huge when you are not feeling well! If you want to help, then cook and prepare meals, especially ones that can be frozen or eaten throughout the week. Soups, stews, casseroles and salads are excellent choices. However, when people are sick, they often need to be quite strict with their diet—or they just can't tolerate or digest certain foods—so make sure you check what they are allowed to eat (and can actually eat and tolerate) before you spend the time doing it!

Helping with Jobs: You can also help with basic chores like mowing the lawn, cleaning, washing, walking the dogs, etc. Even if they say that they are fine, be a good friend and do it anyway! If your friend is really sick, they won't be able to do these things for themselves, and if they have a partner or are living with their family, it can take some pressure off their immediate loved ones! If you are the immediate loved one, you will likely be doing this already!

Telling Them Your Stories—Good and Bad! When I was sick, I loved to hear about my friends' lives. My friend, Jen May, used to always talk about her son, what it was like going back to work, how she was feeling getting back into exercise after having her baby, etc. Don't be afraid to tell your amazing and happy stories; nothing makes people happier than being surrounded by positivity. However, you do need to be sensitive. For example, if your friend was sick and missed a holiday, then you might not want to go on and on about how amazing your holiday was (Personally, I would still want to hear about it.) On the other hand, a lot of my friends stopped confiding in me when they had problems. They thought I had enough problems of my own, and in the scheme of things, they also thought their issues were insignificant com-pared to mine. People with Lyme disease (or any illness or injury) are human, and believe it or not, it's nice to know that everyone has their problems. When you are sick, it's easy to get bogged down in your own issues, but when someone opens up to you about their problems, whether they're big or small, it makes you feel normal and it takes your mind off your own problems for awhile, which can be very heal-ing! So the bottom line is to continue to treat your friend as your friend. Share the good, the bad and the ugly, because at the end of the day, even when someone is sick, they still want to be a good friend and support you, too! Sometimes the role reversal from sick person to support person, if only for a minute, can be healing! Help them and help you! It's a win-win situation!

Appearance: Don't be fooled by their appearance. When people didn't see me very often, they would comment, "How can you be sick when you look so good?" or "You look normal." Unless you live with the person or see them every day, don't expect to see them when they are looking terrible! People tend to hide themselves away when they are sick. Often their weight will fluctuate and they tend to be very sensitive about how they look, especially when they feel so terrible on the inside! To be safe, it is best not to comment on their appearance unless you are very close to the person.

The Little Things Are the Big Things: If you don't have the time or energy to visit, cook or clean (or even if you do), there are little things you can do to show you care. Text or call. Text some positive quotes. Post them some photos. Send them flowers, or even better, pick some flowers from someone's garden and drop them by the house. Share a positive song with them. Text them a joke. Forward them something funny on Facebook. You don't have to spend much money or time to show you care. Just remember that if they don't always reply (especially to phone calls), it's because they probably looked at the message / call / joke and then forgot to reply. I know for me, Lyme disease severely affected my cognitive function, so my short-term memory as well as my concentration and eyesight were affected. If I didn't reply to something straight away, I would often forget until weeks later, but I appreciated EVERY single thing my friends did for me! My friend, Jen, bought me a little book of positivity with quotes about staying strong, and I was so touched by it. It probably seemed so small to her, but it was huge and meaningful to me! I still have it and read it often.

"Extend to each person, no matter how trivial the contact, all the care and kindness and understanding and love that you can muster, and do it with no thought of any reward. Your life will never be the same again."

Og Mandino

Tips for Partners and Family of People Diagnosed with Lyme Disease

Be prepared to be a punching bag. Everyone is affected by illness differently, but it is the people who live with the sick person who generally see the true suffering. *I know I would put on a brave face (as best I could) whenever I had to go out. I might have been a crying mess only hours before, but then I would put on a big smile and plough my way though a social event where no one was any wiser to the fact I was totally struggling. When I was really sick, I was an emotional wreck.* This is very hard for partners who love you and want to take your pain away. Symptoms of Lyme disease include emotional instability and anger outbursts. *I found it really hard when I would get frustrated or angry at the drop of a hat and then feel really guilty and emotional about it afterwards.* It's really hard for the partner, as they always have to be the bigger person and not react. It's hard not to get offended when your loved ones lash out (and they will), so you need to keep telling yourself "This isn't the real (their name) talking. This is the disease talking." The people closest to someone who is sick and who spend the most time with them are usually the ones who see this side the most. *I am usually a very positive person, but even I hit rock bottom and thought "Why me?" "Life isn't worth living." "No one cares about me." "You wouldn't understand."* If your sick partner gets to this point, you just have to show more love and less judgment, even though it's hard and you just want to say, "Everything will be ok." "It could be worse." "Things aren't that bad," etc.

My husband was amazing, and I really feel he was a huge part of why I recovered quicker than most people, as he didn't let me wallow or have too many pity parties, but he also didn't try and oppose what I said or pretend he knew what I was going through either. He would say things like, "I could never possibly understand what you are going through. All I do know is that I love you and I am here for you, so just tell me what I can do to make this easier for you" or "This is a really tough thing you have to go through, so let's think of some positive things you can get out of this experience" or "Today you need to rest. Don't worry about the party we are missing. There will be plenty more parties and fun times ahead because we are going to be together forever!" When we couldn't attend functions, he would always ask, "How are you feeling today? Would you like me to stay with you instead of going to the party?" It was so nice, as he never once made me feel like I was a burden to him or made me feel bad that he was putting his life on hold to help me. He asked me what I wanted. Sometimes I just wanted to sleep, so he would go out on his own. Sometimes I wanted company or was too sick for him to leave me alone, and he would stay. Once again, the key is to ask rather than assume what your partner wants.

Surprises are always nice to break the monotony of being sick! If your partner is having a "good" day, then have something fun up your sleeve every now and again. Plan a picnic or a candlelit dinner at home. Have a friend come over or take them to the movies. At the end of the day, the fact that you are there is the best thing ever, but remind your partner regularly how much you love them and how proud you are of them (if it's true of course!). Sometimes when people are sick, they don't like to be touched, so work out what your partner likes so you can still show signs of affection (I think love is the real healer of all disease and negativity). It might be a wink, using hand gestures to say I love you, blowing a kiss, a head pat, leaving something nice on their pillow, a foot or head massage or a simple cuddle. Once again, all the little things are big things when you are sick and sad!

> *"Love is the most powerful and still is the most unknown energy in the world."*
>
> *Pierre Teilhard de Chardin*

SUPPORT GROUPS

Support groups can be the best or the worst thing, so choose wisely. Many people go to online chat and support groups. These are great to get information, hear other people's stories and get insights into different treatment strategies for various symptoms that you may have. They can be a place of hope and help. They can also be a place of extreme negativity. I personally stayed away from online support groups, as people are often there to unload, blame and feel sorry for themselves, which I felt did not serve me on my healing journey. Unfortunately, some people may not have an amazing and supportive husband, family and friends like I do, so they need to unload somewhere, as this is important for healing. If you are one of those people, then please continue to offload and heal, but do so in a way that doesn't affect other people's healing. If you are lucky enough to have a supportive network, then surround yourself with as much positivity as you can! It's always great to have people who understand each other and can help each other in a loving and healing environment.

"Whether humanity will consciously follow the law of love, I do not know. But that need not disturb me. The law will work just as the law of gravitation works, whether we accept it or not."

Gandhi

SUPPORTIVE THERAPIES

Kinesiology

Please refer to the Kinesiology section in Chapter 6 for in-depth information on kinesiology. NET is a particularly powerful technique for emotional blockages, emotions affecting the physical body, phobias, addictions, breaking through barriers, and relieving stress and anxiety, just to name a few. A good example is when a person who had previously been in a car crash hears the screech of brakes, their neck spasms. Consciously, they know they are safe and they're not in the car this time; however, the screech of the brakes reactivates the emotional trauma and sets off their physical response (neck pain). NET gets to the cause of the emotional blockage and clears it so that the body is no longer physically affected by emotional experiences. Often recurrent pain / injury / emotions stem from a previous experience where your body, for whatever reason, did not integrate a stressful situation. Remember, as your physical body starts to heal and feel stronger after an illness, this is often the time for your stored emotions and trauma to release. This can be a very scary time, as you physically feel the best you have in a long time (possibly ever), yet you may have feelings of anxiety, fear, sadness or grief. You may even wake up feeling like something bad is going to happen, even though there is nothing physical you can put your finger on to explain your strong emotions. Remember, your body has not been able to integrate these emotions and trauma whilst you were sick, and although not pleasant, it is absolutely necessary for them to be released. NET and other techniques can really support and super charge this process of emotional clearance.

Emotional Freedom Technique (EFT)

EFT draws on information from acupuncture, NLP, energy medicine and thought field therapy and was designed to reduce therapy time with psychotherapists. EFT is based on the premise that imbalances in the body's energy system have profound effects on one's personal psychology. Dr. Mercola calls EFT *psychological acupressure*, and he believes that it doesn't matter how devoted you are to eating a proper diet and implementing healthy lifestyle options, if there are emotional barriers in your way, you will never be truly healthy. Correcting these imbalances is done by tapping on certain energy meridian points whilst voicing positive affirmations. This is believed to clear the short-circuit caused by the emotional block from your body's bio-energy system and restore mind-body balance, basically, the body's innate healing capacity. You can Google *EFT* to find a practitioner, go to a seminar and learn it for yourself, or even get the basics from the internet if you want to try it first. Dr. Mercola has a great resource at http://eft.mercola.com. (Basic Steps to Your Emotional Freedom n.d.)

Psychotherapy

Psychotherapy is a broad term and involves a person with an emotional and/or psychological disorder talking to someone in the mental health profession (such as a counsellor, psychiatrist, or psychologist). There are many different practitioners under various banners who can help you get on top of any mental or emotional issues. Psychotherapy can work really well for some people. The key is to ask around and get a good recommendation. There are professionals who specialise in helping people with certain health concerns, so I recommend starting there. They will have tools specific to helping you cope and gain control over your health, and subsequently your life!

Cognitive Behavioural Therapy (CBT)

CBT is a form of psychotherapy that combines cognitive therapy with behavioural therapy in the belief that healthy thoughts lead to healthy feelings and behaviours. Cognitive therapy aims to change the way the person thinks about the issue that's causing concern, whereas behavioural therapy teaches the person techniques and/or skills to change their behavioural response to that issue. CBT focuses on helping the person to change habits, feelings, patterns and behaviours that are not serving them and are affecting the quality of their health and life. It generally involves the use of self-help strategies to overcome automatic or learned beliefs, create positive beliefs and modify their behaviour in order to create more positive feelings, thoughts and behaviours.

> *"To love oneself is the beginning of a lifelong romance."*
>
> *Oscar Wilde*

DEALING WITH YOUR THOUGHTS AND EMOTIONS

Emotional Guidance Scale

All living things have a frequency, and when you are in optimal vibration, you feel happy, free, loving, powerful, positive and purposeful. Your emotions are indications of your well-being and your frequency. Think of your emotions as a scale like a fuel gauge, where the higher the reading on the gauge, the further you can go and the more energy you will have, and vice versa. The following emotional scale is an excerpt from the book *Ask and It Is Given: Learning to Manifest Your Desires* by Ester and Jerry Hicks. (Hicks and Hicks 2004)

- ❖ Joy / Knowledge / Empowerment / Freedom / Love / Appreciation

- ❖ Passion

- ❖ Enthusiasm / Eagerness / Happiness

- ❖ Positive Expectation / Belief

- ❖ Optimism

- ❖ Hopefulness

- ❖ Contentment

- ❖ Boredom

- ❖ Pessimism

- ❖ Frustration / Irritation / Impatience

- ❖ "Overwhelment"

- ❖ Disappointment

- ❖ Doubt

- ❖ Worry

- ❖ Blame

- ❖ Discouragement

- ❖   Anger

- ❖   Revenge

- ❖   Hatred / Rage

- ❖   Jealousy

- ❖   Insecurity / Guilt / Unworthiness

- ❖   Fear / Grief / Depression / Despair / Powerlessness

When the scale of emotions was explained to me, I found it helpful because I realised that sometimes when you have a negative emotion which changes into another negative emotion, you may see this as a snowballing of negativity, but in reality, you may have progressed UP the emotional scale and are actually healing.

For example, at one point I felt completely depressed about the state of my health and my life. I had doubts about myself and began to worry if I would ever be well. I started to get very frustrated because I could not seem to implement all the principles and advice I had given over the years to help my clients ease their pain and suffering in order to help myself. I felt I had all the tools to get well, but for some reason, I couldn't apply them to work for me. When I learnt about the emotional guidance scale, I felt hopeful, as I could see how I was actually moving up the scale—from depression to worry to doubt to frustration, and now to hope! I was actually moving forward!

Use this scale not only to give yourself encouragement that you are improving, but also to guide you in ways to help yourself get to the emotions you want to feel. *I started focusing on optimism, then positive expectation. Then I started to feel eager. My passion for life returned and I started to appreciate and feel appreciated, and love flowed back into my life. There were still times during that healing phase that I went up and down the scale, but I used it to ensure I was filling my tank up with as much positive and loving energy as I could, and it gave my mind a great focus.*

"Do not waste one moment in regret, for to think feelingly of the mistakes of the past is to re-infect yourself."

Neville Goddard

"Sometimes challenges and struggles are exactly what we need in our lives. May you welcome every effort, every struggle, and every challenge and appreciate all your blessings...May you open your wings and fly."

Miranda Kerr

Letting Emotions Out Constructively

Holding onto emotions is a deadly practice. The sicker or more toxic you are, the more damage it will cause. Have you ever thought to yourself, "I can't believe that person died of cancer? They were so kind and caring and patient. How does that happen?" Or, "How does such a positive and energetic person die of such a negative and degenerative disease?" I know I had thoughts like these many, many times when I was younger. The more I learnt about releasing emotions and how much damage they can cause when they remain bottled up inside you, the more I realised that these gorgeous, kind, patient and positive people clearly did not have an outlet for their negative emotions. Now I am not saying that it's okay to be rude and obnoxious by "telling it like it is," but you do need to find a healthy outlet for your emotions. You can see a therapist, meet with a friend to talk or have kinesiology like NET. You could also journal, cry, and scream into a pillow or even punch the pillow. This may sound crazy, but holding onto anger, negativity or hatred will eat away at you, and even worse, you could release it onto someone you love and who doesn't deserve it (Don't worry. We have all been there!).

"Hatred paralyses life; love releases it.

Hatred confuses life; love harmonises it.

Hatred darkens life; love illuminates it."

Martin Luther King, Jr.

Crying is an important way to release emotions, so if you don't cry (and many people have been taught that it is a sign of weakness), I urge you to open your mind to do this very cleansing act, or at least have another way of releasing your emotions. Next time you have any negative emotions, I challenge you to try something different: cry, yell your feelings out loud (into a pillow if you don't have the luxury of wide open spaces) or punch your mattress or pillow (if you have the energy, do a boxing class, and with each punch, release whatever you are feeling with that physical action). I bet you will feel so much better straight away, and long-term, your health will thank you for it!

"Holding onto anger is like grasping a hot coal with the intent of throwing it at someone else; you are the one getting burnt."

Buddha

Living in the Moment

Living in the moment does not mean that you don't remember your past or think about your future. It's about appreciating life as it is, not taking things for granted and avoiding focusing on things that are out of your control. It's letting go of your stress and worry and the "what-ifs" so that you don't keep projecting (and attracting) the same negative outcomes from the past into your future. It's very hard to live in the moment when you are sick and in pain, as your illness is a constant reminder that everything is not okay in your life. However, if you continue to focus on how sick and awful you feel, then it's likely that you will keep feeling sick and awful. To break the pattern, you must be grateful for the good in your life in order to attract more good into your life (Law of Attraction)! Start now. Each day, write five things that you are grateful for (this helps you appreciate life now). Then, set some positive goals for yourself. What do you want to do when you're well again (this gives you hope and excitement for the future). It's never too late to release the negative and embrace the infinite possibilities.

"Every moment is like a blank canvas; it's our emotions and thoughts that colour what we see. When you are in the present moment, it's easier to accept the reality of the situation you are in. When you embrace the way things are in the moment, you start the process of change, and you allow new possibilities to emerge."

Miranda Kerr

Thoughts Affect Physiology

Dr. Masaru Emoto, a Japanese author and entrepreneur, did a study to determine how human consciousness (energy, thoughts and words) would affect the molecular structure of water. The study involved many facets, but he claimed that thoughts and words (written and spoken) could change the water's structure: positive words created beautiful patterns like a snowflake, and negative words created a murky structure. Wouldn't it be amazing if this were true?

At the end of the day, we are 70% water, so everything we say, see, think or write directly affects our physiology. Programming positive thoughts, feelings, emotions, affirmations, words and music can help us make positive healing shifts. You should also surround yourself with positive people, as their thoughts, feelings, beliefs, values and anything else they communicate to you consciously or subconsciously has the ability to affect your health and healing. How many toxic people are still in your life?

"The mind is everything. What you think, you become."

Buddha

Workbooks, Journals and Diaries

Writing (as opposed to typing) is very powerful and healing. You can keep a paper journal or diary in your phone or use an empty scrapbook to write your thoughts down each day. Or you can use something more formal. Here are a few suggestions:

Keel's Simple Diary™: A quirky diary like the one my friend, Kesh Seale, gave me. You can buy the hard copy or download a digital version for your iPhone or Android from www.simplediary.com/apps.

The first page reads:

Dear Reader,

There are many reasons why most people, although they have tried, won't keep a diary. Not every day is eventful. It actually takes a lot of discipline. In retrospect, many find what they have written quite embarrassing.

You may use Simple Diary

however you like

whenever you like

wherever you are

randomly or one page at a time

filling in your thoughts or leaving it blank

reading one page or as many as you wish

and putting it aside for awhile

as an assistant for any occasion in life

I hope you find a true friend, a great place or some wisdom through this book.

Good luck, and thank you for your time. It's all yours.

Phillip Keel (Keel n.d.)

The diary asks questions each day in quirky ways, which is exactly what you need when you are sick and can't think straight. The best part is that you can just read it and laugh, write, tick things and use it as much or as little as you'd like!

THE ANXIETY AND PHOBIA WORKBOOK can be bought from Amazon and is a great tool to use if you have any anxiety or phobia-related issues (as the name suggests) such as social anxiety, panic attacks or obsessive compulsive tendencies. It includes information for assessing anxiety-related disorders as well up-to-date research, self-help and therapeutic techniques to help you manage and conquer your anxiety.

It's Not All in Your Head and You Are Not Crazy

If there is one thing that everyone either gets told (usually repeatedly) or thinks to themselves at least once (but usually more), is that their disease must be in their head. Common thoughts are: "I must be imagining it." "Maybe the doctor is right and it's all in my head." "I think I'm losing the plot.""Surely I couldn't have this many symptoms." Common comments from doctors, family and friends include: "Lyme disease doesn't exist in Australia, does it?""My friend said that Lyme disease is a psychological disorder.""Maybe you should get some counseling.""Have you tried antidepressants?""You look fine to me." And so on and so on. It's hard enough when you think you are going crazy, let alone when other people don't believe you or even support you. So do yourself a favour, and don't hang out with those people! If you are reading this and are a friend or family member of someone with Lyme disease, then be sure to support them with positive language and actions, as it will make a world of difference to them.

There are mental, emotional and psychological issues that need to be dealt with when people are very sick (especially for a long time), but these are manifestations of the disease NOT symptoms of a psychiatric disorder. Not all symptoms are visible, but they are just as real as the physical ones.

"People don't care how much you know,
until they know how much you care"

Unknown

Top Tips to Improve Your Mental and Emotional Health

Be Positive – Think of your life like a garden with your thoughts being the seeds. If your garden isn't thriving, you have either forgotten to water it and give it TLC, or you have been watering the weeds! So if you aren't thriving in your life, what are you missing, what can you add or what are you spending time on that isn't serving you right now? Add a little positivity and watch your garden flourish.

The grass is always greener on the other side – why don't you spend more time watering your own garden and see how green it really is or can be?

Adapted by Kate Wood

Associate with Positive People – Have you ever noticed that when you spend time with certain people you feel energised, but with others you feel totally drained? When you are sick, you can't afford to spend time with people who suck your energy. Pick people who are positive and energetic and inspire you to be a better you! Be careful, though, as positive energy in big groups can be draining, so socialise in small groups and for small amounts of time.

Change the Channel – When you are always reading and talking about something, it can become overwhelming, and you can actually create more of it in your life (works well for the positive stuff but not so well for disease). So change the channel often. Don't get bogged down in always talking about, researching, chatting on forums and reading books about Lyme or chronic disease. You need to get a balance of learning and knowledge to beat your disease, but not be so focussed on it that you never have a chance to actually break free and heal yourself.

Smile – As you have learnt it takes less muscles to smile than frown and it releases endorphins. Sometimes the "fake-it-'til-you-make-it" attitude can help you forget your worries for awhile. I'm not saying to ignore your problems, but always concentrating on them isn't going to help either. Think of proactive things you can do to solve your problems, and SMILE!

Breathe – Just increasing your intake of oxygen can help you feel calmer, and it's FREE! See Breathing in the Physical Treatment chapter for breathing tips and tricks, and how it can help release anxiety!

Meditate – Meditation provides an effective way to improve your mental state. Try thinking of a place or person that you love. Go through your photo album and imagine yourself during happier times and in peaceful places, and project them to your future. See the Spiritual Strategies chapter for more meditation tips.

Sleep and/or Rest – A rested body is a calm body. Allow your body time to heal and restore. Your body as well as your mind will thank you.

Have an Attitude of Gratitude – Gratitude is everything. Even when the worst thing possible happens, there is ALWAYS something to be grateful for, so look for it. Say "Thank you" three times in a row to intensify your gratitude. See more information on gratitude in the Spiritual Strategies chapter.

Do Something to Actively Release Endorphins – Smile, exercise, do a back bend, or get a massage or an adjustment (Google *endorphin-releasing activities* and see what you find!)

Get Regular Treatments – Get a massage or a facial, or any treatment that makes you feel better about yourself. You deserve it!

Be Prepared for the Emotional Aftermath

No matter how well you deal with your emotions during your illness, be prepared for an emotional clearance after you start to get well. The body is often unable to totally integrate or release emotions when it is very sick. As your body starts to heal and strengthen, you are physically strong enough to release the rest of the stored up emotions. This may have a gradual onset or hit you like a ton of bricks one day.

The emotional aftermath hit me like a ton of bricks and I was suicidal at the thought that my physical pain had been transformed into emotional pain. It wasn't until my naturopath Kelly Galvin pointed out to me that releasing negative emotions was a wonderful sign that my physical body was finally strong enough to process the last of the emotional trauma caused from being sick for so long. Knowing that I was actually healing as I felt so emotional helped me understand the purpose of the release and embrace it.

> *"Your emotions affect every cell in your body. Mind and body, mental and physical, are intertwined."*
>
> ### *Thomas Tulko*

I had anxiety that set in over months, and it started very mildly. I would feel anxious and sweaty when I woke up in the morning. It felt like something bad was going to happen (or had happened), but I couldn't consciously identify the cause of the anxiety. This anxiety built up over months into full-fledged depression. It was the worst I had ever felt emotionally, and I just couldn't put my finger on why I was feeling so blue. I had come through a horrible disease, was feeling physically well, exercising daily, seeing my friends again and was about to go back to work. In my mind I should have been the happiest person in the world, not the saddest as I was.

One day I started to cry and pretty much did not stop for about 3 ½ weeks. I did not leave the house for even a second for two of those weeks. I felt suicidal and my husband had to take time off work to look after me. He was too scared to leave me alone, and I refused to let him tell anyone or get help for me. I would go for a run in the bush but would cry the entire way. In the end, my husband pleaded with me to call my naturopath, Kelly Galvin (who was also someone we considered our spiritual guide and support), and I slowly got myself back on track using kinesiology, meditation, homeopathics and Bach flower remedies.

I urge you to continue using emotion-releasing techniques so this doesn't happen to you. If it does, do not stick your head in the sand like I did. Reach out for help straight away.

"Wisdom is the serenity to accept the things you cannot change, the courage to change the things you can, and the wisdom to know the difference."

Reinhold Niebuhr

CHAPTER 9 –
SPIRITUAL STRATEGIES

"Destiny is no matter of chance. It is a matter of choice."

William Jennings Bryan

WHY ARE YOU HERE?

Purpose

I believe we are all put on Earth for a purpose. If you stray too far from your core truth or values, you will receive signs along the way that can help get you back on track, if you listen. This could be a health symptom, an emotional symptom, a symbol, a dream, déjà vu or even a "gut feeling." The more you listen and are guided by your intuition, the more likely you will be able to fulfil your purpose and live a happy, healthy life.

"We can only be said to be alive in those moments when our hearts are conscious of our treasures."

Thornton Wilder

Learning Life's Lessons

Life would be very boring if everything went to plan, if we were all friends, if there were no wars, if there was no disease. Don't get me wrong, that's a world that I'd vote for, but at the end of the day, life is all about balance—what goes up must come down. It's the law of nature! So good comes with bad and success comes with failure, and most of our growth occurs not when we are winning and successful and at the top of our game, but from all the lessons learnt getting there. We have all heard the saying "Happiness is a journey, not a destination," so if you can take a step back and look at your life as a journey, it is easier to put things in perspective. Life gives us lessons to learn along the way, and if we miss or ignore the lesson, another lesson will come along. This will keep happening until the universe believes you have learnt that lesson or lessons.

I was one of those people who tended to race through life fast. I was so focussed on the end result that I was completely inflexible and often missed the fun of the journey itself. So while I was successful at almost everything I put my mind to, it came at a cost. I was a yes-woman. I found it very hard to say no to people, so I often found myself going places and doing things that I didn't really want to. Of course, in life, you sometimes have to do the things you don't want, but again, at what cost. When you sacrifice your own beliefs and energy for the sake of others, not only do they take advantage of you, but there is no longer an even exchange of give-and-take and balance is disrupted! The universe will always try to restore balance. Some of the lessons I had to learn in order to grow and heal were:

❖ I can't help anyone else if I can't help myself. As a member of a healing profession, I must first spend time on my own health by eating well, exercising (balanced exercise), getting adjustments and other treatments regularly, doing yoga and meditating so I can stay healthy and lead by example.

❖ Slow down! I always thought that when I had children I would slow down, but life had other plans. It slowed me down with a disease in order to show me it would take a lot more than a child for me to find the right balance. It took me a long time to learn this lesson. Every time I would slow down and start to heal, I would return to work and start running, and then get sick again.

❖ I don't have to run EVERYDAY to maintain my ideal weight. I have always been active and run at a competitive level; I've trained seven days a week since I was eight years old. It's all I knew, and I had this fear that I would get fat if I didn't continue to do this. Being sick and resting my body showed me that there are other healthy ways to maintain my weight (and my sanity).

❖ It's okay to be successful. I was aware that I had this subconscious self-sabotage pattern. It started in athletics. Just as I was about to reach my goal or run my fastest time or get picked for a team, I would get injured. Every single time! It then spread to my social life and my work life. It was brought to my conscious awareness when I did some life coaching during my illness. I believe Lyme disease was my biggest self-sabotage. I did some Time Line Therapy™, NET, positive affirmations and visualisations around breaking these patterns, and it made a huge difference!

❖ I don't have to be the most successful person in the world to still have purpose. When I was unable to work, cook or even get out of bed some days, I felt like I had no purpose, and then I lost hope. If you don't have hope or purpose, you don't have anything to live for.
I started writing this book in order to give me purpose. Later, I realised that sharing this information with you was part of my healing journey.

❖ Before every rainbow is a storm. Life isn't always about waiting for the storm to pass; it's about learning to dance in the rain and appreciate the magnificent rainbow at the end! In her book *The Lyme Disease Survival Guide*, Connie Strashiem outlines some life lessons of chronic illness. So be proactive and start learning your lessons now so you can enjoy the wondrous rainbow of health. Look for these lessons that I have learnt and/or summarised from Connie's book in your own life. (Strasheim 2008):

Slow down: Start finding balance now instead of waiting until you have to slow down. Life is just as much about *being* as it is *doing*.

Fuel your body: You can't put rubbish in and expect energy out. Don't wait until you are sick to eat the right foods and look after your body. Eat and drink well now and enjoy your health and life.

You have control over making well-informed decisions about your habits and lifestyle: As much as we like to think things happen by chance, taking the time to research and understand how certain actions affect our lives, in a big part, is in our control.

Your worth is not directly related to your productivity: You don't have to be saving the world to have purpose and joy. Fulfilment needs to come from within.

Have empathy and compassion for others: After being sick, depressed and poor, you will be able to understand and empathise with those in need without judgment.

Cultivate new talents and habits: When you can no longer run around like a mad person (you simply don't have the energy), you will often take the time to do things you would never have thought or allowed yourself the time to do in the past, such as knitting, scrapbooking, cooking, reading, making jewellery, playing cards and board games.

Learn more about health and how to help others with your knowledge: You have been through it and learnt some things that have worked (or not worked, for that matter) for you, so sharing this information can not only be very helpful for others, but very healing for you.

Money is not everything: Chronic illness empties the budget like nothing else. You will learn how to manage money better, and you'll realise that money does not buy anything that's important in life, like happiness, health or love.

Health is your greatest wealth: Once you have lost your health, you realise that it is, by far, your greatest wealth, and you will pay any amount of money and travel any distance to get it back. Value your health now so you don't have to learn this lesson the hard way!

Learn who your real friends are: When you are sick and can't always be at social events and/or return calls, you will truly learn who your real friends are. The people who were there for what you could give them will disappear, and the people who truly care about you will always be there for you in some form. Learning this lesson means you can focus your energy on the people who matter most in your life, because at the end of the day, you can't be friends with everyone!

"When I started counting my blessings, my whole life turned around."

Willie Nelson

Grounding Yourself

In the Physical Treatment chapter, I talked about the physical nature of grounding and earthing yourself. In a spiritual sense, there are also visualisations you can do to ground yourself. Here is my favourite: you can record and play it with music in the background or just memorise the practice and perform it daily. Even better try to get your bare feet on the ground at the same time.

Stand with your bare feet on the earth (I love doing this at the beach). Gently close your eyes and take note of how your body is feeling. Feel your feet attached to the ground and imagine roots extending from your feet deep down into the ground. Like tree roots, it will stabilise you, connect you to the earth and provide energy from Mother Earth. Imagine lots of twisting and twining roots going wider and deeper into the earth. A feeling of heaviness comes over your body as you feel totally stable and still. Now imagine the sun shining white light down onto your body. Lift your arms and head up towards the sun and welcome its white, healing light and warmth. Welcome that light through the top of your head, through your fingertips and down your arms. Allow the white light to fill your chest cavity and your heart space, and then run down your legs and down through the roots attached to your feet. As this light comes down, it is exchanged in the earth for grounding energy, which then soars back up through the roots, into your feet, up your legs, into your chest and heart space, back up through your arms and head, and out the top of your fingertips. Repeat this cycling of energy as many times as you want.

"I am still determined to be cheerful and happy, in whatever situation I may be; I have also learned from experience that the greater part of our happiness or misery depends upon our dispositions, and not upon our circumstances."

Martha Washington

WHAT DO YOU SEE?

Is the Glass Half-Full or Half-Empty?

How we look at the world determines the outcomes we receive. Positivity is a big part of how successful, how healthy and how amazing your life is and will be. When things aren't going your way, it's very easy to see the glass as half-full; the less you see, the less you get. However, have you ever noticed how positive people always seem to have things go their way? They always get "lucky." The first part of your healing journey is to see the glass as half-full. Even better, imagine how you are going to fill up the glass! You can fill a glass of water halfway and set it where you will see it often as a constant reminder of the choice you have in how you see the world. Of course, what comes back to you is the result of your choices!

"Luck is where preparation meets opportunity."

Seneca

"All the principles of heaven and earth are living inside you."

Morihei Ueshiba

WHAT DO YOU BELIEVE AND HOW DO YOU LIVE?

The Eternal Principles

Dr. Carmen Harra wrote the spiritual book *The Eleven Eternal Principles: Accessing the Divine Within,* which outlines 11 of life's many laws or principles. My husband and I based part of our marriage ceremony on these principles, as they were principles we wanted to build our marriage on and live our lives by. We called the special ceremony Take This Step with Me. I would like to share with you the eight readings from our ceremony that were inspired by these principles as well as the other three principles from Dr. Harra's book, as I believe they are great principles to help you heal yourself and create the life of your dreams. (Harra 2009)

"If we find meaning in the challenges that confront us, we can break through to a life of growth, mission, and ongoing miracles."

James Redfield

The Law of Totality

All people and all creatures are one, united with the Divine.

The Law of Karma

What you do and what happens to you is the result of your soul's choice to come to Earth and learn the lessons it needs to learn. Karma was originally defined as actions, thoughts and deeds. It is the collection of memories of everything you have ever felt, thought, experienced, done or suffered. You can deal with karma in two ways—through suffering fruitlessly, or by courageously choosing to experience love, forgiveness and acceptance, even when it may be difficult to do so. May you choose to look at challenging situations as an opportunity to be more loving and positive towards yourself and others. Remember each small kind act toward a neighbour is an act of good karma that changes the energy of the matrix of your life.

The Law of Wisdom

Wisdom is the serenity to accept the things you cannot change, the courage to change the things you can, and the wisdom to know the difference, as well as accepting your limitations and maximising your strengths. It's about choosing to use your mistakes and triumphs as a tool for learning about yourself in order to grow into a more balanced individual.

The Law of Unconditional Love

We are here on Earth to love each other unconditionally, no matter how challenging that may be. Genuine, divine, authentic love is never demanding or domineering, and it does not have any conditions placed on it. To be capable of true love, you must also be able to love yourself unconditionally.

The Law of Harmony

Harmony is an energetic state in which there is alignment and balance. When you are in harmony, you are happy, healthy and creative. If you are in alignment with the universe, everything seems to work perfectly, and you recognise that problems are just learning curves along your journey. Harmony within a relationship requires a commitment to put that relationship ahead of your personal fears and needs as well as agreeing to serve the partnership more than yourself. A romantic soulmate is someone who complements you energetically. May you have harmony in all your relationships, always give as much as you take and love as much as you are loved.

The Law of Abundance

Abundance is not something you lose or have taken away from you, but something you create. Both abundance and lack exist simultaneously in our lives as parallel realities. It is always your conscious choice which secret garden you will attend. When you choose to be grateful for all the abundance that is present rather than focussing on what is missing in your life, the wasteland of illusion fades away and you will experience heaven on Earth! May you always be grateful for your blessings and give to others even when it calls for a sacrifice. May you enjoy an abundance of love for yourself and others and be joyful no matter what your circumstances.

The Law of Attraction

The law of attraction is how the universe works with you to bring you what you desire! What you think about comes about—good or bad! However, there is often a big gap between what our conscious mind desires and what our subconscious mind attracts. May you always continue to have a positive outlook on life, seeing only the good in everything. May you feel grateful and confident in your ability to attract all that you need, and be content and thankful even when there is a gap between what you desire and what you attract.

The Law of Evolution

The law of evolution states that we will continuously evolve to a higher state of consciousness.

The Law of Manifestation

The law of manifestation is the ability to make things happen in the physical world through our thoughts, feelings, words and actions. You must have total well-being to manifest. May you continue to balance not only your own health, but the health of all the people around you— mentally, physically, biochemically, spiritually and emotionally. May you manifest and create well-being so you are able to be creative and envision ways to improve your life and the world.

The Law of Destiny

The law of destiny states that we are all flawed creatures, driven to unite ourselves with a higher good or being to end our suffering, and that we choose to take human form in order to purify our souls, rid ourselves of bad karma, and reunite with a higher being for all eternity.

The Law of Infinite Possibilities

Physical reality uses the left brain and contains things you can measure, contain, count and limit. In the reality of infinite possibilities, all is one and ever-changing. Nothing is fixed, not form, space or time. The more you use your right brain, let go of any manmade limitations and align yourself with the law of infinite possibilities, the better you open yourself up to opportunities that have no boundaries. You can defy the laws of time and space, and participate in the co-creation of the seemingly impossible. No dream is too big. May you have patience and trust in divine timing, be open to opportunities that come along, and watch for all the doors that are opening, allowing infinite possibilities to flood into your life.

"What this power is I cannot say; all I know is that it exists..."

Alexander Graham Bell

WHAT CAN YOU DO?

Life Setting

Over the years, I have created something which I call life setting. It incorporates your purpose, dream setting, goal / dream board(s), goal setting, affirmations, visualisations, ideal day, and a power up process

/ routine. I do this for myself and with my husband at the start of each year and re-adjust as necessary throughout the year. I also implement life setting with many of my open-minded staff members where we focus on business-related topics such as our ideal client (i.e., who do we want to attract into our business so we can help them?) and our ideal day (how would our ideal day play out?). As an athlete in high school, I naturally set goals and did visualisations long before I was actually taught how to do it or knew the meaning behind it; it's just something I naturally did. I find it very motivating and rewarding, so I would like to share how I do my life setting in the hope of inspiring you to do the same. You wouldn't build a house without a blueprint, so how do you expect to have a great life if you don't plan it! All the information you will need is in Appendix E:14-21.

"Success is peace of mind which is a direct result of self satisfaction in knowing you did your best to become the best you are capable of becoming."

John R. Wooden

Gratitude

The power of gratitude dates back centuries and is found in all cultures, religions and traditions. Rhonda Byrne, in her book *The Magic* (she also wrote *The Secret* and many other fabulous books), says the magic formula to health, happiness and success is gratitude. The two simple words of thank you can and will create magic in your life. You must say it, believe it and feel it. Thank you is the bridge between where you are now and the life of your dreams! (Byrne 2012)

Rhonda Byrne's Magic Formula (Byrne 2012):

❖ Deliberately think and say the magic words – *Thank you*

❖ The more you deliberately say the magic words *thank you*, the more gratitude you will feel

❖ The more gratitude you deliberately think and feel, the more abundance you will receive

"Gratitude is a vaccine, an antitoxin, and an antiseptic."

John Henry Jowett

In Rhonda's book, there are 28 daily magical practices to help you use gratitude to create the life of your dreams. The first 12 practices focus on what you need to be grateful for now and in the past. The next 10 practices focus on using gratitude to attract and achieve your desires, dreams and future goals. The final 6 practices focus on dissolving negative circumstances that you have or may encounter in your life and also helping others to do the same.

By rewiring your brain to practice gratitude not just consciously but subconsciously, you become automatically grateful and express gratitude in all areas of your life. Learning to be grateful in all areas of your life will revolutionise your health, finances, career, relationships, material possessions, personal desires and self-esteem as well as dissolve and transform any negative experiences you have created in the past or present.

Gratitude practice is best done after you have done your life setting (mentioned at the beginning of this section). If you are very clear on what you want, then gratitude will help you achieve it. If you practice gratitude a little, it will change your life a little. If you practice gratitude regularly, it will help your life immensely. I have summarised a few of the practices to get you started, but I highly recommend that you buy and read the book. (Byrne 2012)

GRATITUDE PRACTICE 1: COUNT YOUR BLESSINGS

One of the easiest steps you can take is to count your blessings. This can be done on a whiteboard, in your diary or in an app on your phone. Rhonda recommends writing 10 things you are grateful for every day. Start with one thing a day, and by the end of 28 days, you will have written at least 28 things you are grateful for.

1. First thing in the morning, make a list of blessings in your life and what you are grateful for.

2. Write why you are grateful for each blessing.

3. At the end of each day, review your list and say the magic words *Thank you, Thank you, Thank you,* feeling as much gratitude as you can for each blessing.

4. Repeat for 28 days (and beyond!).

> *"He who enjoys good health is rich, though he knows not."*
>
> *Italian Proverb*

MAGICAL PRACTICE 4: MAGICAL HEALTH

1. On a piece of paper, write the words *THE GIFT OF HEALTH IS KEEPING ME ALIVE* and place it where you will see it often.

2. Set an alarm or a time (e.g., with every meal) where you will hold the paper and carefully and gratefully read the words. Visualise yourself in full health.

3. Just before you go to sleep at night, say the magic words *Thank you, Thank you, Thank you for the gift of health that is keeping me alive,* and visualise your body healing and completely healthy.

> *"Miracles are not contrary to nature,*
> *but only contrary to what we know about nature."*
>
> *Saint Augustine*

MAGICAL PRACTICE 16: MAGIC AND MIRACLES IN HEALTH

Our birthright is full health. Unfortunately, at some point, we all take our health for granted. It is important to be grateful for our past, present and future health. As Virgil said, "Health is our greatest wealth."

❖ Remember three times in your past or childhood where you felt healthy, happy and on top of the world. Visualise how you felt, and give thanks for each of those amazing times in your life.

❖ Think about each of the functions that your body automatically performs, and give thanks to every organ, system and physical sense that is currently working in your body. Say *Thank you* three times after you visualise each organ and function. You might like to choose a few each day and work through the body that way.

❖ Choose one thing about your health that you want to improve, and spend time visualising yourself with the ideal state of body and health. Once you have a full vision of that optimal state, then give thanks three times.

"No duty is more urgent than that of returning thanks."

Saint Ambrose

Meditation

People have various perceptions about mediation. Some people think of meditation as something hippies, monks and weirdos do! I, however, believe meditation has come full circle. Although it has powerful spiritual connections, there is now research that supports its use to heal and improve well-being. Dr. Craig Hassed, a GP and lecturer at Monash University, says that 1 in 6 doctors now teach some type of meditation, and over 80% of GPs now include meditation practices as part of their patients' recommended treatment. Research also supports its effectiveness in helping with a range of conditions including stress-related cardiovascular disease, depression, anxiety, chronic pain and cancer. (Hassad 2012)

There are so many different forms and types of meditation; it's just a matter of finding the right style for you. I love guided meditation, as it helps keep my mind focussed. However, even within the bracket of guided meditation, there are so many different styles.

I meditate every day without fail, and when I was sick, I meditated even more. In this world, it is so easy to go on autopilot and be influenced by everyone with whom you come in contact. More than ever before, people are spending more and more time in sympathetic dominance, which is our "fright, flight or fight" mode. It is designed for survival, like running away from bears, which I imagine is very stressful! Research shows that stress can kill brain cells, decrease the ability of the immune system, affect digestion, decrease sex drive, increase ageing and damage DNA. Let's face it, when we are running for our lives, we need as much blood, nutrition and oxygen as possible running to our muscles in order to keep us moving and to keep our brain alert so we can survive. Hence, we don't need to send blood and energy to our digestive, reproductive or immune systems; you don't need to digest food, fight off pathogenic microbes or procreate when you are running for your life! So it makes sense that when you are stressed, these systems come under the most strain. However, to heal we need to return the body to a parasympathetic dominant state so that our body can rest and digest. Meditation helps you to achieve this.

Hassed argues that too often our thoughts slip into a default mode. This involves replaying the past, worrying about the future and experiencing other negative thoughts, which leads to the over-activation of the body's stress response.

This stress response is designed to help you deal with dangers or threats, but when it is too frequently over-activated by threats existing only in your mind, it can cause wear and tear on your body over time. According to Hassed, this wear and tear can increase your risk of illnesses such as heart attacks, strokes, high blood pressure and diabetes.

He also cites studies that show prolonged stress can kill cells in our brains and damage DNA in ways that predict illnesses associated with ageing, including cancer. Learning to switch off through meditation, which has been shown to significantly benefit those already suffering from poor health, can reverse those effects. Meditation can help your body revert from that sympathetic state to a parasympathetic state where it can rest-and-digest and heal. (Hassad 2012)

Dr. Sarah Edelman is a clinical psychologist who uses mindfulness meditation to teach people how to "... watch with curiosity but without judgment, so you don't activate the secondary distress system." Attachment or resistance to unpleasant emotions or sensations causes your body to actually experience the stress or pain, so learning detachment through meditation is a great tool. (Edelman 2013)

Meditation can:

❖ Decrease stress and promote relaxation

❖ Manage and even eliminate anxiety

❖ Help cope with illness and pain

❖ Halve the chance of relapse for depression sufferers

❖ Accelerate healing and well-being

❖ Improve mood, energy and feelings of well-being

❖ Increase production of substances that boost immunity while reducing so-called pro-inflammatory chemicals that help cancer cells replicate and form their own blood supply

My Favourite Meditation Apps

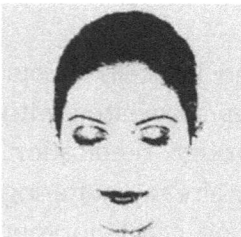

Relax and Rest ($1.99) – Different meditations of varying lengths allow you to relax deeply regardless of how much time you have available. No previous meditation experience is required.

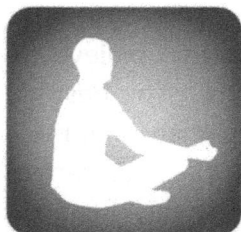

The Mindfulness App ($1.99) – This app can be used by everyone. It is easy to use, and you can choose your favourite type of meditation (e.g., guided, meditation in silence and guided introductions) as well as how long you want to meditate.

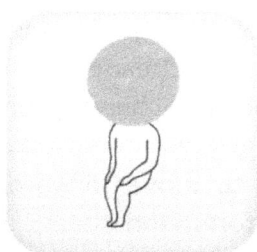

Headspace (Free)– This app contains bite-sized techniques to help you sleep better, focus more and get some relief from a busy mind.

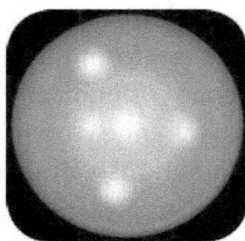

Happiness—A guided meditation (Free)—Happiness is not something you are born with, nor is it outside of your control. It comes from within. This guided meditation helps you to calmly focus on improving your mood and outlook on life. Each 15-minute session brings you to a relaxed state where you more easily consider and rehearse practical ways to be a happier person.

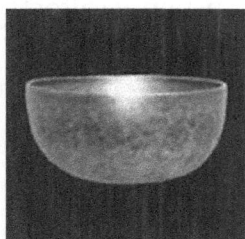

The Insight Meditation app ($2.99) – Featuring guided meditations by Tara Brach, Jack Kornfield, Jon Kabat-Zinn, Sharon Salzberg and many more amazing teachers.

I cover all the Louise Hay apps in more detail in Chapter 9.

Life Coaching

Just like you need an athletic coach and a business coach, I believe we actually all need a life coach. How can you expect to have the best life without some guidance? Although anyone can benefit from one, most people seek out a life coach when they need help making changes in their lives. Those changes might be related to career, finances, relationships or health. A life coach can help you to achieve goals, maximise your potential, attain self-mastery, and break through limiting beliefs and patterns in order to create the life of your dreams. Just like any coach, a life coach can give you a framework to achieve your goals, keep you accountable, provide strategies and give you feedback. A life coach can give you confidence and support to move forward in a positive manner when you crave change and transformation.

Children generally don't have the same limitations when it comes to what they can do, be or have in life. According to the sociologist Morris Massey (ChangingMinds.org n.d.), all of your core values are formed by 21 years of age and will not change unless you experience a significant emotional experience or make a conscious effort to change them, as with life coaching (http://changingminds.org/explanations/values/values_development.htm). By the time you're an adult, many things have influenced your belief patterns, such as family (first you model your parents), your friends (they have the largest impact during the socialisation period), religion, school (teachers, friends and lessons), geography (where you were raised), economics and prosperity (affects your beliefs about money), major historical events (e.g., growing up during a war) and, of course, the media.

We know that whatever you believe is what you create in your life. Your values will determine what motivates you, and your attitude will affect how you behave and respond to events that occur in your life. A life coach can help you explore the motivations, values, beliefs and attitudes that have become your identity. Then they can guide you to overcome any limiting beliefs and behaviours, and help you reprogram those beliefs to maximise your potential.

There was a time when my negative thoughts about my body prevented it from doing its job—healing itself. So I did a six-month program of life coaching. I worked through some generational patterns and past life sequences that were creating a clash between my subconscious beliefs and my current conscious thoughts. I wrote down my KPIs (key performance indicators) and how I would know when I had achieved them. Now that I finally understood how my negative thought patterns, learned behaviours and values had impacted my natural instincts, I used affirmations, kinesiology, meditation and Time Line Therapy™ to restore my core values. I related everything back to a cellular level and visualised and gave thanks for my body's miraculous and natural self-healing ability. I put faith back in myself and my innate ability to heal and be healthy. I made huge breakthroughs in my health during this time and continue even now to apply many of the practices I learnt to my everyday life. I can't recommend life coaching highly enough, especially my coach, Sarah Nonclares, of Equilibro coaching in Sydney.

Reiki

The word Reiki comes from two Japanese words: *rei* which means God's wisdom and *ki* which means life force energy. It is used for a variety of purposes but primarily for stress reduction, relaxation and optimising the body's natural healing ability. Reiki is a safe, natural method of spiritual healing that has been shown to help virtually every known disease and also offset the side effects from modern medicine in order to promote recovery and supercharge healing.

I had a beautiful client, Kuve Bradley, who treated me weekly for six months and then fortnightly, then monthly all the way through my journey. She cleared my house, balanced my energy, tapped into my guides and helped give my body the life force it needed to heal itself. Sometimes she would place her hands on me and other times she wouldn't. During the treatment, I would often feel energy moving through my body and a glowing radiance inside and around me. I would often have visions or dreamlike states where I would receive information or messages. I would always feel very calm and centred afterwards, and it was much easier to meditate, stay focussed and be positive.

Shamanism

The word shaman originates from the Tungas tribe of Siberia and means "one who sees in the dark / with a heart." Shamanism is the way of the heart—a way of life that empowers, delivers and embodies truth, integrity, personal healing and interconnectedness. It is the oldest form of healing. A shaman works with the spiritual aspect of an illness / disease / life block(s), and therefore, looks after and cares for the spirit of the person and the land. A shaman reaches altered states of consciousness, also known as the shamanic state of consciousness (SSC), to travel and journey out of their body into different spirit realms. They can communicate and interact in the spirit world to connect with nature and past loved ones, retrieve parts of the soul, communicate with spirit or power animals or act as a psychopomp (a person who assists souls to cross over). In a shamanic healing, a space is created for you to reach a level of altered consciousness where you can reconnect with your inner truth. Shamanic healing can incorporate cellular memory healing, vibrational / sound healing, soul retrieval and hands-on healing. Each shaman, depending on how and where they were trained, will have different techniques. The shaman's healing unlocks the ancient power that is stored within you, as it is believed that YOU are the true shaman in your life.

I had my first experience with a shaman when I did Module 4 of the TBM course in 2007. The shaman was from America and had grown up and trained with African-American tribes. My first session was in a group, and the power of his presence was unbelievable. He taught us how to enter our body's biocomputer to scan and become aware of blockages that stop us from achieving optimal health. He taught us how to clear and reset those patterns. He then took each person individually through to their "secret garden," and whilst that happened, the rest of the group would all hold the space for that person. I could often see what the person described in their garden before they would actually say it aloud, like having déjà vu or being psychic. It was incredible! He then went through all the chakras, and never have I done a visualisation with so much detail and colour. Each time I would see the colour of the chakra long before he would tell us what the colour was (even though at that stage of my life,

I had never even heard of chakras having colours!). The power of these visualisations and healings lasted a very long time afterwards, and I have used many of the skills I learnt every day since then.

There are a few shamans in Sydney. One shaman who I have been particularly attracted to but have not physically met is Samantha Corrie. I have also had some healing done by an Aboriginal healer known as Gary, and I believe his style of healing is the aboriginal version of shamanism. If you want to experience shamanic healing, the right person for you will come at the right time.

Louise Hay

I came across Louise Hay when I first watched the movie The Secret *in my early twenties. Her work really resonated with me, even though I didn't exactly understand all the principles at the time. I started reading her books and applying her concepts to my life and saw a huge difference. I now had control of my destiny and was able to channel the positivity I was born to share even more than before. Then I used her related apps which made her work even more easily accessible.*

Louise Hay is an American motivational author and the founder of Hay House. Her journey began as an impoverished child who suffered years of abuse. In her teens she ran away to New York where she forged a modelling career and married a rich businessman. It was after the collapse of her 14-year marriage that she really delved into the mind-body connection and used her own tormented upbringing to help herself and others. She became a speaker and eventually a popular workshop leader at her church. When she began counselling people, she noticed a link between mental and physical ailments. She then created positive thought patterns for people to apply to their lives and found ways to reverse illness and regain optimal health. She released her first book, *Heal Your Body*, in 1975 and began traveling throughout the United States to share her findings and heal lives.

During this journey, she created an intensive program of affirmations, visualisations, nutritional cleansing and psychotherapy that she was also able to apply to her own life when she was diagnosed with "incurable" cancer. Using the principles she had created to heal and help others, she healed herself from cancer in just six months! After this she began to put her methods onto paper, which resulted in her second book, *You Can Heal Yourself,* released in 1984. She was a pioneer of the self-help movement in the 70s, long before self-help methods were really known about or accepted in mainstream health. Her second book was revised and expanded in 1988 and has been sold in 33 countries around the word and translated into 25 different languages! She started a support group in 1985 for six men diagnosed with AIDS, which grew to a gathering of 800 people by 1988 and led her to write *The AIDS Book: Creating a Positive Approach.* Her publishing company, Hay House, Inc., began as a small venture in the living room of her home and is now a super successful, non-profit organisation that has sold millions of books, DVDs and apps worldwide for both herself and other notable self-help authors. This organisation also financially supports organisations that provide food, shelter, counselling, hospice care and money to people with AIDS, women who have suffered abuse, and people who have faced other crises and need help. She has now released the movie version of *You Can Heal Your Life,* which I highly recommend that you watch whether you have read her books or not! (order at http://www.louisehay.com./products-events/)

My Favourite Louise Hay Apps (Apple n.d.)

MORNING AND EVENING MEDITATIONS ($5.99) – A collection of positive audio affirmations accompanied with soothing music intended to be heard the moment one awakens and just before sleep at night. These affirmations begin each day with hope and positivity, while later concluding the day with contentment. This app will ensure calm outlooks at sunrise and settling resolutions at sunset.

AFFIRMATION MEDITATIONS: ESSENTIAL AFFIRMATIONS FOR HEALTH, LOVE, SUCCESS, SELF-ESTEEM (free) – Unleash your full potential for love, health, success and self-esteem.

410

HEAL YOUR BODY A-Z ($4.99) – Based on the bestselling book, this fresh and easy step-by-step guide is set up in an A-Z format. Just look up your specific health challenge to find the probable cause as well as the information and affirmations you need to overcome it by creating new thought patterns.

I CAN DO IT! 2015 CALENDAR ($3.99) – So many exciting adventures are waiting for us each year! We need to trust that life will bring to us all that we need, and what better way is there to do that than with the I CAN DO IT 2015 Calendar! Filled with 365 days of wisdom and glorious photographs from world traveler Daniel Peralta, this gorgeous calendar helps you focus on that "I can do it attitude" that will make this a year of exploring like no other. This beautifully designed calendar is the perfect gift for friends, family members and, of course, you, because you can do it...no matter what "it" is! Each year there is an updated calendar available.

LOVING YOURSELF ($3.99) – Experience 52 loving cards that you can swipe between, shuffle, view "face up" or "face down" with the choice of which cards to flip over to read messages. You can email these inspiring cards to friends or save them to your Photo Library and use as wallpaper and screen savers.

AFFIRMATIONS FOR A STRESS-FREE LIFE (0.99c) – A deck of 24 affirmations to help you create a stress-free life! Living a stress-free life means letting go of the past, so be willing to release the need to be right about how stressful your life is. Every day gets easier and easier when you know that you're doing the best you can.

AFFIRMATIONS FOR HEALTH (0.99c) – A deck of 24 affirmations to help you create good health in every part of your mind and body! When you take care of yourself in the best way you can, you radiate beauty and happiness...and the world responds in an appreciative way. Good health comes from within, and it's a reflection of the thoughts you think and the words you speak. When you combine uplifting inner dialogue with good nutrition and regular exercise, you create all the tools you need to be...healthy, from head to toe! Choose a card each morning, and it will be your positive message for the day!

AFFIRMATIONS FOR SELF-ESTEEM (0.99c) A deck of 24 affirmations to help you create self-esteem in your life! "It doesn't matter what other people say or do. What matters is how I choose to react and what I choose to believe about myself." This is the most powerful affirmation you can ever say. And it's just one of many in this card deck designed to assist you in knowing that you're perfect, whole, and complete—right here, right now. Our thoughts create our future. When we think we're not good enough, we give away our power. Be willing to see life in a new and different way by beginning each day with a positive affirmation.

POWER THOUGHT CARDS ($3.99) – Beautifully illustrated deck of 64 inspirational cards to help you find your inner strength and guidance. They contain 128 unique pieces of art exquisitely illustrated by five artists. Each vibrant card contains a powerful affirmation on one side and a visualisation on the other to enlighten, inspire, and bring joy to your life. Close your eyes, ask for guidance, and then choose a card. Follow the message and watch what happens. Enjoy!

FEELING FINE AFFIRMATIONS ($5.99) – A compilation of positive audio affirmations set with motivating music created to help you lift your spirits and feel more joy in your life. It will reveal self-appreciation and release the past programming of expectation and negativity. Listening to these affirmations with receptive ears and consistency will induce you to change long-standing, negative thoughts into ones of self-love, self-worth, and self-esteem. Positive feelings of health, energy, and well-being will soon leave you feeling better than fine.

AFFIRMATIONS FOR JOB SUCCESS (0.99c) – A deck of 24 affirmations to help you create job success in your life! What does job success mean to you? More money? A loving, nurturing environment where your talents are recognised and used to their fullest? Mastering a new skill? All of this can be a reality for you. The key is to practice success, and stop practicing failure.

I THINK, I AM! ($3.99) – This app teaches kids the power of affirmations so they can learn and understand the powerful idea that they have control over their thoughts and words, and in turn, what happens in their lives.

The happiness and confidence that come from this learning is something children will carry with them their entire lives!

So download an app that appeals to you and get started. There are many more apps produced by Louise Hay and Hay House. Sometimes a little guidance goes a long way, which is why I have included my favourites for you! Even if you fall asleep listening to them, don't worry. Your subconscious will still hear them and reprogram itself!

Spiritual Protection, Clearing and Cleansing Techniques

Negativity can come in many forms. Your energetic and emotional strength and how well you are protected will determine how that energy affects you. Have you ever noticed that some days, people just really drain you, whilst other days you are much more resilient despite the negativity around you? Fear, anger, resentment, guilt, depression, anxiety, stress, fatigue, overwhelm, negative places or people, and arguments, to name a few, carry negative energies that can cling to you and build up in your environment (work or home). Over time, they can cascade to cause even more problems. No matter what your spiritual beliefs are (or lack thereof), you should know how to protect yourself from negative energy and entities. Spiritual cleansing and protection are a very important part of maintaining your space and health. The sicker you are, the more important these strategies are.

Grounding Yourself

Firstly, it is important to be grounded and centred for optimal health, as it brings together your physical, emotional and spiritual self within your earthly body and helps to literally keep your feet on the ground!

White Light Protection

Most people have at least heard of the concept of white light protection. It is a very easy visualisation to do and can be done for as little or as long as you like. Just imagine yourself surrounded by white light from head-to-toe. Really focus on the continuity of the white light, and keep increasing the brightness until it is SUPER bright and you are glowing. Imagine this bright light as a barrier of protection that negative energy can't penetrate. This is all you have to do, although you can say a prayer or some affirmations whilst doing this. You could say something simple like, "Please protect me from negative energy. Send my angels to protect me and my spirit guides to guide me, and protect me from all negative influences." You can do this protection for yourself, your loved ones, your pets and your belongings (e.g., for your car, you can imagine white light around the whole car and say, "Please protect me whilst I drive to and from work" or something similar). At night you can imagine the white light surrounding your whole house and protecting you and your family. Ideally, this sort of practice is done regularly. Over time the white light acts like a shield that constantly protects you regardless of how you are feeling or what you are doing. I recommend doing it morning and night, and as many times during the day as you need.

Wearing Purple Around Your Wrists

At TBM kinesiology seminars, there is as much focus on protecting yourself as a healer as there is in healing others. At the end of the day, if you aren't protected and optimally healthy, then it's very hard to help and heal others, especially long-term. A really easy thing to do is to wear purple around your wrists. Purple is a very protective colour, so it not only protects your inner energy, but also blocks the negative energy of others. You can wear purple beads, a string or plastic wrist bands. You can even draw on your wrist with a purple pen (it must be a continuous line of purple to work). Purple clothes can be useful in protecting yourself from negative energy in general, too.

Clearing Your Home of Negative Energy

Clearing your home is also important. Because negative energy can attach to anything and linger in any dwelling, it can cause issues with the people living there as well as with items in the home, such as appliances. The best thing to do is to clean the house and declutter it as much as possible. Then you can work on clearing it. I have someone else clear my house, but there are various ways this can be done if you want to do it yourself (or can't afford to have someone else to do it). Some ideas include:

Get a packet of salt or your salt grinder. Open the front door, turn right and start sprinkling or grinding the salt from the edge of the front door moving clockwise around your entire house. Once you reach your front door (don't put a line of salt across the front door yet), go inside and sprinkle some salt in each room (especially where you feel there might be negative energy). Focus mentally or verbally on releasing negative energy from your home. After at least an hour (you might need to leave it longer), you can finish the loop of salt by sprinkling some across the front door and closing it. You may choose to leave a cup of salt at all the doors and windows that lead to the outside, to keep the house protected. This needs to be done regularly and depends on how much negative energy there is, but I would recommend at least once a month. If you or your kids have bad dreams, this can be very helpful. You can even put a cup of salt in the doorways of the room or at the head of the bed to protect you and your family from negative energy during the night.

A friend gave me this clearing technique that I'd like to share with you. To begin, dissolve sea salt in two cups of warm water. Imagine charging the cups of salt water with the energy of white light. Now, take a shower and pour one cup of salt water over your head. As it runs down your body, imagine the salt and white light cleansing you. When you get out of the shower, do the white light visualisation (surround yourself with a bubble of bright white, cleansing light). Before you get dressed, you can also rub sandalwood oil above your brow, over your heart and on both shoulders. In each room as well as at each entrance to the house, light a white candle and one stick of incense (myrrh, sandalwood or sage is best). Get the other cup of salt water and thoroughly sprinkle it in each room, including behind doors, in corners, in cupboards, above cupboards or anywhere that negative energy can linger. Have the intention to clear negative energy either mentally or verbally. "I release negative energy away. In my house negative energy may not stay." Let the candles and incense burn completely in every room of your house. You might choose to write an intention on a piece of paper that states what you would like to attract as you release the negative energy. *We did a clearing like this with the intention of love and creating a family using pink rose quartz. We conceived that very week and on our first try (once we were healthy, of course).*

Put lavender flowers, fennel seeds or basil around the house, on dishes or in little hanging bags. You can also sprinkle herbs across doorways or hang bags of herbs in the cupboards, at work or in your car for protection. These herbs are great at removing the negativity around the house and should be replaced every few months by sprinkling them outside or on your garden to return to Mother Earth.

Herbs for Protection and Purification

Just as herbs have healing properties, they also have cleansing and purifying properties. The following list of herbs are great for removing negative energy and preventing negative energy from returning: aloe, anise, barley, basil, bay leaf, cactus, carnation, cedar, chamomile, cinnamon, clove, cumin, curry, dill, dragon's blood, eucalyptus, fennel, fern, flax, frankincense, garlic, ginseng, ivy, lavender, myrrh, onion, parsley, pepper, peppermint, rosemary, sage, thyme and violet. *I use frankincense to clear my aura by rubbing it on my hands and moving my hands as if to cover the space around my body. I do this regularly, particularly if I am feeling anxious or overwhelmed for no conscious reason.*

Smudging

Smudging is done by lighting the end of a bunch of dried sage leaves until it begins to smoke, and then waving the sage and smoke around your house (or body) to remove negative energy. *If you are sensitive to smoke, make sure to leave the house afterwards so you can let it air out. I made the mistake of doing it just before bed one night, and the smoke irritated my throat. I found it very hard to breathe and, of course, to sleep! My Reiki master also taught me to sage myself by setting the smoking sage bundle on the ground (or in some tin foil), then walking over it three times to clear myself, so give it a go!*

Burning Incense

Incense has similar properties to herbs and can achieve the same effect of clearing negative energy. Frankincense, sandalwood, myrrh and sage are the best for removing negativity.

Sea Salt Protection and Purification

Water has a negative charge, so that's why you often feel invigorated and calm after a swim in the ocean. Just as the ocean works to balance us when we swim via its negative ions, sea salt has this power as well. Sea salt is great for neutralising the body, mind, soul and environment. You can bathe in it, drink it, sprinkle it and place cups of it around or in your home (or workplace or car) in order to protect and purify.

Charging Objects with Your Intent

To charge something is to infuse it with your energy and intention. Choose an object and imagine that it is being infused with white light from your hands. As the object soaks up the energy, it begins to glow bright white from the inside out. Now you can state your intention (silently or aloud). For example, you can say, "I infuse white light, love and energy into this crystal. May it continue to spread energy, love and light through our home and protect us from any negative energy."

You can charge things like jewellery, belongings, candles, crystals, gratitude stones, gemstones and metals. Metals and crystals tend to hold energy for a long time, especially agate, amber, amethyst, black onyx, citrine, coral, emerald, garnet, obsidian (Apache tears), ruby and tourmaline. Gemstones and jewellery can then be worn as protection with the intent or charge that was placed on them.

Angels and Spirit Guides

We are all assigned angels and spirit guides who look over us and guide us, regardless of whether we know, believe or understand their role. However, we all have free will, so asking our spirit guides to help us can be very powerful. You can ask for their help and protection daily or for specific purposes in your life. Respect and gratitude are essential to get the most from your spirit guides. They are not our slaves, and there must be an even exchange of gratitude and love for the help they provide us.

Gold Light Smudge

Jenna Sifonis shared a protection method on her blog that I have sum- marised and want to share with you (Sifonis 2013):

1. Get comfortable and start to tune into your breath. Breathe in through the nose and out through your mouth. Allow your breath to slowly deepen, and visualise the air passing through your chakra centres, including the throat, the heart and the sacral chakra (5–7cm below your belly button). As the air reaches deep into your abdomen on the inhale, hold the breath for four seconds before releasing the air back up through the chakra centres and back out through the mouth. Repeat this process for a few cycles.

2. Now close your eyes (if they aren't already) and continue to breathe while focusing deep inside your solar plexus. Look even deeper inside your solar plexus for the smallest possible cell and imagine that it is a gold speck. See that gold speck expand into a ball of "beautiful, restorative, rejuvenating gold light." (Sifonis 2013) Imagine this gold light saturating every cell of your being.

3. Now move this golden light out from your body and into your auric field. Imagine cleansing this field and locking in that beautiful, cleansing protective energy.

As you practice this method, you may find that the gold light, which is initially chosen for its warming, calming, nurturing, healing and protective qualities, becomes a different colour for you.

TBM Personal Protection Technique

I first learnt to protect myself with a shaman and have continued to do so every morning and night since then. My version of the visualisation follows, and I recommend that you tape yourself saying it first so you can follow it until you have it down pat! Using music in the background is a great idea, too!

1. Close your eyes and get comfortable.

2. Concentrate on your heart centre and visualise a bright light emitting from the centre of your chest.

3. Focus closely on that light, and allow the light to shine beyond the body on the inhalation and return to the glowing heart centre on the exhalation.

4. Keep focussing on this light as it gets brighter and brighter while your breaths get deeper and deeper (continue this for as long as you'd like).

5. On your next breath out, allow the light to linger outside the body rather than returning to the heart centre.

6. On the next breath in, slowly aim the bright light up towards the head, saturating the upper body and cleansing it with white, purifying light.

7. As you breathe out, slowly aim the light towards the lower body, drenching it in beautiful, white, cleansing light

8. On the next breath, breathe in and hold all the white light inside your heart centre

9. As you breathe out, spread the white light up inside the entire chest, up towards the head and down the arms into the fingertips

10. As you breathe in again, continue to spread the white light down through the abdomen, both legs and into the feet until the whole body is glowing from the inside out with this gorgeous white light

11. As you breathe out, let go of any negative feelings, thoughts or emotions and feel your body as light and glowing white

12. Take another deep breath in, hold, and as you exhale, allow the light to gently penetrate through your skin into your auric field by a few centimetres. Hold for a second at the end of the out breath

13. Take another deep breath in and hold it. See the bright light just pouring out from your luminous body to the very edges of the skin

14. As you breathe out, allow the light to flow out beyond your skin and your aura (opening up your divine chakra) to encompass your whole body like a bubble of golden shining light

15. Breathe and observe the bubble around you for any holes. Patch up any holes that may have occurred in your energy field in order to protect your energy from within and also any negative energy from outside

16. Take as many breaths here as you need. Make repairs and energise by drawing healing energy in from the earth

17. Once you are done, exhale deeply and fully, and on the next breath, complete a fast, sharp inhalation. As you do this, pull all the light back into your body

18. Let your breathing just happen without too much focus now as you look up and see a bucket above your head. You reach up and pull a rope that tips the bucket upside down to release a light green, gooey coating that lands on your head and runs down your body. You spread this protective layer over your whole body—your head, behind your ears, down your neck and back, down your arms, your fingertips, over your chest, your stomach, your back, your groin, between your butt cheeks, down your legs and eventually the soles of your feet and your toes. You notice how light and flexible this coating feels and the immediate sense of safety and protection you feel.

19. You look up and see another bucket. You again reach up and pull the rope, which turns the bucket upside down. The same light green, gooey coating hits your head and runs down your body. Again, you spread this protective layer over your whole body, which still has amazing agility under this protective coat. You feel calm and grounded.

20. You look up again and see another bucket above your head. You reach up and pull the rope again, but this time a pink, foamy mixture comes down on top of your head (pink is the colour of unconditional love). You use your hands to spread and pat this foamy pink substance all over your body, just like before. You can feel that barrier giving you the strength to protect your inner energy and love. This layer also protects you from negative energy and converts any negative energy aimed at you into unconditional love. Then it sends it back to the sender with love. You are now protected from negative energy and filled with love, and you may choose to visualise or say affirmations that will help you through your day, night or specific activity.

Music

Music has the ability to heal you physically, chemically, emotionally and spiritually. Some healing music I listen to includes:

❖ Bruce Lipton – Music for a Shift in Consciousness

- ❖ Budapest Strings – Bach for Meditation

- ❖ Healing Touch

- ❖ Xavier Rudd

- ❖ Pops Mohammed – Healing Sounds of Mother Africa

CHAPTER 10 –
OTHER HANDY DIAGNOSES AND TREATMENT TIPS & TRICKS

(for those who want to go the extra mile or have had treatment failures)

LYME TREATMENT AND PROTOCOLS TO CONSIDER

As you well know, I truly believe that attending the St. Georg Klinik (SGK) in Bad Aibling, Germany kickstarted my healing journey. Not only do they have state-of-the-art treatment protocols, but they have alternate and modern medicine working side-by-side as well as staff and doctors who are 100% committed to helping you and treating Lyme disease. They believe it exists and that with the right treatment, it can be cured. Having such positive people around you is a big part of the healing process. That, in combination with extreme heat hyperthermia and their advanced detox therapies, is the reason why people get better from Lyme and cancer after going to this clinic. Here is important information if you are interested in going to St. Georg. This information is correct at the time of writing but please confirm with the Klinik or me if you are thinking of going.

St. Georg Klinik (SGK)

Center for Internal Medicine, Oncology, Immunology & Environmental Medicine

Medi-Therm Kliniken GmbH & Co. KG Rosenheimer Str. 6-8, 83043 Bad Aibling 08061-398-0 - Fax 08061-398-200

What Is SGK?

The St. Georg Klinik (SGK) is a place where people with Lyme disease and cancer go for treatment. It is an integrative therapy concept which combines conventional, alternative and scientifically-based therapies in one location.

What Sets SGK Apart from Other Places That Treat Lyme Disease?

In my opinion, the WBHT (Whole Body Hyperthermia) in combination with ozone therapy, detoxification and an immune biological support program is the key to healing from Lyme disease. Treatment includes IV vitamins and antibiotics, magnetic therapy, singlet oxygen, detox foot baths, colonic irrigation, enemas, herbal supplements and even Reiki, meditation and yoga. The fact that the medical staff and alternate therapists work together under one roof with a true belief that they can cure Lyme disease is truly amazing and unique.

Where Is the SGK Located?

The SGK is located in a gorgeous town called Bad Aibling, which is just under an hour from Munich.

What Are the Contact Details?

Phone: +49-8061-398-233

Fax: +49-8061-398-454

E-Mail: info@klinik-st-georg.de

Website http://www.klinik-st-georg.de/en/

How Do I Get There?

The nearest airport is Munich (MUC), and it is about a one hour drive from the clinic. On the way over, many patients find that it's easier to stopover for a day or two in order to break up the flight and preserve their health. If you live in Australia, I highly recommend a stopover for a day or two on the way over to help prevent jet lag. I also recommend Etihad Airways with a stopover in Abu Dhabi. Once you arrive in Munich, you can have the clinic organise a private transfer for you for about 85 euros, or you can just catch a cab (which is about the same amount). I recommend organising the transfer so that you can just relax and not stress about where to go.

Organising Transport from the Airport to the St. Georg Klinik

You can find precise directions on the website www.cancerclinicstgeorg. com under Contact. You can get there easily by public transport, but I highly recommend that you allow the SGK to arrange for a pickup by a shuttle company (do this when you leave as well). Again, all info including pricing can be found on the website.

The Director of Admissions, Gabi Rudolph (Gabi.Rudolph@klinik-st-georg. de) can arrange the shuttle pick up for you.

Will I Need Accommodations in Bad Aibling Before or After the Treatment?

You are more than welcome to arrive early or stay longer. However, the package includes your accommodations at the SGK the night before your treatment starts. On the day you are assigned to checkout, you should be ready to leave by about 10 a.m. This should help you with booking flights, accommodations and timing.

I've provided some links to hotels and apartments in Bad Aibling for you, if you decide to stay longer, and/or accompanying guests:

*Most patients like Hotel Lindner and Pension Helga

http://www.lindners.net/ (across from the clinic)

http://www.lindl-hof.de/

http://www.sanktgeorg.com/de/

http://www.schmelmer-hof.de/cms/

http://www.hotel-bihler.de/

http://www.ferienwohnungen-gallinger.de/

http://www.hotel-pension-maier.de/

Pension Helga – Rosenheimer Strasse 25, 83043 Bad Aibling. Five minute walk from the clinic.

TEL: +49 (0)8061 36171 (no website)

HYPERTHERMIA

The following information is taken and summarised straight from the SGK's website and includes my opinion along with extra information. (Lieberman n.d.)

Introduction

Malignant cells, cancerous tissues and microbes are heat-sensitive, and under certain conditions, they can be selectively destroyed by heat. Systemic whole body hyperthermia (SWBH) heats the body up to a temperature of 41.6°C (106°F) and above. SWBH is used principally in the advanced stages of cancer and is also used as a metastatic prophylaxis in high risk patients (e.g., young premenopausal women with breast cancer, lymph node involvement and negative hormone receptor status). SWBH also enhances the effects of adjuvant chemotherapy or radiation treatment and has been found extremely useful in the treatment of Lyme disease as well. SWBH cannot be compared to the fever therapy that is used in natural medicine. During fever therapy, bacterial lysates are injected, which then induce the release of cytokines, which then brings about a fever reaction. This fever only reaches a maximum of 39°C (102°F), which is not sufficient to induce enough thermal damage within the cancerous tissue. It must however be stated that the immunological effect of this treatment can improve the general condition of the patient, resulting in a positive response.

What are the different types of hyperthermia?

Superficial hyperthermia is specifically for small tumours located near the surface, that are often inoperable.

Local regional hyperthermia involves heating a larger and more deep-seated area of the body and is combined with chemotherapy.

Systemic whole body hyperthermia heats the entire body to a core temperature of 41.6°C+ (106°F+) using a specially developed device.

Extensive hyperthermia and extreme hyperthermia are great treatment options for oncological medicine and to treat Lyme disease. The treatment is carried out under sedation with oxygen saturation, pulse rate, blood pressure, core temperature, and electrolyte and blood gases strictly supervised and controlled. This allows the treatment to be carried out either on an inpatient or outpatient basis.

❖ Extreme Hyperthermia: From 41.5°C to 42.2°C (106°F–107°F) used at St. Georg Klinik

❖ Extensive Hyperthermia: Between 40.5°C and 41.5°C (104°F–106°F)

❖ High Hyperthermia: Between 39.5°C and 40.5°C (103°F–104°F)

❖ Medium Hyperthermia: Between 38.5°C and 39.5°C (101°F–103°F)

❖ Mild Hyperthermia: Between 37°C and 38.5°C (98°F–101°F)

How and why does whole body hyperthermia work for Lyme disease?

From my understanding and research, there are two main reasons why hyperthermia works well for Lyme disease (and cancer). The obvious reason is that a whole body fever is beneficial in killing bacteria, in this case Borrelia and co-infections (especially co-infections that are bacterial in nature). It is understood that Borrelia bacteria die at 105°F (40.5556°C), so to get maximum results, the body's core temperature must ideally reach this heat or higher for a significant period of time. At the SGK, they use extreme hyperthermia of 106°–107°F (41.1°-41.7°C). When I had extreme hyperthermia treatment, my body reached a top temperature of 107.8°F (42.11111°C). You are only at the top heat for a short period of time, hence the importance of going well above 105°F so that a significant amount of the treatment is hot enough to kill the Borrelia and its co-infections as well as release the cysts. On top of this, the Borrelia and other bacteria try to flee the heat, and the antibiotics in the bloodstream assist in the destruction of these bacteria.

The second and, in my opinion, the most effective part of the whole body hyperthermia is the way it supercharges the antibiotics. The day before you have your hyperthermia treatment, you will fast and have a colonic irrigation. You will have an enema on the morning of your hyperthermia to ensure that there is little food or waste in your digestive tract. You will be hooked up to monitoring equipment and a sedative will be administered through your temporary drip (you will also be hooked up to an antibiotic drip simultaneously). As your body temperature rises, the body looks for glucose to feed the cells and the brain. However, all it can find are the antibiotics, so it is believed that the antibiotics are up-regulated allowing them to be drawn into the cells and tissues, and across barriers that antibiotics would not usually be able to penetrate. This is the same process that occurs with cancer treatment, except chemotherapy drugs are supercharged and can penetrate the tumour / cancer at a much more aggressive rate.

Is whole body hyperthermia safe?

People always ask if hyperthermia is safe (I did as well before going to SGK). Before any patient is accepted for systemic whole body hyperthermia, stringent physical examination controls are carried out, including ECG, pulmonary function test, blood coagulation, blood count and blood gases. The patient is only accepted upon completion of these controls.

SWBH is carried out in a specially developed unit (WBH 2000 – Onco Therm, Germany) with intensive care control. Together with fever-stimulating substances (by injection), cytokines (interferons, interleukins) are introduced to modulate the immune system. Infrared light is introduced, which then brings the body temperature up to at least 41.1°C (106°F) and often higher. The patient's head (outside the unit) is cooled. In addition to the thermal damage and PH-shift, the increased heat has been shown to enhance the effect of the chemo drugs for cancer patients and IV antibiotics for Lyme patients without having to use high dosages. Thus the strong and often toxic side effects of these drugs can be overcome (when compared to regular chemotherapy treatment in cancer patients and long-term antibiotic use in chronically ill Lyme disease patients) using SWBH.

It is important that your body is detoxing as effectively as possible before you start treatment to ensure that your body can tolerate the heat. You are very closely monitored and have a nurse with you 100% of the time. If your body is not adapting and tolerating the heat, then the heat will not be increased any further, so it is a very safe and well-monitored procedure.

How Long Is the Lyme Program at SGK?

The treatment cycle is 14 days.

How Much Does It Cost?

15000 EUR

What Does the Lyme Disease Package Include?

Infusions and detoxification programs are established according to the individual situation, but everyone will receive:

- ❖ Daily care charge (around-the-clock nursing and doctor care)

- ❖ Initial and final lab controls

- ❖ Dark field blood analysis (if indicated or may be substituted with other tests such as VCS)

- ❖ CRS

- ❖ Infusions with vitamin C, chelation, selenium, procaine, antibiotics

- ❖ Ozone therapy

- ❖ Singlet oxygen therapy

- ❖ Laser therapy (red and green)

- ❖ Magnetic field treatment

- ❖ Detox foot baths

- ❖ Colon cleansing

- ❖ Systemic whole body hyperthermia x 2

- ❖ Detoxification program

- ❖ Daily oral medications and supplements

Other Services Available

Other services that are optional and cost extra may be recommended by the physicians based on a patient's individual clinical condition and wishes.

- ❖ Stress diagnostic or Lüschertest

- ❖ Dr. Douwes mouth hygiene – Detox set

- ❖ Reiki

- ❖ Physical therapy and massages

- ❖ Hormonal modulation

- ❖ Cell therapy for regeneration

- ❖ Yoga and meditation

    * Pricing can be provided upon request.

- ❖ **Are There Any Extra Expenses?**

- ❖ When needed, the cost for a central line is approximately 80 euros. It is not part of the package price, so it will be charged separately.

- ❖ Room and Board Accompanying Person (non-patient) / A day in the patient's room is 67.85 euros.

- ❖ Wi-Fi

Can I Bring a Friend or Family Member?

Yes, you can, and I highly recommend that you do. The program is quite intense, and it's nice to have someone there to comfort you and hang out, as there is a lot of sitting and lying around (usually hooked up to a machine or an IV). They can share a room with you or have a separate room for 68 euros a day (includes accommodations and meals).

How Do I Pay?

You can pay with certified bank cheques, traveler cheques (not smaller than $100 bills) or wire transfers. For a wire transfer, they will need a bank confirmation of the outgoing transaction. You can also pay by credit card (add an additional fee of 3% for Visa and MasterCard, and an additional 5% for American Express). However, with such a large amount of money, I don't recommend using a credit card!

Bank details for payment:

Account holder: St. George Hospital, Medi-Therm Kliniken GmbH & Co. KG

Bank: VR Raiffeisenbank Rosenheim eG, Tegernseestr. 20, 83022 Rosenheim

SWIFT Code: GENODEF1VRR

Branch Code No.: 71160000

Account No.: 7 249 470

IBAN: DE 31 711 600 00 000 72 494 70

It is important that they receive your payment before you check in. Please fax or email a copy of the payment and include your name and the address of your bank as well as the accountholder name (if different from your name). Have the bank write your name in RE.

Do I Need to Do Anything Before I Go?

Before, during and after my trip to Germany, I documented all the steps I took to successfully get well again. Over the years, the pre- and post-protocols for the STK have changed. Although each person will have a slightly different protocol (as we are all different), everyone should follow these general steps, which I believe need to be included in order to have the best chance of a full recovery.

<u>STOP MEDICATIONS AND ANTIMICROBIALS</u>

If possible, come off all antibiotics and antimicrobials for 2–3 months prior to going to SGK to give your body a rest and see what bacteria are just hiding in cyst form. Only do this if it doesn't make you feel worse or relapse. I kept taking some of mine until a week or two before my arrival. For example, I kept taking Byron White Formula A-Bab right up until we left for Germany, as my Babesia symptoms were too severe if I didn't. Some people feel better when they stop taking antibiotics (like me) and others deteriorate rapidly. It's important for this step to be managed by your primary care practitioner to ensure that it's safe and effective for you.

<u>DIET AND NUTRITION</u>

It is recommended that you follow *The Patient's Detoxx™ Book* by Patricia Kane (find it at BodyBio). I recommend that my patients stick to a Paleo-like diet. The basic rules are as follows: no caffeine, no sugar (even keep fruit to a maximum of one piece per day), no alcohol, no gluten, no processed foods, no vegetable oils, no grains (or soaked/sprouted if you are eating them), minimal corn or corn based products, minimal dairy (1-2 serves per week maximum if you can tolerate it), GMO free, ideally certified organic and drink filtered water. It sounds very restrictive, but eating clean is important. Because you're ingesting fewer toxins, your body is better able to detox the current toxins and die-off that are already overloading it. There are many great Paleo recipes including yummy salads and soups, so you don't need to go hungry or eat plain foods. I have actually kept eating this way since recovering, and I love it!

<u>SUPPLEMENTS</u>

Although supplements will be prescribed individually, the following supplements are recommended for everyone.

Supplement	Dose	Where to get it
BodyBio Phosphatidylcholine (PC): caps or liquid (detoxifier) *take on non-PC IV days*	Caps: 6 caps 1x day building to 6 caps 2x day Liquid: 1 tsp 1x day building to 1 tsp 2xday	order on http:// healthygoods.com or amazon.com
Ortho Molecular – Candicid Forte (antifungal)	1 cap 3x day and work up to 2 caps 3x day	order on www.iherb.com
Bioray™ NDF® (heavy metal chelator / detoxifier) *optional (I loved this supplement and highly recommend it)*	2 drops on an empty stomach before breakfast, working up to a full dropper (increase dose no quicker than every 3 days)	order on www.iherb.com

IVs

1–2 times per week for 2–3 months prior and 2–6 months post-treatment.

❖ Phosphatidylcholine (PC) – from Switzerland is the best (2 amps per IV)

❖ Glutathione –500mg per IV

❖ Vitamin C –50g per IV

There is a lot of debate as to which IV's should be infused together or if they should all be done separately. I had all three IV's infused together in 500ml of saline, and that worked well for me. Work with your team to work out the best combinations for you.

Kingsway Compounding (I had my IVs compounded here)

40/9 Powells Road

Brookvale NSW 2100 Australia

Tel: 1300 564 799

Fax: 1300 564 899

compounding@kingswaycompounding.com.au

Hours: Mon-Fri only, 9am to 5pm

What you need for the IVs?

- ❖ 500ml saline bags ($7 each)

- ❖ Giving sets ($10 each) – connect saline bag to the cannula in your arm or gripper needle

- ❖ Cannulas – 22G with a 25mm length ($5 each)

- ❖ 50ml syringe to prepare the mixture

- ❖ 19G and 21G needles to prepare

- ❖ Cotton balls and Band-Aids – use once the needle is removed

- ❖ Gloves – keep everything sterile whilst preparing

- ❖ Alcohol spray / wipes – to clean the point of entry for the needle

- ❖ If you have a portacath, you will also need gripper needles, 10ml syringes and heparinised saline

DAILY INFRARED SAUNAS

See the Infrared Sauna section in the Physical Treatment chapter

What Should I Pack?

❖ Comfortable clothes – the temperature inside is nice all year round

❖ Toiletries – toothbrush, toothpaste, soap, shampoo, conditioner, tampons, etc.

❖ Bathrobe / dressing gown

❖ Joggers – there is a beautiful park where you can stroll and get some fresh air

❖ Slippers / UGG® boots

❖ Nightgown / pyjamas / underwear / socks or stockings

❖ Reading material / reading glasses

❖ Stationery / pens

❖ Needlework or other recreational items

❖ Laptop / iPad with DVDs and games – There is TV, but it is in German. You will have a lot of downtime in your room, so it's super handy to have lots of movies or TV series to help pass the time

❖ Camera

❖ Supplements / medications, if required

**Recommend leaving any expensive jewellery at home

*** Make sure any gel nails are removed before leaving as you can't have them on for the whole body hyperthermia

Once I Return from Germany, What Do I Need to Do?

You will be given a full report from the STK when you leave the clinic.

You will need to do 2–6 months worth of IVs when you get home to help you detox properly. I recommend having it all ordered and ready so you can start straight away. I was delayed by six weeks and feel that this slowed my recovery.

I also recommend:

❖ A good whole food supplement (I take Juice Plus)

❖ A strong probiotic (either Metagenics, Bioceuticals® Ultrabiotic or VSL#3) – ideally dosed after stool testing for specificity (I used Bioscreen)

❖ High dose fish oil (once again Metagenics or Bioceuticals®)

❖ Fermented cod liver oil (I use Greener Pastures)

❖ Magnesium (best in powder form and my favourite for taste, quality and price is Bioceuticals® Ultra Muscleze)

❖ Adrenal support (if indicated via saliva or blood cortisol testing, e.g., Metagenics Adrenotone)

❖ Enzymes (I swear by VitälzymX www.worldnutrition.info, but it is expensive)

❖ Good liver support (I take DefenCELL® by Cell-Logic http://www.enduracell.com/defencell-capsules-1/defencell-capsules and Seeking Health Liver Formula)

❖ Fermented foods to heal your gut – e.g., sauerkraut, kefir, kombucha (they are easy to make, but you can order fermented foods and beverages online [e.g., GPA Wholefoods]), or if you live in Sydney, you can buy them at many health food and whole food stores, including our very own Health Space Wholefoods in Potts Point and Mona Vale.

Even as you start to feel better, don't overdo it! Keep your diet as clean as possible and drink lots of water. Sleep as much as possible and don't overdo it with exercise! Slowly and progressively get back to your old life! My rule is that it's better to do less and feel good than to overdo it and have to go back to square one! There may be times you need to give your body a rest from all supplements, too.

Is There Anything Else I Can Do to Prepare?

I understand that Lyme disease is very costly, both physically on your body, emotionally on your relationships and financially on your back pocket. It would be great if we could afford to have treatments every day. In an ideal world, I would recommend regular treatments with holistic health care practitioners such as chiropractic, massage, acupuncture, kinesiology, reflexology and naturopathy.

While nothing can take the place of having a Lyme-literate primary health care practitioner support your healing physically, biochemically and emotionally, there are many easy and inexpensive things you can do to help at home (as outlined in this book) such as skin brushing, keeping hydrated, making bone broths, Epsom salt baths, meditating, earthing (getting your bare feet on the earth) and, more importantly, rest and sleep!

Dr. Klinghardt's Lyme Disease 4-Step Treatment Protocol

One of my clients was under the care of Dr. Klinghardt, who is very well respected in the Lyme community, so I did some research on his protocols and really liked the way he addressed the disease. Dr. Klinghardt hypothesises that Borrelia could be "the bug that opens the door for all other infections to enter the system." He also believes that "microbes often invade tissues that have been injured: your chronic neck pain or sciatica really may be a Bb infection. The same may be true for your chronic TMJ problem, your adrenal fatigue, your thyroid dysfunction, your GERD and many other seemingly unrelated symptoms." In addition, "Many Bb symptoms are mistaken for problems of natural or premature ageing." Dr. Klinghardt believes that "the severity of symptoms correlates most closely with the overall summation or body burden of coexisting conditions and with the genetically determined ability to excrete neurotoxins." (Dr. Klinghardt's Treatment of Lyme Disease 2009)

Dr. Klinghardt's method is not a treatment that I am personally familiar with, but I wanted to add some information here so you can decide for yourself whether this option is worth further exploration. Please DO NOT use this information to self-treat.

1. *Decreasing the Toxic Body Burden / Unloading the System*

ESSENTIAL TOXIN ELIMINATION SUPPORT

❖ Quality and quantity sleep, including non-toxic bedding and the elimination of noise and light pollution

❖ Minimise / eliminate EMF

SHORT FORM OF TOXIN ELIMINATION AND ANTIMICROBIAL TREATMENT: "LE COCKTAIL"

❖ Freeze-dried garlic (for microbes, toxins, sulfur), chlorella (for viruses, bacteria, toxins, nutrients), cilantro (for bacteria, viruses, toxins) and fish oil (for microcirculation and cell wall flexibility)

LONG FORM OF TOXIN ELIMINATION

❖ Remove intestinal biofilm: 1 tsp clay followed by 1 tbsp fibre laxative for six weeks, prior to starting anything else

❖ Address genetic glitches (methylation, sulfation, acetylation—B12, B2, Folic acid, SAM-e, Methionine, Taurine, MSM)

❖ Mercury and metal detox: Phospholipid Exchange (EDTA, phospholipids, alpha lipoic, magnesium, energy), Matrix Metals, CVE and CGF, DMEP (ORS), sound cracked chlorella, nanonised chlorella and cilantro, EDTA, DMSA, DMPS

❖ Solvent and carbon-based detox: glycine, laser-or homeopathy aided detox

❖ Consider the UNDA remedies (243 is best)

SELF-HELP TOXIN REMOVAL

❖ Colon hydrotherapy and lymphatic drainage, rhythmic cranial and liver compression

❖ Dry skin brushing and warm / cold showers

❖ Swedish sauna and Toxaway Ionic Foot Bath

TOXIC INTERFERENCE FIELDS

❖ Jaw infections and devitalised teeth

❖ Chronic localised infections (tonsils, appendix, sinuses, etc.)

❖ Dysfunctional autonomic ganglia (superior cervical, sphenopalatine, pelvic ganglia, etc.)

REMOVE TOXIC, ALLERGENIC TRIGGERS FROM THE ENVIRONMENT

❖ Food allergies

❖ Volatile organic compounds (VOC's) from carpets, furniture and paint

❖ New car smell (phthalates and off gassing)

❖ Newspaper and office printing

❖ Work / profession-related compounds

REMOVE PSYCHOLOGICAL TOXINS

❖ 20 minute writing exercise to overcome past trauma

❖ Family constellation work to resolve trans-generational issues

❖ Applied psycho-neurobiology to resolve conflicts and severe trauma

❖ Regular time spent in nature

❖ Regular massage

❖ Qi Gong, Tai Chi or meditation

REMOVE STRUCTURAL TOXIC BLOCKAGES

❖ Optimise the dental occlusion to restore cranial lymphatic pump

❖ Cranio-sacral therapy to improve fluid dynamics in cranial nerves

❖ Visceral manipulation to improve organ function

2. *Improving Disturbed Physiology and Biochemistry*

(vitality, detox, immune responses, tissue repair)

BIOCHEMISTRY

Always start with KPU urine test and address it!

➢ Assessment via lab work or ART: correct what is missing and what is too much (hormones, minerals and electrolytes, glutathione, sulfur, etc.).

➢ Genetic testing: find minimal bypass nutrition to correct for SNPs or gene deletions / mutations.

➢ Diet: gluten and casein-free diet, Specific Carbohydrate Diet, metabolic typing, blood group diet or ART-based diet.

➢ Common deficiencies in Lyme: magnesium, which has to be given transdermally (through the skin) or via injection. Oral magnesium feeds spirochetes.

➢ Copper, zinc and iron are spent by macrophages and appear in oxidised form in hair and serum, giving the wrong appearance of excess.

➢ Over 80% of our Lyme patients have developed HPU (hemo-pyrrol-lactam-uria). The term incorrectly used in most U.S. literature is KPU (krypto-pyrrol-uria).

➢ HPU disarms the immune system by catastrophic depletion of zinc, manganese, arachidonic acid, histamine, taurine.

➢ These losses are hard to detect with any current technology. Only bone and CNS biopsies are reliable.

LABS TO CONSIDER

➢ KPU urine test (Vitamin Diagnostics)

➢ alkaline phosphatase low normal

➢ copper: zinc ratio in hair and urine

➢ low omega-6 in red cell membrane fatty acid test

➢ white blood cell zinc, red cell copper level.

If KPU is treated first and the system is restored to normal levels (4–8 months), Borrelia, Bartonella-like organisms and Babesia respond to much milder interventions without significant Herxes or problems.

<u>NEUROPHYSIOLOGY</u>

➢ Gives your brain healthy rhythms: KMT technology

➢ Listen to Lyme entrainment CD

➢ Spend time in nature

➢ Avoid EMFs: cordless phones, cell phones, wireless technology, home near airport (radar), computer

<u>EXERCISE</u>

➢ Stretching

➢ Weightlifting

➢ Movement (dance, Tai Chi, Qi Gong, etc.)

➢ Aerobic exercise – avoid post-exercise fatigue and pain

3. Decreasing the Microbial Count Using Rizols

Rizols (ozonated castor oil treated with high voltage electrolysis) have strong and specific antimicrobial properties, no known adverse long-term effects, are relatively inexpensive and are pleasant to take. They have been used successfully since 1905.

TREAT PARASITES, MOULD AND ANAEROBES

Step 1 Rizol Gamma (effective dose: 15–20 drops)

Step 2 Treat Viruses – Continue Rizol Gamma. To address both RNA (Borna, etc.) and DNA (HHV-6, EBV, etc.) viruses, add Rizol Zeta (20 drops).

Step 3 Treat Babesia – A full dose of Rizol Gamma and Zeta (from Steps 1 and 2) for two months will address Babesia.

Step 4 Bartonella – after two months of a full dose of Gamma and Zeta, stop or reduce Rizol Gamma and use Rizol My (20 drops), i.e., use Rizol Zeta and My together.

Step 5 Spirochetes – After another two months, reduce the dose of Rizols Zeta and My to 10 drops tid and add Rizol Epsilon and Jota (10 drops each)

Note: *Always follow Rizol with absorbent (biosorption): chlorella (20 tbl), chitosan (1–2 caps), zeolite (1 tsp) or charcoal (2 caps).*

Rizol recipes

Rizol-Gamma 70% Rizol-raw material (ozonated castor oil treated with high voltage electrolysis), 10% clove oil, 10% oil of artemesia, 10% black walnut oil

Rizol-Zeta 69.3% Rizol-raw material, 10% oil of artemesia annua, 10% clove oil, 5% black cumin oil, 5% moxa oil, 1.8% walnut oil, 0.9% oil of marjoram

4. *Immune Modulation*

❖ Use the CD-57 test (Labcorp's Stricker panel) to monitor immune status.

❖ Enderlein remedies: treat immune responses to mould – Pleo Nig, Not, Muc, Fort, Pef, Ut and UT-S, Lat

❖ Auto-hemotherapy or auto-urine therapy (2 ml biw)

❖ Buhner herbs (Quintessence from BioPure) 8–10 dropperfuls in 1 liter of water

❖ Adjunctive physics-based immune modulation tools:

  ➢ KMT frequency-based biofield treatment

  ➢ Health Light super LED treatment of focal areas

❖ Valkion: singlet oxygen energy delivery via inhaled air or drinking water

  ➢ Photon Wave or Jae Laser immune modulation

❖ Medical drugs: Occasionally the use of medical antimicrobials is beneficial in addition to this program (ILADS recommendations). These may include:

  ➢ Antivirals (Valtrex and Valcyte)

  ➢ Antifungals (Itra– and Voriconazole)

  ➢ Antiparasitics (Alinia and Biltricide)

  ➢ Antibiotics (with program mentioned earlier, minocycline, and antimalarials)

Buhner Core Protocol for Lyme Disease Treatment (Buhner n.d.)

Note: *Please refer to Buhner's website www.buhnerhealinglyme.com for his regularly updated protocols. They are not to be used to self-treat.*

Here are some of the herbs he recommends for Lyme disease: Japanese knotweed, Cat's claw (*Uncaria tomentosa*), Eleuthero (*Eleutherococcus senticosus*), Astragalus (*Astragalus membranaceus*) and Ashwagandha (*withania*)

For my clients and I, I use a prevention protocol that I learned from Steven Buhner of a minimum of 1,000 mg of astragalus daily if you live in a Lyme-endemic area. It is believed that this will keep the necessary immune markers at the right level in order to prevent infection, or if you are infected, to keep the disease symptoms as minimal as possible.

New Tick Bites

For new tick bites, he recommends taking 3,000mg of astragalus daily for 30 days and 1,000 mg daily thereafter, indefinitely.

Babesia

Buhner generally recommends the use of a *Sida acuta, Alchornea cordifolia*, and *Cryptolepis sanguinolenta* herbs either in isolation, as a blend or rotated for the treatment of Babesia. Stephen no longer recommends artemisinin or artemisia for Babesia infections. He believes they *can* work, but feels that *Sida acuta* will work better, especially for Babesia or Bartonella.

Bartonella

❖ Use of herbs such as *Sida acuta* tincture

❖ Hawthorne tincture

❖ Japanese knotweed

❖ EGCG

❖ Houttuynia (Yu Xing Cao powder)

❖ L-arginine and milk thistle seed

DO NOT USE L-ARGININE if you have active herpes, chicken pox, or shingles.

Mycoplasma

❖ Use of herbs such as Serrapeptase: 1 capsule daily on an empty stomach. This will help break the mycoplasma cell walls open and make them more vulnerable to the herbs.

❖ Raintree Nutrition Myco formula

❖ Cryptolepis, Bee pollen, Muscle tone blend, Eleutherococcus tincture, a general multivitamin supplement plus extra C, D, E, CoQ10, beta-carotene, quercetin, folic acid, bioflavoids and biotin in combination with a gluten-free diet (mycoplasma love gluten).

Candida

Stephen suggests reading his book, *The Fasting Path,* as fasting has shown some of the best results with tough-to-treat Candida. (Buhner 2003) He has also had success with a tincture combination of desert willow and chapparo amargosa.

OTHER TESTING TO CONSIDER

Pyrroluria

Many Lyme patients suffer from Pyrroluria (aka pyrrole disorder, krypto-pyrrol-uria), a metabolic illness where abnormal porphyrins carry out significant amounts of needed zinc and vitamin B6. Even though it is assumed that this illness is hereditary, every single Lyme sufferer I have met, (myself included) and anyone who is chronically ill for that matter, have at least a degree of it. Dr. Mercola has his doubts about its direct hereditary nature, too, and suspects that the appearance of kryptopyrroles in the urine can be "induced" by the illness, which I tend to agree with! Klinghardt believes that the correct term is actually HPU (hemo-pyrrol-lactam-uria) and that more than 80% of Lyme patients develop HPU. He says it disarms the immune system by depleting essential vitamins and minerals such as zinc, manganese, arachidonic acid, histamine and taurine. (Klinghardt 2009)

Genetic Testing

There are many options you can choose for genetic testing. Although genes can't be changed, their expression can be. Genes can be up- and down-regulated by our lifestyle and environment. So genetic testing is handy information to have, not just to improve your health but to give your body the best fighting chance, especially when you are already sick. In an ideal world, we would test our kids when they were young, then tailor their lifestyle to include exercise, nutrition and supplementation in order to support and optimise the genes they have inherited, which would give them the best chance at a healthy quality of life. There are some genes and SNPs discussed in the Detoxification and Methylation section, but I've included some here that, if mutated, can impact your health, particularly if you are already sick with a chronic disease like Lyme disease! Every little bit helps!

MAOA (monoamine oxidase A)

The MAOA gene codes for the enzyme active in serotonin breakdown as well as degrading other amine neurotransmitters such as dopamine and norepinephrine. A mutation in this breakdown can create mood swings, OCD or even aggressive behaviour.

COMT (catechol-O-methyltransferase)

COMT helps to break down important neurotransmitters and catechol-amines such as dopamine, epinephrine and norepinephrine. COMT is important in controlling brain functions, such as planning, short term memory, personality traits, attention and emotion, so a mutation (especially if homozygous [two mutated genes]) will cause symptoms and abnormal behaviours such as hyperactivity, irritability, erratic behaviour, poor attention span, short-term memory issues and even a lower threshold of pain. COMT is also important for processing estrogen.

NOS (nitric oxide synthase)

NOS is an enzyme that detoxes ammonia from the urea cycle, and a mutation will down-regulate this enzyme's activity. Therefore, a mutation in this enzyme leads to excess ammonia, and when CBS mutations are also present, it can have a compounded effect in the body.

SUOX

SUOX is an enzyme located in the mitochondria. Its job is to oxidise sulfite to sulphate as the last step in the metabolism of sulphur-containing compounds so the sulphur can be excreted. Sulfites can be generated as a byproduct of the methylation cycle, from foods containing sulphur that we ingest, food preparation and packaging, and certain preservatives in food and drinks. Sulphites give off the gas sulphur dioxide, which can cause irritation to the lungs, so the most common symptom of a mutated SUOX gene is difficulty breathing, as in wheezing and asthma.

ACE (angiotensin-converting enzyme)

If this gene is working properly, then your blood pressure will be well-maintained (as long as you have a healthy lifestyle, of course). The changes that affect this gene activity are caused by a deletion that can then contribute to high blood pressure, as ACE indirectly increases blood pressure by causing blood vessel constriction. Imbalances in this pathway have also been associated with anxiety and decreases in learning and memory. The essential mineral balance may also be affected. This causes increased excretion of sodium and potassium in the urine (provided the kidneys are functioning optimally), which has been linked to decreased energy production and, hence, fatigue.

Functional Medicine Testing

I use Healthscope and sometimes Nutripath to refer for functional testing for my clients and, of course, monitor my own health. These companies provide a range of tests including stool parasite tests, Helicobacter pylori, gut permeability, IgA, IgG food allergy / intolerance tests, base hormone tests, adrenal tests, thyroid tests, liver function tests and tests for heavy metals, to name a few. Work with your primary health care practitioner to get these test referrals, interpret the results and make necessary changes. I believe that doing this testing and working with my doctor and natu-ropath to make specific changes to MY lifestyle was one of the KEY parts of my recovery from Lyme disease. Instead of just guessing which supple-ments and doses to take, we worked out what would be best for MY body.

I have added some tests that may be useful for you. The information comes directly from the Healthscope website (Tests 2015):

Baseline Hormone Profiles—Male & Female

The Baseline Hormone Profile is a salivary test that provides valuable information on an individual's hormonal status and the potential impact that this may have on their physical and emotional health. Hormonal imbalance may result in a symptom picture that includes weight gain, mood swings, night sweats, disturbed sleep pattern, loss of libido and hot flushes. This testing is unique in that it helps identify the hormonal imbalances that may be causing chronic health problems. Results obtained from the test make it possible to individualise treatment in order to reestablish optimal hormone balance. The Baseline Hormone Profile is a non-invasive test which requires the collection of one saliva specimen, from which multiple hormones are tested including:

In males: Testosterone (TT), Oestradiol (E2), DHEA-S, Cortisol

In females: Oestrone (E1), Oestradiol (E2), Oestriol (E3), Progesterone (P4), Testosterone (TT) and DHEA-S

Adrenal Hormone Profile

The Adrenal Hormone Profile can be done in combination with the Baseline / Female Hormone Profile (I recommend this), and is a non-invasive saliva test which monitors the levels of the stress hormones cortisol and DHEA-S over the course of a day (6 a.m., 12 p.m., 6 p.m. and 10 p.m.). This is an important test to determine adrenal function in patients presenting with symptoms such as anxiety, depression, mood swings, insomnia, headaches, low energy, stress, hormonal imbalance and poor immune function. Altered levels of cortisol and DHEA-S are indicative of acute and/or chronic mental and/or physical stress. Prolonged stress causes increased secretion of cortisol and can eventually lead to hypertrophy of the adrenal cortex, adrenal exhaustion and immune suppression.

DHEA-S is the main androgen in both men and women and its levels naturally decline with age. Reduced levels of DHEA-S may result in fatigue, poor immune function, weight gain, increased ageing, memory loss and poor concentration. When you understand which time of day your adrenals are under the most stress, you can alter your lifestyle accordingly. You can also determine which adrenal support would be best for you, and the best time to take it.

Melatonin Profile

Melatonin is a neuropeptide predominantly produced by the pineal gland. Melatonin is secreted in a distinct circadian rhythm; it is stimulated by darkness, inhibited by light and independent of sleep. The phase of the circadian rhythm is influenced by day length (increasing in amplitude in the winter and decreasing in spring) or artificial light. The levels of melatonin in the body tend to decrease with age, and low levels may result in sleep disturbances such as insomnia, poor immune function, depression and other mood disorders. Due to its circadian rhythm, melatonin must be collected at midnight in the dark and again upon rising (6:00–8:00 a.m.). This test is helpful in combination with the Adrenal Hormone Profile for people who are stressed and find that it affects their sleep.

Thyroid Hormone Profile

Thyroid-stimulating hormone (TSH) is produced by the pituitary gland and activates the thyroid gland to produce thyroxine (T4) and triiodothyronine (T3). T4 is converted to T3 in the liver and requires the presence of selenium and zinc. T3 and T4 regulate the body's basal metabolic rate, influence heart and nervous system functions, and are essential for growth and development. The thyroid gland also produces calcitonin which is essential in the regulation of calcium balance in the body. The Thyroid Hormone Profile measures the levels of unbound, free hormones which are available to the tissues and reflects a true measure of the body's metabolic rate. Disorders of the thyroid are among the most common diseases of the endocrine glands, particularly in women. Thyroid function naturally decreases with age; an under-active thyroid or hypothyroidism (myxoedema) is most common in menopausal and postmenopausal women. Symptoms of an under-active thyroid include dry and coarse skin, weakness and lethargy, constipation, weight gain, a slow pulse, heavy and irregular periods and depression. Symptoms of an overactive thyroid, or hyperthyroidism (thyrotoxicosis), include a fast metabolic rate, a rapid heartbeat, nervousness and palpitations, and weight loss despite an increased appetite and frequent bowel movements.

Functional Liver Detoxification Profile (FLDP)

The Functional Liver Detoxification Profile (FLDP) challenges the liver's Phase I and Phase II detoxification capacity with low doses of caffeine, aspirin and paracetamol. Saliva and urine specimens, collected at timed intervals, are then analysed for metabolites of the three compounds to determine the efficiency of the liver in their conversion and clearance from the body. Phase I reactions utilise the Cytochrome P450 mixed-function oxidase (MFO) enzymes. The primary function of these enzymes is to oxidise endogenous and exogenous chemicals for excretion. This provides a mechanism of protection from a wide variety of toxins. Phase I is followed by an intermediate phase where oxygen-free radicals may be generated in substantial quantities, which in some instances may change harmless compounds into potentially toxic substances. Phase II reactions involve the addition of a small polar molecule to the substance, a conjugation step that may or may not be preceded by Phase I. Several types of conjugation reactions occur in the body, including glutathionation, sulphation, glucuronidation and glycination.

The results of an FLDP will support the accurate identification of the individual's detoxification profile and assist in the direction of treatment. The FLDP may provide particularly valuable information in the management of patients who suffer from food allergies, multiple chemical sensitivities, chronic fatigue syndrome, leaky gut and hormonal imbalances (e.g., premenstrual syndrome and menopausal symptoms). If your liver enzymes are affected on blood tests, then this is a great test to do.

FMA (Faecal Microbial Analysis)

In my opinion, Bioscreen Laboratories is the best lab available to perform a stool analysis. They perform a detailed quantification and qualification of intestinal microflora along with a detailed review based on laboratory research. The Bioscreen stool analysis is the most useful test available for determining microbial imbalances of the gut—whether they are a result of "bad" bugs or because of an imbalance of "good" bugs. Bioscreen tests are useful for patients with any kind of gut irritation or abnormality in stool consistency or frequency. Those diagnosed with or who have symptoms of autism, IBS, CFS or IBD usually find this test particularly useful. Because gut bacteria can produce amines / natural chemicals, the test may also be useful for those with food intolerances. Having specific information about your gut flora means you can address your treatment with specific protocols and probiotics, rather than just guessing with broad-spectrum probiotics!

I have done this stool test a few times. After six months of antibiotic therapy for Lyme disease and an 11-month healthy eating and supplementation program, my GIT was still a mess. My test results showed that I had low E. coli, very high Streptococcus and very high bifidobacterium. I was also taking very high doses of probiotics throughout my antibiotic therapy. Although this was better than having no good bacteria in my GIT, it did throw out the balance; some strains were actually too high, which is just as bad as having low levels. This is an example where not all natural supplements work well with your body. Because my bifidobacterium was so high and I continued to supplement with it, it did not allow my gut flora to restore. Once I received the results, I supplemented with Mutaflor® (prescription E. coli which, despite how it sounds, is actually quite safe), eliminated bifidobacterium from my diet and supplements, and changed my probiotics to target the good bacteria that were low in my GIT. It is essential that you work with someone who knows what they are doing because getting the GIT right is a game changer!

UEE Test (Urine Essential Elements) and UTM Test (Urine Toxic Metals)

It is essential for your health that you maintain an optimal trace mineral balance in your body. When you are chronically ill, stressed, have gene mutations or are taking medications, these trace levels can be affected. Many people already know the importance of supplementing, but the best way to know exactly what your levels are is to do a UEE test. Then you can monitor your progress and efficacy of supplementation using a weekly spot UTM test. Leave it to your doctor to interpret this testing. However, Amy Yasko has some general guidelines (Yasko 2008) that may help you when reviewing your results. Remember, when reviewing them, you are looking for "optimal" levels rather than just being "normal" range.

Optimal levels:

❖ Calcium and copper in the low / normal range

❖ No detectable iron on a urine essential element test

❖ Magnesium, molybdenum and selenium in the high end of normal

❖ Zinc levels should be slightly above 50% but lower than magnesium levels.

❖ Chromium and boron in the mid-range

❖ Sodium, potassium and phosphorus should be in a similar range on either side of 50%.

❖ You should have more zinc than copper. Look for the zinc / copper ratio to be greater than one.

CHAPTER 11 –
TRAVEL TIPS

PROTECT YOURSELF FROM JET LAG AND THE HARMFUL EFFECTS OF FLYING TBM STYLE!

Flying in an airplane brings a whole set of stressors that often derail the process of healing unless you are as prepared as possible. Those problems are primarily caused by radiation, dehydration, prolonged sitting, time zone changes, sleep deprivation, air sickness, neck strain, and the adrenaline surge from the excitement or stress of visiting new places. Many of my recommendations come from Kevin Millet and the TBM kinesiology study I have done as follows:

Dehydration – Drink more water than normal a few days before the flight so you are super hydrated. Bring your own drink bottle (empty if need be) so you can fill it up on board. If you can't bring your own drink bottle then ask the flight attendant for extra water at each meal. Drink ONLY water while flying. Remember, you need to drink a minimum of 43ml of water per 1kg of body weight every 24 hours. Calculate your minimum and then drink a litre more than that while flying if you can. I always ask for one of the big water bottles the flight attendants have in their onboard kitchen to save having to keep asking for water.

Prolonged sitting – Get up from your seat frequently, which will happen, more or less, automatically because of all of the water you're drinking. Spend some time moving around while you are up. Take a stroll to the back of the plane, do some stretching, move your body around. If you find that on long flights, you tend to have fluid pool in your lower limbs, you may want to purchase support stockings at a chemist or medical supply store before you fly and do the recommended exercises to prevent DVT (deep vein thrombosis), as this will help keep the fluid moving. Even just doing simple calf raises whilst sitting, or pointing and flexing your toes are easy ways to improve lower limb circulation.

Sleep deprivation – Sleep on the plane. Take a light-blocking eye mask. If you forget, most airliners have them. Try and go to bed and get up in the new time zone straight away to maintain your sleep cycle. Take a short nap in the day if needed.

Air sickness – If you experience air sickness, firmly tap a point halfway between the bottom of your sternum and your belly button for 30 to 60 seconds. Repeat as necessary to decrease nausea / sickness. This can be used for any nausea anytime.

Neck strain – Invest in a neck pillow. It can be a lifesaver. They are always available in airport gift shops but significantly cheaper if you buy one before you get to the airport. I often take my contour memory foam pillow as hand luggage and use it to sleep on. It's especially handy if the plane isn't full and you can lie down across a few seats!

Adrenal excitement or stress – Traveling is fun and exciting for some, yet the preparation and flight may be stressful, too. If you are super busy, stressed or sick leading up to your flight, I highly recommended that you take an adrenal supplement (for recommendations, see the table in Chapter 7 Overview of Supplements for Specific Systems Directly and Indirectly Affected by Lyme Disease, and Opportunistic and Co-infections). See your naturopath or TBM practitioner, if possible, for the correct prescription. If you support the adrenal glands before and during your flight, you will likely have more energy to enjoy your holiday once you get there! If you are taking adrenal support already then just continue!

Circadian rhythm disruption – Crossing time zones can significantly upset your circadian rhythm (also known as your body clock) and is one of the biggest contributors to jet lag. The NET homeopathic remedy #24 Day & Night Vitals is great to prevent and treat jet lag. You can take 9–12 sprays under the tongue as often as needed whilst on the plane and 3x a day afterwards until body clock is back in synch.

Following I have outlined some more tips for radiation protection and jet lag that are best implemented by a qualified TBM or NET practitioner.

Dealing with Radiation – *You will need two flying protection vials from your TBM practitioner. They can be used as many times as you like (best stored in salt between trips).*

Once you get above the atmosphere, you are exposed to a lot more radiation. There are flying protection vials and a kinesiology protocol that can help protect you from the harmful effects of radiation.

Before getting on the plane

Take two flying protection vials and put them on your body within five minutes of getting on the plane (pockets, bra or socks are ideal, so there is one on each side of your body).

Once in your seat, complete the following body tapping combinations:

1. Place five fingertips together and tap the mid-forehead once

2. With the back of your hand, tap the top of your head once

3. With five fingertips together, tap the mid-forehead again

4. Cross your arms and tap across your chest with your fingers extended and thumbs pointing away from you

5. Finish with your left hand holding your right wrist and making a light thrust downwards over the pubic region

It sounds confusing on paper, so it is best to get someone who knows the protocol to show you!

Getting off the plane

(ideally done within five minutes off getting off the plane)

1. Within five minutes of getting off the plane, remove the vials and store them away safely

2. Repeat the tapping combinations that you used when you got on the plane

* *Repeat this with every boarding and disembarking of an airplane.*

Dealing with Time Zone Changes

To program your body to the local time zone, rub the Spleen 21 point (left rib cage halfway between the armpit and the bottom of the rib cage) for 30 seconds. Immediately following, rub both ears beginning at the bottom and working toward the top as if you were trying to uncurl or flatten the ears (use the thumb on the front of the ear and the index finger on the back of the ear). Do one pass up and one down. If you arrive less than three hours away from going to bed, then wait to do this in the morning, preferably prior to your feet touching the ground. Anyone who experiences broken sleep (e.g., shift workers and mums) and wants to reprogram their body clock can use this technique, too.

**Radiation protection and time zone procedures in combination with hydration eliminate jet lag in virtually all cases.*

CHAPTER 12 –
PETS AND LYME DISEASE

Don't forget that your furry friends are also susceptible to Lyme disease and other co-infections. Many animals are closer to the ground and have more hair than the average human, so not only is it easier for ticks to get on them and attach, but it's harder to see and find them. The easiest way to prevent Lyme in your pets is to avoid woody, tick-infested areas. It's important to routinely check your pet for ticks, particularly if you live in high-risk areas or have visited any recently. If you pull a tick off your pet, you can always have the tick tested for Lyme if your pet displays any of the common signs and symptoms of Lyme. This is more accurate than testing the animal itself (just like in humans!). Vets can also check your pet for Lyme disease. Remember that if your pet comes inside, it can potentially carry ticks inside that may later attach to you or your family.

It's not just pets that carry ticks, but also other animals and pests. If you have animals like possums or rats in your roof, then your best bet is to try to get rid of them humanely so they don't carry ticks into your house. I had a possum living in our roof and believe this is how the ticks were getting into my home.

INFORMATION AND SYMPTOMS FOR VARIOUS ANIMALS

Dogs

There is a vaccine against Lyme disease for dogs, but the vaccine is somewhat controversial. Most veterinarians only recommend vaccinating dogs that live in tick-infested areas. For more information about tick control products, consult your veterinarian.

Symptoms: arthritis (sudden lameness), pain, fever, lack of appetite, dehydration, inactivity, and swollen lymph nodes and joints.

Cats

Lyme disease in cats is rare but not unheard of. In most cases, Lyme is diagnosed only when an infected tick is discovered.

Symptoms: pain, stiffness in limbs and joints, lameness, fever, loss of appetite, fatigue, sudden collapse, a zombie-like trance, and in cases of heavy infestation, severe anaemia

Horses

Lyme disease is quite common in horses. I have been told that it is believed that 50% of horses in high-risk areas will contract Lyme disease during their lifetime. Horses are at a higher risk than other animals because ticks often go unnoticed. An adult tick is usually large enough to be detected during grooming, if you are particular. Check for ticks around the head, throat, and belly, and under the tail. To decrease the chance of infection, check the horse regularly and remove ticks quickly and safely.

Symptoms: chronic weight loss, erratic lameness, laminitis (inflammation of the tissues inside the hoof wall), fever, swollen joints, muscle tenderness, eye inflammation and stiffness.

Neurological signs: depression, dysphagia (difficulty swallowing), head tilt and encephalitis.

DIAGNOSIS

It's difficult to accurately diagnose animals with Lyme disease. In most cases, a Lyme diagnosis is based on whether the pet lives in a tick-infested area, has signs of arthritis and/or responds to treatment.

TREATMENT

Similar to humans, pets can be treated with antibiotics and usually respond quite quickly if they do have Lyme disease. If there is no improvement, let your vet know. Just like humans, if Lyme disease is left untreated in your pet, then the disease is likely to progress to chronic Lyme, which is not only harder to treat, but can cause kidney damage or even death.

WORKS CITED

[FDA], U.S. Food and Drug Administration. "Parabens." 2015.

ACIDS. *Australian Chronic Infectious Disease Society Guidelines.* PDF, Sydney: ACIDS Limited, 2014.

American Academy of Environmental Medicine. 2015. https://www.aaemonline.org/gmo-pressrelease.php (accessed June 15, 2015).

Anglesey, Debby. "Hidden Names for MSG." *Battling the MSG Myth.* April 2014. http://msgmyth.com/hidden_names_for_msg.html (accessed 2014).

Apple. "iTunes Apps."

Asokan, Sharath, et al. "Effect of oil pulling on Streptococcus mutans count in plaque and saliva using Dentocult SM Strip mutans test: a randomized, controlled, triple-blind study." *J Indian Soc Pedod Prev Dent* 26, no. 1 (2008): 12-17.

Asokan, Sharath, P Emmadi, and R Chamundeswari. "Effect of oil pulling on plaque induced gingivitis: a randomized, controlled, triple-blind study." *Indian J Dent Res* 20, no. 1 (2009): 47-51.

Asokan, Sharath, R S Kumar, P Emmadi, Raghuraman, and N Sivakumar. "Effect of oil pulling on halitosis and microorganisms causing halitosis: a randomized contolled pilot trail. [PubMed Abstract]." *J Indian Soc Pedod Prev Dent* 29, no. 2 (2011): 90-94.

Barwick, Steve. "Colloidal Silver Cures MSRA Infections." *Colloidal Silver Secrets.* February 4, 2008. http://colloidalsilversecrets.blogspot.com/2008/02/does-colloidal-silver-really-cure.html (accessed 2014).

"Basic Steps to Your Emotional Freedom." *Mercola.com.* http://eft.mercola.com (accessed 2014).

"Biofilm: Background." *Fry Laboratories, L.L.C. Tomorrow's Diagnostics Today.* http://frylabs.com/services-list/biofilm/.

"Bone Broth, Broths and Stocks." *Nourished Kitchen.* 2015. http://nourishedkitchen.com/bone-broth/.

"Bowen technique." *Wikipedia: The Free Encyclopedia.* July 22, 2015. https://en.wikipedia.org/wiki/Bowen_technique.

"Brain ." *Florida Action Network.* http://fluoridealert.org/issues/health/brain/.

Bransfield, Robert. "Lyme Disease and Cognitive Impairments." *Mental Health and Illness.* September 2013. http://www.mentalhealthandillness.com/Articles/LymeDiseaseAndCognitiveImpairments.htm.

Buhner, Stephen. *The Fasting Path: The Way to Spiritual, Physical and Emotional Enlightenment.* New York: Penguin Publishing Group, 2003.

"The Protocols." *Buhner healing lyme.* http://buhnerhealinglyme.com/the-protocols/ .

Burrascano, James J. "Advanced Topics in Lyme Disease: Diagnostic Hints and Treatment Guidelines for Lyme and Other Tick Borne Diseases. 16th ed." *International Lyme and Associated Diseases Society (ILADS).* October 2008. http://www.ilads.org/lyme/B_guidelines_12_17_08.pdf.

Byrne, Rhonda. *The Magic.* New York: Atria Books, 2012.

ChangingMinds.org. "Values Deveolopment." *Changing Minds.* http://changingminds.org/explanations/values/values_development.htm.

Chenggang Jin, Deanna J. Fall, Diana Roen, Gottfried Kellerman. "iSpot Lyme: A New Generation of Lyme Disease Testing." *NeuroScience Assess & Address.* April 2013. https://neurorelief.com/index.php?p=cms&cid=486&pid=149 (accessed 2014).

"Chiropractic FAQs." *Chiropractors' Association of Australia.* February 6, 2015. www.chiropractors.asn.au (accessed 2014).

"COWDEN SUPPORT PROGRAM: Protocol for Borrelia and Lyme Co-Infections & Most Chronic Conditions." *BIONATUS News and Research: NutraMedix.* 2011. http://www.nutramedix.ec/ns/lyme-protocol (accessed 2014).

"Diagnosis." *Lyme Disease Association of Australia.* 2015. http://www.lymedisease.org.au/about-lyme-disease/diagnosis/#testing.

"Diagnosis." *Lyme Disease Association of Australia.* 2015. http://www.lymedisease.org.au/about-lyme-disease/diagnosis/#testing (accessed 2015).

"Do you experience symptoms from EMR? ." *EMR Australia Pty Ltd.* 2014. http://www.emraustralia.com.au/EMR_symptoms.html.

"Dr. Klinghardt's Treatment of Lyme Disease." August 4, 2009. http://articles.merco-la.com/sites/articles/archive/2009/08/04/Dr-Klinghardts-Treatment-of-Lyme-Disease.aspx (accessed 2014).

"Dr. Ron's Ultra-Pure: the additive free company." *Grassfed New Zealand Freeze-Dried Organs & Glands.* 2015. http://www.drrons.com/organ-and-glandular-supple-ments/index.html (accessed 2014).

Edelman, Sarah. *Change Your Thinking [e-book].* 3rd ed. ABC Books, 2013.

EPA. "Drinking Water Contaminants." *EPA United States Environmental Protection Agency.* October 29, 2014. http://water.epa.gov/drink/contaminants/index.cfm.

"Exercise Physiology." *Wikipedia: The Free Encyclopedia.* https://en.wikipedia.org/wiki/Exercise_physiology.

"Fact Sheet-Is Chiropractic Safe?" *Chiropractors' Association of Australia.* http://chiro-practors.asn.au/images/stories/Files/Chiropractic Fact Sheets/Fact Sheet - Safety.pdf (accessed 2015).

"Fact Sheet-Neck Adjustment Safety and Benefits." *Chiropractors' Association of Australia.* www.chiropractors.asn.au (accessed 2014).

Fife, William. "Lyme Disease and Hyperbaric Oxygen Therapy." *Hyperbaric Therapy Center of Rome.* January 29, 1998. http://hyperbarictherapycenterofrome.com/condi-tions/lyme_disease.shtml.

"FM Criteria Work Sheet. PDF." *National Data Bank for Rheumatic Diseases.* 2015. https://www.arthritis-research.org/sites/default/files/FM%20Criteria%20Work%20Sheet.pdf (accessed 2015).

Forsgren, Scott. "From a Source of Profound Insight Comes Hope: A Master's Update on the Treatment of Lyme Disease." *Public Health Alert: Investigating Lyme Disease & Chronic Illness in the USA.* Vol. 5. no. 4. April 2010.

Gardner, Cindee. "Treating Lyme Disease Naturally & Effectively." Revised 2012. http://www.cindeegardner.com/articles/9545617127/treating-lyme-disease-naturally.

Gladstein, J. "Headache." *Med Clin North Am* 90, no. 2 (2006): 275-90.

Goldman, L R, and S Koduru. "Chemicals in the Environment and Developmental Toxicity to Children: A Public Health and Policy Perspective." *Environ Health Perspect* 108, no. Suppl 3 (2000): 443-448.

Golightly, Marc G., and Josephine A. Thomas. "Lyme Borreliosis serologies in per-spective." *Clinical Immunology Newsletter.* Vol. 11. November 8, 2002. 113-118.

Harra, Carmen. *The Eleven Eternal Principles: Accessing the Divine Within.* Berkeley: Crossing Press, 2009.

Hassad, Craig. "Mindfulness @ Monash: The health benefits of medication and being mindful." *Foundation 49: Men's Health.* May 8, 2012. www.49.com.au/wp-content/uploads/The-health-benefits-of-meditation-and-being-mindful_v21-2.pdf (accessed June 15, 2015).

"Health Benefits of Bone Broth." *The Paleo Mom.* 2012. http://www.thepaleomom.com/2012/03/health-benefits-of-bone-broth.html.

"Health Risks." *Institute for Responsible Technology.* 2010. http://www.responsible-technology.org/health-risks (accessed 2014).

Healthy, Get Living. "Do We Live In A Toxic World? Lost in Toxic World of Warcraft... NO." October 7, 2010.

Hicks, Esther, and Jerry Hicks. *Ask and It Is Given: Learning to Manifest Your Desires.* Carlsbad: Hay House, 2004.

"Home Test Kit." *EMF Australia Pty Ltd.* 2014. http://www.emraustralia.com.au/EMR_meters.html.

Horowitz, Richard. *Why Can't I Get Better? Solving the Problem of Lyme and Chronic Disease.* New York: St. Martin's Press, 2013.

Horowitz, Richard, and Ann Corson. "Byron White Formulas Brochure." *Why Byron White Formulas?* Victoria: John Coleman.

"How To Make Bone Broth." *Wellness Mama [Blog].* http://wellnessmama.com/5888/how-to-make-bone-broth/.

humanERGETIC THERAPIES. "What can Hyperbaric Oxygen therapy do for you?" *Hyperbaric Oxygen Therapy.* 2015. http://www.humanergetics.com.au/hyperbaric.php.

Infectolab Australia. "Overview of the many frequent co-infections accompanying Lyme Disease." *Infectolab Australia.* 2014. http://www.infectolab.com.au/Pages/Coinfections.aspx.

International College of Applied Kinesiology Australian Chapter. www.icaka.org.au (accessed 2014).

Izikson, L. "The flushing patient: differential diagnosis, workup, and treatment." *J Am Acad Dermatol* 55, no. 2 (2006): 193-208.

Jaminet, Paul. "The PHD Food Plate." *PerfectHealthDiet.* August 14, 2011. http://perfecthealthdiet.com/2011/08/the-phd-food-plate/ (accessed 2014).

Johnson, Larry E. "Vitamin D." *Merck Manual: Professional Version.* October 2014. http://www.merckmanuals.com/professional/nutritional_disorders/vitamin_deficiency_dependency_and_toxicity/vitamin_d.html (accessed 2014).

Keel, Phillip. "Keel's Simple Diary App."

Klinghardt, Dietrich. "Dr. Klinghardt's Treatment of Lyme Disease." *Mercola.com.* 2009. http://articles.mercola.com/sites/articles/archive/2009/08/04/Dr-Klinghardts-Treatment-of-Lyme-Disease.aspx.

Klippel, John. "Chronic Fatigue Syndrome and Fibromyalgia." *Arthritis Foundation.* http://www.arthritis.org/living-with-arthritis/tools-resources/expert-q-a/fibromyalgia-questions/chronic-fatigue-syndrome-fibromyalgia.php.

Kresser, Chris. "9 Steps to Perfect Health." *Chris Kresser: Let's Take Back Our Health.* 2015. http://my.chriskresser.com/wp-content/uploads/membership-files/free/9-Steps-To-Perfect-Health.pdf.

Kumar, S S, P Emmadi, and R Raghuraman. "Mechanism of oil-pulling therapy – in vitro study." *Indian J Dent Res* 22, no. 1 (2011): 34-37.

Lieberman, Shari. "Hyperthermia." *Klinik St. Georg: Bad Aibling.* Townsend Letter. http://www.klinik-st-georg.de/en/klinik/therapies/hyperthermia/.

linkin. "Benefits of the salt/vit.C protocol [Blog]." *CureZone.* October 28, 2005. http://www.curezone.org/forums/am.asp?i=478977 (accessed 2014).

Lombard, Robert M. "Lyme Disease." *The Robert M. Lombard Hyperbaric Oxygenation Medical Center, Inc. Lyme Disease and Treatment with HBOT.* 2008. http://hboxygen.freeyellow.com/id36.html (accessed 2014).

Lourie, Bruce, and Rick Smith. *Toxin Toxout. 2013. St. Lucia: University of Queensland Press.* St. Lucia: University of Queensland Press, 2013.

Lu, Z, S Wang, Z Sun, R Niu, and J Wang. "In vivo influence of sodium fluoride on sperm chemotaxis in male mice ." *Archives of Toxicology* 88, no. 2 (February 2014): 533-9.

Lynch, Benjamin. *MTHFR.Net.* www.mthfr.net.

Lynch, Diahanna, and David Vogel. "Council on Foreign Relations." *The Regulation of GMOs in Europe and the United States: A Case Study of Contemporary European Regulatory Politics.* April 5, 2001. http://www.cfr.org/agricultural-policy/regulation-gmos-europe--united-states-case-study-contemporary-european-regulatory-politics/p8688.

Makman, Maynard H. "Morphine receptors in immunocytes and neurons." *Adv Neuroimmunol* 4, no. 2 (1994): 69-82.

Mansour, H H, and S S Tawfik. "Efficacy of lycopene against fluoride toxicity in rats." *Pharmaceutical Biol* 50, no. 6 (June 2012): 707-11.

Mayne, Peter. "Emerging incidence of Lyme borreliosis, babesiosis, bartonellosis, and granulocytic ehrlichiosis in Australia." *Int J Gen Med* 4 (Dec 2011): 845-852.

McFadzean, Nicola. *Lyme Disease in Australia: Fundamentals of an Emerging Epidemic.* South Lake Tahoe: BioMed Publishing, 2012.

The Lyme Diet: Nutritional Strategies for Healing from Lyme Disease. South Lake Tahoe: BioMed Publishing, 2010.

Mercola, Joseph. "Guidelines for Safe Usage of Colloidal Silver: Dr. Mercola's Comments." *Mercola.com.* February 2009. http://articles.mercola.com/sites/articles/archive/2009/02/07/new-guidelines-released-for-safe-usage-of-colloidal-silver-supplements.aspx (accessed 2014).

"Important Facts You Need to Know About Water Fluoridation." December 7, 2014. http://articles.mercola.com/sites/articles/archive/2014/12/07/important-facts-water-fluoridation.aspx.

"The Most Dangerous Types of Water You Can Drink." *Dr. Mercola Healthy Home.* December 20, 2010. http://waterfilters.mercola.com/drinking-water-filter.aspx (accessed 2014).

"Why Walking Barefoot Might Be an Essential Element of Good Health." *Mercola.com.* September 20, 2012. http://articles.mercola.com/sites/articles/archive/2012/09/20/barefoot-on-electron-deficiency.aspx (accessed 2014).

Metcalfe, D D. "Food allergy." *Prim Care* 25, no. 4 (1998): 812-29.

Moorjani, Anita. *Dying to Be Me: My Journey from Cancer, to Near Death, to True Healing.* Sydney (Australia): Hay House, 2012.

Morones-Ramirez, Jose Ruben, Jonathan A Winkler, Catherine S Spina, and James J Collins. "Silver Enhances Antibiotic Activity Against Gram-Negative Bacteria." *Science Translational Medicine* 5, no. 190 (June 2013).

"National Research Council, 2006." *FLUORIDEALERT.ORG: Florida Action Network.* http://fluoridealert.org/researchers/nrc/findings/.

Nickerson, Krista. "Environmental Contaminants in breast milk ." *J Midwifery Women's Health* 51, no. 1 (2006): 26-34.

Nixon-Livy, Michael J. "Mercola.com." *Gentle Hands Can Restore Your Health.* January 2015. http://www.mercola.com/nst/neurostructural-integration-technique.htm (accessed 2014).

"Nutrigenetics." *Wikipedia: The Free Encyclopedia.* July 20, 2014. https://en.wikipedia.org/wiki/Nutrigenetics.

"Nutrigenomics." *Wikipedia: The Free Encyclopedia.* June 17, 2015. https://en.wikipedia.org/wiki/Nutrigenomics.

"Organic Claims." *Australian Competition and Consumer Commission.* http://www.accc.gov.au/consumers/groceries/organic-claims (accessed 2014).

Oschman, James L. "Can electrons act as antioxidants? A review and commentary." *J Altern Complement Med* 13, no. 9 (November 2007): 955-967.

Pavia, Charles. "Preliminary in vitro and in vivo Findings of Hyperbaric Oxygen Treatment in Experimental Bb Infection [PDF]." *The HYPERBARIC Therapy Center.* March 2000. http://www.hypertc.com/articlepage.cfm?id=51.

Pollan, Michael. *Food Rules: An Eater's Manual.* New York: Penguin Books, 2009.

Researched Nutritionals: solutions for life. 2015. https://www.researchednutritionals.com (accessed 2014).

RestorMedicine. 2015. http://shop.restormedicine.com/main.sc.

Return to Stillness. "BYRON WHITE FORMULAS: General Usage." Victoria .

Romero-Franco, M, et al. "Personal care product use and urinary levels of phthalate metabolites in Mexican women." *Environ Int* 37, no. 5 (July 2011): 867-71.

"Room Air Purifiers." *Breathing Easy.* http://www.breathing-easy.net/iqair/room-air-purifiers.

Rosa, Gabriela. *The Awful Truth About Cleaning Products and Fertility Revealed.* U.S.: Edes Publishing Company, 2008.

Rosner, Bryan. *When Antibiotics Fail: Lyme Disease and Rife Machines.* South Lake Tahoe: BioMed Publishing Group, 2005.

Roy, Sabita, and Horace H Loh. "Effects of opioids on the immune system." *Neurochem Res* 21, no. 11 (1996): 1375-1386.

Sarah. "How to Turn Baking Soda into Washing Soda ." *Nature's Nurture.* May 8, 2012. http://naturesnurtureblog.com/2012/05/08/ttt-turn-baking-soda-into-washing-soda/ (accessed 2014).

Schaller, James. *A Laboratory Guide to Human Babesia Hematology Forms. .* Naples: Hope Academic Press., 2008.

Shaeffer, Michelle. "Naturally Frugal Cleaning." *FrugalFun.com.* http://www.frugalfun.com/cleansers.html (accessed 2014).

Sifonis, Jenna. "Spiritual Protection and Unwanted Negative Energies." *Memory Release Therapies.* 2013. http://www.memoryreleasetherapies.com.au/spiritual-protection-unwanted-negative-energies/.

Singleton, Kenneth. *The Lyme Disease Solution.* South Lake Tahoe: BioMed Publishing, 2008.

Strasheim, Connie. *The Lyme Disease Survival Guide.* South Lake Tahoe: BioMed Publishing , 2008.

Stricker, R B, and E E Winger. "Decreased CD57 lymphocyte subset in patients with chronic Lyme disease." *Immunol Letters* 76 (2001): 43-48.

Stricker, R B, Joseph J Burrascano, and Edward E Winger. "Longterm decrease in the CD57 lymphocyte subset in a patient with chronic Lyme disease." *AAEM,* 2002: 111-113.

Sylver, Nenah. *The Holistic Handbook of Sauna Therapy.* Glendale: Center for Frequency Education, 2003.

"Table 1: Characteristics of epidemiological studies of fluoride exposure and children's cognitive outcomes." *Environ Health Perspect* 120, no. 10 (October 2012): 1362-1368.

"Tests." *Healthscope Pathology.* 2015. http://www.healthscopepathology.com.au/index.php/functional-pathology/tests/ (accessed 2014).

"The 2014 International Congress on Natural Medicine Conference (Metagenics)." Sydney.

"The Breathing Well Program: Re-learning Breathing and Posture." *Breathing Well Pty Ltd.* 2015. http://www.breathingwellopt.com/ (accessed 2014).

"Top tips for safer products." *EWG's Skin Deep Cosmetics Database.* http://www.ewg.org/skindeep/top-tips-for-safer-products/ (accessed 2014).

Vandenberg, L N et al. "Human exposures to biphenol A: mismatches between data and assumptions [info from metagenics detox seminar] Rev Environ Health." *Rev Environ Health* 28, no. 1 (2013): 37-58.

Viebahn-Haensler, Renate. *The Use of Ozone in Medicine.* 4th English. Iffezheim, Germany: Odrei Publishers, 2002.

"Vitamin D Insufficiency." *Healthscope Pathology.* http://www.healthscopepathology.com.au/files/2213/3341/7754/HPG-1051_W_Vitamin_D_Insufficiency.pdf (accessed September 12, 2015).

An Inconvenient Tooth. Directed by Guy Wagner. 2012.

Wang, S, R Niu, J Wang, and Z Lu. "In vivo influence of sodium fluoride on sperm chemotaxis in male mice." *Archives of Toxicology* 88, no. 2 (Feb 2014): 533-9.

"What Do I Do?" *Surviving Mold.* http://www.survivingmold.com/treatment.

"What Tests to Order." *IGeneX, Inc.* http://www.igenex.com/Website/ (accessed 2014).

"What's In a Bone?" *Paleo Leap.* 2015. http://paleoleap.com/eat-this-bone-broth/.

Whitmont, Ronald. "Homeopathy and Lyme Disease." *Ronald D. Whitmont, M.D.* 2012. http://www.homeopathicmd.com/2012/04/homeopathy-and-lyme-disease/.

"Why Certified Organic." *The Divine Company.* (accessed 2014).

Yasko, Amy. *Autism: Pathways to Recovery [PDF].* 2008.

Zhang, Qingcai, and Yale Zhang. *Lyme Disease and Modern Chinese Medicine: An Alternate Treatment Strategy Developed by Zhang's Clinic.* New York: Sino-Med Research Institute, 2006.

APPENDIX A:
RECOMMENDED READING

LYME-SPECIFIC

Beyond Lyme Disease by Connie Strasheim

"Evidence Based Guidelines for the Management of Lyme Disease." The International Lyme and Associated Diseases Society. Expert Rev. Anti-infect. Ther.2(1), Suppl. (2004)

Insights into Lyme Disease Treatment by Connie Strasheim

Lyme Disease and Modern Chinese Medicine by Dr. Quingcai Zhang and Yale Zhang

Lyme Disease and Rife Machines by Bryan Rosner

Lyme Disease in Australia: Fundamentals of an Emerging Epidemic by Dr. Nicola McFadzean

Sauna Therapy by Dr. Lawrence Wilson

Supplements and Advanced Treatments for Lyme and Associated Diseases by Marty Ross and Tara Brook

The Lyme Disease Survival Guide by Connie Strasheim

The Top 10 Lyme Disease Treatments by Bryan Rosner

Please note there are many other great Lyme based recommended books in the Appendix.

HEALTH AND LIFESTYLE

Ask and It Is Given: Learning to Manifest Your Desires by Esther and Jerry Hicks

Dying To Be Me: My Journey From Cancer, to Near Death, to True Healing by Anita Moorjani

Fat Chance: Beating the Odds Against Sugar, Processed Food, Obesity and Disease by Robert H. Lustig

Food Rules: An Eater's Manual by Michael Pollan

Grain Brain: The Surprising Truth about Wheat, Carbs, and Sugar – Your Brain's Silent Killers by David Perlmutter

Hero, The Magic, The Power and The Secret by Rhonda Byrne

I Quit Sugar: Your Complete 8-Week Detox Program and Cookbook by Sarah Wilson

Mental Health and Illness: The Nutrition Connection [Paperback] by Patrick Holford and Carl C. Pfeiffer

Nourishing Traditions: The Cookbook That Challenges Politically Correct Nutrition and the Diet Dictocrats by Sally Fallon, Mary Enig and Marion Dearth (Illustrator)

Perfect Health Diet: Regain Health and Lose Weight by Eating the Way You Were Meant to Eat by Paul and Shou-Ching Jaminet

Recipes for Repair: A Lyme Disease Cookbook by Laura and Gail Piazza

Ringing Cedar Series by Vladimir Megre

Slow Death by Rubber Duck: The Secret Danger of Everyday Things and *Toxin Toxout: Getting Harmful Chemicals Out of Our Bodies and Our World* by Bruce Lourie and Rick Smith

Spontaneous Evolution: Our Positive Future and a Way to Get There from Here by Bruce Lipton and Steve Bhaerman

Sweet Poison/The Sweet Poison Quit Plan by David Gillespie

The 4-Hour Body /The 4-Hour Chef/The 4-Hour Work Week by Timothy Ferriss

The Awful Truth About Cleaning Products and Fertility Revealed by Gabriela Rosa

The Biology of Belief: Unleashing the Power of Consciousness, Matter and Miracles by Bruce H. Lipton, Ph.D.

The Brain That Changes Itself: Stories of Personal Triumph from the Frontiers of Brain Science by Dr. Norman Doidge

The Chemical Maze: Your Guide to Food Additives and Cosmetic Ingredients by Bill Statham (Book and App)

The Force by Lyn McLean

The Honeymoon Effect by Bruce H. Lipton Ph.D.

The Transformational Power of Fasting by Stephen Harrod Buhner

Wheat Belly by William Davis MD

RECOMMENDED WEBSITES

LYME WEBSITES

www.buhnerhealinglyme.com

www.healthspaceclinics.com.au/service/lyme-disease-consulting

www.ilads.com

www.karlmcmanusfoundation.org.au

www.lyme-disease-research-database.com

www.lymedisease.org.au

www.sydneylymeclinic.com

www.whatislyme.com

OTHER WEBSITES

www.mcmasteryourhealth.com (this is a blog site my sister and I run with amazing health tips, recipes, parenting tips and Lyme disease information)

www.1stchineseherbs.com/lyme_disease.html

www.23andme.com

www.barefoothealing.com.au (Earthing information)

www.bearcreekherbals.com/

www.chriskresser.com

www.drrons.com/organ-and-glandular-supplements/index.html

www. greendragonbotanicals.com

www.healthspaceclinics.com.au

www.healthspacewholefoods.com.au

www.herb-pharm.com/

www.iherb.com

www.juvenaire.com/pics/Australian_Mold_Guidelines_2005-1.pdf

www.lymeprotocol.com/assets/pdf/rife%20freaks%20appendix.pdf

www.mercola.com

www.mthfr.net

www.netmindbody.com

www.neurolinkglobal.com

www. paleologix.com

www.professionalbotanicals.co/?s=ADR+Complex

www.shokos.com/science.htm

www.simplediary.com/apps

www. smartdna.com.au

www.stopthethyroidmadness.com/mthfr/

www.survivingmold.com/store1/online-screening-test

www.tbmseminars.com

www. theorganicbeautyshop.com.au.

www. woodlandessence.com

APPENDIX C:
LYME DISEASE FACEBOOK PAGES

Dr. Richard Horowitz – www.facebook.com/drrichardhorowitz

Global Lyme project – www.facebook.com/WorldwideLymeProtestAustralia

Karl McManus – www.facebook.com/pages/Karl-McManus-Foundation/115391818529455

Lyme Australia and Friends – www.facebook.com/lymeaustraliafriends

Lyme Disease Association of Australia – www.facebook.com/LymeDiseaseAustralia

St. Georg Lyme Patients – www.facebook.com/groups/245388828991898/?fref=nf

APPENDIX D:
LABS AND TESTING

Australian Biologics in Sydney – www.australianbiologics.com.au

Fry Labs Test for Lyme and Co-infections – www.frylabs.com/

Igenex in California – www.igenex.com.au

Infectolab in Germany – www.infectolab.com.au

APPENDIX E:
SUPPLEMENTAL MATERIALS

*Please log onto www.drkatewood.com.au for free access
to Appendix E: Supplemental Materials and http://
healthspaceclinics.com.au/service/lyme-disease-consulting for
our Lyme and consulting information.*

1. Lyme and Its Co-infections Symptoms Table

2. Health Space Information for St. Georg Klinik Treatment

3. Health Space Application Process for St. Georg Klinik in Germany

4. Chronic LD Assessment Tool – Schloeffel

5. Mayne's Chronic Lyme Disease Assessment Tool – 2

6. Symptom and Diagnosis List – Horowitz

7. Lyme Log Template

8. Examples of my Schedules

    a. Eat, Think, Supplement + Extra's Schedule

    b. Move, Think and Work Schedule

GLOSSARY

adjuvant chemotherapy. The use of anticancer drugs after or in combination with another form of cancer treatment. The method is used when there is a significant risk that micrometastasis may still be present. It is most commonly used in treating breast cancer.

Adrenal Cortex and Liver Capsules. A supplement of freeze-dried, New Zealand grass-fed, bovine adrenal, adrenal cortex & liver (an alternative to eating fresh organ meat).

amines. Organic compounds that contain nitrogen.

anaerobic. Lacking molecular oxygen; living, growing or occurring in the absence of molecular oxygen.

aspergillus. A genus of fungi that includes many common moulds.

atmosphere absolute. A unit of absolute pressure (also known as barometric pressure) expressed in atm.

auric field. The energy that emanates from our physical body.

basophil. Cells or cell contents easily stained by basic dyes

carrier oil. An oil used to dilute essential oils for use in massage and other skin care applications.

cat scratch disease. An infectious disease that may follow the scratch or bite of a cat, producing localised inflammation or lymph nodes and a low-grade fever. Also called *benign inoculation lymphoreticulosis, cat scratch fever.*

CBS (& Methylation). The CBS gene provides instructions for making an enzyme called cystathionine beta-synthase. This enzyme acts in a chemical pathway and is responsible for using vitamin B6 to convert building block of proteins (amino acids) called homocysteine and serine to a molecule called cytathionine. Another enzyme then converts cystathionine to the amino acid cysteine, which is used to build proteins or is broken down and excreted in urine. Additionally, other amino acids, including methionine, are produced in this pathway. (http://ghr.nlm.nih.gov/gene/CBS).

codons. A sequence of three adjacent nucleotides constituting the genetic code that determines the insertion of a specific amino acid in a polypeptide chain during protein synthesis or the signal to stop protein synthesis.

compounding chemist. A chemist who creates tailor-made medications for patients.

conjugation. The combination, especially in the liver, of certain toxic substances formed in the intestine, drugs, or steroid hormones with glucuronic or sulfuric acid; a means by which the biologic activity of certain chemical substances is terminated and the substances made ready for excretion.

cystathionine. An intermediate in the conversion of methionine to cysteine.

Dark-field therapy. Using darkfield microscopy, the shape and condition of blood cells can be seen, as well as the by-products and other micro-organisms associated with various diseases. (http://www.health911.com/darkfield-micoscopy).

dental foci. An area anywhere in the mouth—whether a tooth or an extraction site—that is chronically irritated and/ or infected. These "dental focal infections" can include impacted wisdom teeth, incompletely extracted wisdom (and other) teeth, failed root canals, failed dental implants, and devitalised teeth (from deep fillings, crowns or physical trauma). (http://www.westonaprice.org/holistic-healthcare/dental-cavitation-surgery/).

dirty energy. Energy sources (e.g., gas, oil and coal) that leave waste products that pollute the environment.

diverticulitis. Inflammation of a diverticulum in the intestinal tract, causing fecal stagnation and pain.

DMSA. Is used to help mobilise heavy metals stored in body tissues (and therefore not typically present in the circulation) and increase the excretion of heavy metals in the urine.

dominance. In genetics, the full phenotypic expression of a gene in both heterozygotes and homozygotes.

dysbiosis. An imbalance in the intestinal bacteria that precipitates changes in the normal activities of the gastrointestinal tract or vagina, possibly resulting in health problems.

encephalopathic. Degeneration of brain function, caused by various disorders, including metabolic disease, organ failure, inflammation and chronic infection. Also called *cephalopathy, cerebropathy.*

endogenous. Produced within or caused by factors within the organism.

epigenetics. The study of heritable changes in gene expression that are caused by factors such as DNA methylation rather than by a change in the sequence of base pairs in DNA itself.

estradiol. The most potent naturally-occurring estrogen.

estriol. A relatively weak human **estrogen**, being a metabolic product of **estradiol** and **estrone** found in high concentrations in urine, especially during pregnancy.

etiology. The science and study of the causes or origins of disease.

exogenous. Originating outside or caused by factors outside the organism.

febrile. Pertaining to or characterised by fever.

fermentable fibres. A type of fibre that acts as food for good bacteria in the gut. (http://www.nyrnaturalnews.com/food/2014/01/dietary-fibre-protects-against-asthma/).

fibrin. The last step in the coagulation process. Fibrin forms strands that add bulk to a forming blood clot to hold it in place and help plug an injured blood vessel wall.

filaments. A fibril, fine fibre, or threadlike structure.

(hexa) fluorosilicic acid. It is commonly used as a source of **fluoride** for **water fluoridation**. Concentrated hexafluorosilicic acid is corrosive and can attack the skin.

genome. The complete set of genes in the chromosomes of each cell of a specific organism.

Gram-negative bacteria. Gram-negative bacteria cause infections including pneumonia, bloodstream infections, wound or surgical site infections, and meningitis in healthcare settings. Gram-negative bacteria are resistant to multiple drugs and are increasingly resistant to most available antibiotics. These bacteria have built-in abilities to find new ways to be resistant and can pass along genetic materials that allow other bacteria to become drug-resistant as well (http://www.cdc.gov/hai/organisms/gram-negative-bacteria.html).

hemoglobinuria. The presence of hemoglobin in the urine.

hemolytic. Destructive to red blood cells.

homeostasis. The ability of an organism or a cell to maintain internal equilibrium by adjusting its physiological processes.

homocysteine. An amino acid occurring as an intermediate in the metabolism of methionine. Elevated levels in the blood may indicate increased risk of cardiovascular disease.

hyperinsulinaemia. Increased levels of insulin in the plasma due to increased secretion of insulin by the beta cells of the pancreatic islets.

hypertrophy. A non tumorous enlargement of an organ or a tissue as a result of an increase in the size rather than the number of constituent cells.

hypocalcaemia. Abnormally low levels of calcium in the circulating blood; commonly denotes subnormal concentrations of calcium ions.

hypoglycaemia. Abnormally low concentration of glucose in circulating blood (i.e.<2.9mmol/L); induced in diabetics by mismatch of administered insulin and food intake in relation to exercise levels; symptoms (triggered by low cerebral glucose levels and reflex autonomic nervous system stimulation) include warning signs (e.g., appearing drunk, slurring speech, poor concentration, behavioural truculence, feeling faint/light-headed, trembling, oral paraesthesia, inappropriate sweating) or rapid progression to coma.

incognitus strain (Mycoplasma fermetans). A strain of Mycoplasma linked to AIDS.

innervate. (1) To supply an organ or a body part with nerves. (2) To stimulate a nerve, muscle, or body part to action.

insufflations. (1) The act of blowing powder, vapour, or gas into a body cavity. (2) Finely powdered or liquid drugs carried into the respiratory passages by such devices as aerosols.

insulin. (1) A polypeptide hormone that is secreted by the islets of Langerhans, helps regulate the metabolism of carbohydrates and fat conversion of glucose to glycogen, and promotes protein synthesis and the formation and storage of neutral lipids. (2) Any of various pharmaceutical preparations containing this hormone that are derived from the pancreas of certain animals of produced through genetic engineering and are used parenterally in the medical treatment and management of insulin-dependent diabetes mellitus.

interleukin. One of a large group of proteins produced mainly by T cells and in some cases by mononuclear phagocytes or other cells. Interleukins participate in communication among leukocytes and are important in the inflammatory response. Most interleukins direct other cells to divide and differentiate. Each acts on a particular group of cells that have receptors specific to that interleukin.

leucocytopenia. Also known as leucopenia. An abnormally low number of white blood cells in the circulating blood.

leucopenia. See leucocytopenia.

leukotrienes. A class of biologically active compounds that occur naturally in leukocytes and produce allergic and inflammatory reactions similar to those of histamine. They are thought to play a role in the development of allergic and auto-allergic diseases such as asthma, rheumatoid arthritis, inflammatory bowel disease, and psoriasis.

lysates. A product of dissolution of matter by lysis (destruction or dissolution of a cell or molecule through the action of a specific agent), as in the destruction of proteins by hydrolysis.

lytic infection. Infection of a bacterium by a phage which replicates uncontrollably, destroying its host and eventually releasing many copies into the medium.

manual therapy. A clinical approach utilising skilled, specific hands-on techniques, including but not limited to manipulation/mobilisation, used by the physical therapist to diagnose and treat soft tissues and joint structures for the purpose of modulating pain; increasing range of motion (ROM); reducing or eliminating soft tissue inflammation; inducing relaxation; improving contractile and non-contractile tissue repair, extensibility, and/or stability; facilitating movement; and improving function.

metabolome. The complete set of small-molecule metabolites (such as metabolic intermediates, hormones and other signalling molecules, and secondary metabolites) to be found within a biological sample, such as a single organism.

microti (B. microti). A rodent parasite which causes human Babesiosis.

micturition. The act of passing urine; urination.

MMS (Miracle Mineral Supplement). Sodium chlorite is being promoted as a miracle mineral supplement with superior antimicrobial activity. Its active compound chlorine dioxide is lethal not only to the malaria protozoa, but also virtually all forms of *bacteria, fungi, parasites,* and a surprising number of *viruses.* (http://www.mmshealthy4life.com/).

navicular bone. The boat-shaped tarsal bone on the medial side of the foot in front of the talus (ankle bone).

nephrotoxic. Toxic, or damaging, to the kidney.

neutropenia. Neutropenia is an abnormally low level of neutrophils in the blood. Neutrophils are white blood cells (WBC) produced in the bone marrow that ingest bacteria.

NutraMedix® range of products. Highly bio-active nutritional supplements, which are bio-available whole plant, broad-spectrum, cost-effective extracts. (http://nutramedix.com/company.asp).

nutrigenomics. The study of how diet influences gene expression and thus health.

orthomolecular psychiatry. A therapeutic approach designed to provide an optimum molecular environment for body functions, with particular reference to the optimal concentrations of substances normally present in the human body, whether formed endogenously or ingested.

pathogen. An agent that causes disease, especially a living microorganism such as a bacterium, virus, or fungus.

PCR (Polymerase Chain Reaction). A test performed to evaluate false-negative results to the ELISA and western blot tests. In PCR testing, numerous copies of a gene are made by separating the two strands of DNA containing the gene segment, marking its location, using DNA polymerase to make a copy and then continuously replicating the copies. The amplification of gene sequences that are associated with HIV allows for detection of the virus by this method.

PCOS (Polycystic Ovary Syndrome). A set of symptoms due to a hormone imbalance in women. Symptoms include: irregular or no menstrual periods, heavy periods, excess body and facial hair, acne, pelvic pain, trouble getting pregnant, and patches of thick, darker, velvety skin. Risk factors include obesity, not enough physical exercise, and a family history of someone with the condition.

piroplasm. Any of several parasitic protozoans of the order Piroplasmida, such as Babesia, that infect red blood cells.

pleomorphic. (also known as polymorphic) Among fungi, having two or more forms; also used to describe a sterile mutant dermatophyte resulting from degenerative changes in culture.

porphyrins. Any of various organic compounds containing four pyrrole rings, occurring universally in protoplasm, and functioning as a metal-binding cofactor in hemoglobin, chlorophyll, and certain enzymes.

proteinuria. Excessive amounts of protein in the urine.

proteome. The complete set of proteins that are produced by the genes of an organism.

prostaglandins. A family of lipid compounds found in various tissues, associated with muscular contraction and the inflammation response.

pyrogen. A substance that produces a fever.

sacroiliac joint. The sacroiliac joint or SI joint (SIJ) is the **joint** in the bony pelvis between the **sacrum** and the **ilium** of the **pelvis**, which are joined by strong **ligaments**. In humans, the sacrum supports the **spine** and is supported in turn by an ilium on each side.

sensorium. (1) The part of the brain that receives and coordinates all the stimuli conveyed to various sensory centres. (2) The sensory system of the body.

serotonin. An organic compound formed from tryptophan and found in animal and human tissues, especially the brain, blood serum, and gastric mucous membranes, and active in vasoconstriction, stimulation of the smooth muscles, transmission of impulses between nerve cells, and regulation of cyclic body processes. Also called *5-hydroxytryptamine.*

singlet oxygen. An excited or higher-energy form of oxygen character-ised by the spin of a pair of electrons in opposite directions, where a selectron spin is unidirectional in normal molecular oxygen. Because of its great reactivity, it is a probable intermediate in most photo oxida-tion reactions.

SNP (Single Nucleotide Polymorphism). The naturally occurring substitution of a single nucleotide at a given location in the genome of an organism, the more interesting of which results in phenotypic variability, including alterations in the organism's physiologic responses to endogenous hormones and neurotransmitters or endogenous substances.

SPECT scan (Single Photon Emission Computed Topography) Tomograph-ic imaging of local metabolic and physiological functions in tissues. The image is formed by a computer synthesis of data that is transmitted by single gamma photons emitted by radionuclides administered to the patient.

TENS (Transcutaneous Electrical Nerve Stimulation). A technique used to relieve pain in an injured or diseased part of the body in which electrodes applied to the skin deliver intermittent stimulation to surface nerves and block the transmission of pain signals.

TGA (Therapeutic Goods Association). Australia's regulatory authority for therapeutic goods. (http://www.tga.gov.au/about-tga).

thermal receipts. Are made from thermal papers (a special fine paper that is coated with a chemical that changes colour when exposed to heat) coated with BPA, a chemical considered to be an endocrine disruptor that can transfer readily to the skin in small amounts.

thrombocytopenia. An abnormal decrease in the number of platelets in the blood. Also called *thrombopenia.*

thrombophlebitis. Inflammation of a vein caused by or associated with the formation of a blood clot.

titers (or titres). (1) The concentration of a substance in a solution or the strength of such a substance determined by titration. (2) The minimum volume needed to cause a particular result in titration. (3) The dilution of a serum containing a specific antibody at which the solution retains the minimum level of activity needed to neutralise or precipitate an antigen.

vectors. An organism, such as a mosquito or tick, which carries disease-causing microorganisms from one host to another.

visna virus. A lentivirus that is the causal agent of a type of pneumonia in sheep.

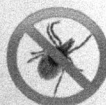

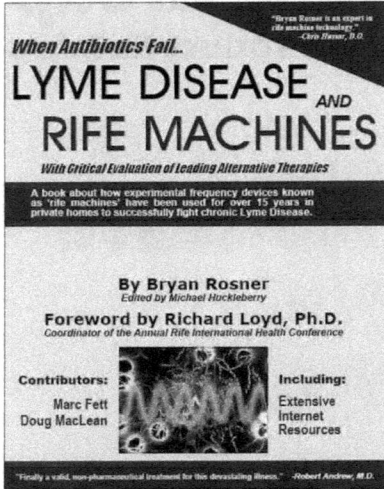

When Antibiotics Fail...

LYME DISEASE AND RIFE MACHINES

With Critical Evaluation of Leading Alternative Therapies

"Bryan Rosner is an expert in rife machine technology."
-Chris Hussar, D.O.

A book about how experimental frequency devices known as 'rife machines' have been used for over 15 years in private homes to successfully fight chronic Lyme Disease.

By Bryan Rosner
Edited by Michael Huckleberry

Foreword by Richard Loyd, Ph.D.
Coordinator of the Annual Rife International Health Conference

Contributors:
Marc Fett
Doug MacLean

Including:
Extensive
Internet
Resources

"Finally a valid, non-pharmaceutical treatment for this devastating illness." -Robert Andrew, M.D.

Book • $35

When Antibiotics Fail: Lyme Disease And Rife Machines, With Critical Evaluation Of Leading Alternative Therapies

By Bryan Rosner
Foreword by Richard Loyd, Ph.D.

There are enough books and websites about what Lyme disease is and which ticks carry it. But there is very little useful information for people who actually have a case of Lyme disease that is not responding to conventional antibiotic treatment. Lyme disease sufferers need to know their options, not how to identify a tick.

This book describes how experimental electromagnetic frequency devices known as rife machines have been used for over 15 years in private homes to fight Lyme disease. Also included are evaluations of more than 25 conventional and alternative Lyme disease therapies, including:

- Homeopathy
- IV and oral antibiotics
- Mercury detox.
- Hyperthermia / saunas
- Ozone and oxygen
- Samento®
- Colloidal Silver
- Bacterial die-off detox.

- Colostrum
- Magnesium supplementation
- Hyperbaric oxygen chamber (HBOC)
- ICHT Italian treatment
- Non-pharmaceutical antibiotics
- Exercise, diet and candida protocols
- Cyst-targeting antibiotics
- The Marshall Protocol®

Many Lyme disease sufferers have heard of rife machines, some have used them. But until now, there has not been a concise and organized source to explain how and why they have been used by Lyme patients. In fact, this is the first book ever published on this important topic.

The Foreword for the book is by Richard Loyd, Ph.D., coordinator of the annual Rife International Health Conference. The book takes a practical, down-to-earth approach which allows you to learn about*:

"This book provides life-saving insights for Lyme disease patients."

- Richard Loyd, Ph.D.

- Antibiotic treatment problems and shortcomings—why some people choose to use rife machines after other therapies fail.
- Hypothetical treatment schedules and sessions, based on the author's experience.
- The experimental machines with the longest track record: High Power Magnetic Pulser, EMEM Machine, Coil Machine, and AC Contact Machine.
- Explanation of the "herx reaction" and why it may indicate progress.
- The intriguing story that led to the use of rife machines to fight Lyme disease 20 years ago.
- Antibiotic categories and classifications, with pros and cons of each type of drug.
- Visit our website to read <u>FREE EXCERPTS</u> from the book!

Disclaimer: *Your treatment decisions must be made under the care of a licensed physician. Rife machines are not FDA approved and the FDA has not reviewed or approved of these books. The author is a layperson, not a doctor, and much of the content of these books is a statement of opinion based on the author's personal experience and research.*

Paperback book, 8.5 x 11", 203 pages, $35

The Top 10 Lyme Disease Treatments: Defeat Lyme Disease With The Best Of Conventional And Alternative Medicine

By Bryan Rosner
Foreword by James Schaller, M.D.

This information-packed book identifies ten promising conventional and alternative Lyme disease treatments and gives practical guidance on integrating them into a comprehensive treatment plan that you and your physician can customize for your individual situation and needs.

The book was not written to replace Bryan Rosner's first book (*Lyme Disease and Rife Machines*, opposing page). It was written to complement that book, offering Lyme sufferers many new foundational and supportive treatment options, based on the author's extensive research and years of personal experience. Topics include*:

"A creative and fascinating book... with many new and clearly described options for hope."
James Schaller, M.D.

THE TOP 10 LYME DISEASE TREATMENTS

Defeat Lyme Disease with the Best of Conventional and Alternative Medicine

The Practical Guide to Understanding Modern Treatments and Building a Comprehensive Treatment Plan

Bryan Rosner

Foreword by
James Schaller, M.D.

Book • $35

- Systemic enzyme therapy, which helps detoxify tissues and blood, reduce inflammation, stimulate the immune system, and kill Lyme disease bacteria.
- Lithium orotate, a powerful yet all-natural mineral (belonging to the same mineral group as sodium and potassium) capable of profound neuroprotective activity.
- Thorough and extensive coverage of a complete Lyme disease detoxification program, including discussion of both liver and skin detoxification pathways. Specific detoxification therapies such as liver cleanses, bowel cleanses, the Shoemaker Neurotoxin Elimination Protocol, sauna therapy, mineral baths, mineral supplementation, milk thistle, and many others. Ideas to reduce and control herx reactions.
- Tips and clinical research from James Schaller, M.D.
- A detailed look at one method for utilizing antibiotics during a rife machine treatment campaign.
- Wide coverage of the Marshall Protocol, including an in-depth discussion of its mechanism of action in relation to Lyme disease pathology. Also, the author's personal experience with the Marshall Protocol over 3 years.
- An explanation of and new information about the Salt / Vitamin C protocol.
- Hot-off-the-press information on mangosteen fruit (not to be confused with mango) and its many benefits, including antibacterial, anti-inflammatory, and anti-cancer properties.
- New guidelines for combining all the therapies discussed in both of Rosner's books into a complete treatment plan. Brief and articulate for consideration by you and your doctor.
- Also includes updates on rife therapy, cutting-edge supplements, political challenges, an exclusive interview with Willy Burgdorfer, Ph.D. (discoverer of Lyme), and much more!

"Bryan Rosner thinks big and this new book offers big solutions."
- **James Schaller, M.D.**

"Another ground-breaking Lyme Disease book."
- **Jeff Mittelman, moderator of the Lyme-and-rife group**

"Brilliant and thorough."
- **Nenah Sylver, Ph.D.**

Do not miss this top Lyme disease resource. Discover new healing tools today! Bring this book to your doctor's appointment to help with forming a treatment plan.

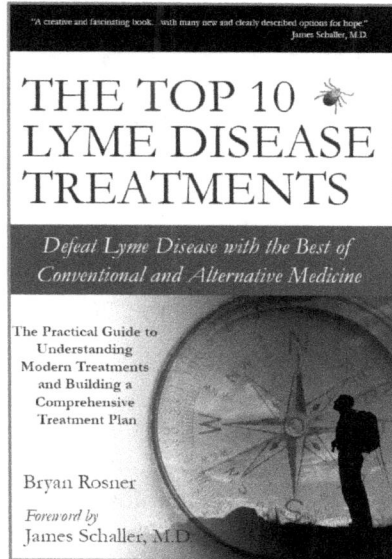

Paperback book, 7 x 10", 367 pages, $35

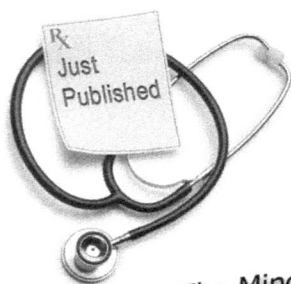

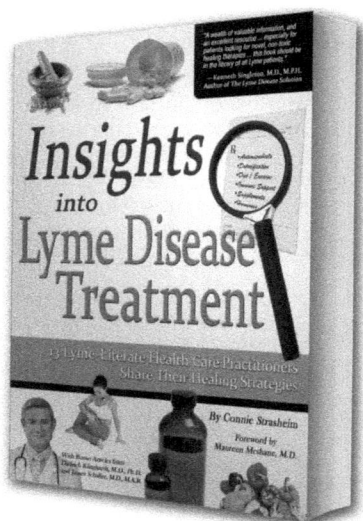

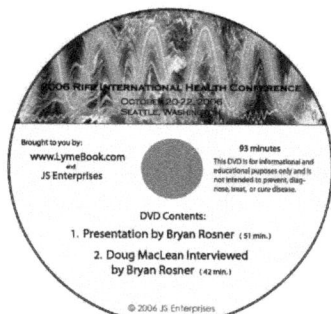

DVD • $24.50

Rife International Health Conference Feature-Length DVD (93 Minutes)

Bryan Rosner's Presentation and Interview with Doug MacLean

The Official Rife Technology Seminar Seattle, WA, USA

If you have been unable to attend the Rife International Health Conference, this DVD is your opportunity to watch two very important Lyme-related presentations from the event:

Presentation #1: Bryan Rosner's Sunday morning talk entitled *Lyme Disease: New Paradigms in Diagnosis and Treatment - the Myths, the Reality, and the Road Back to Health.* (51 minutes)

Presentation #2: Bryan Rosner's interview with Doug MacLean, in which Doug talked about his experiences with Lyme disease, including the incredible journey he undertook to invent the first modern rife machine used to fight Lyme disease. Although Doug's journey as a Lyme disease pioneer took place 20 years ago, this was the first time Doug has ever accepted an invitation to appear in public. This is the only video available where you can see Doug talk about what it was like to be the first person ever to use rife technology as a treatment for Lyme disease. Now you can see how it all began. Own this DVD and own a piece of history! (42 minutes)

Lymebook.com has secured a special licensing agreement with JS Enterprises, the Canadian producer of the Rife Conference videos, to bring this product to you at the special low price of $24.50. Total DVD viewing time: 1 hour, 33 minutes. We have DVDs in stock, shipped to you within 3 business days.

Price Comparison (should you get the DVD?)

Cost of attending the recent Rife Conference (2 people):
Hotel Room, 3 Nights = $400
Registration = $340
Food = $150
Airfare = $600
Total = $1,490

Cost of the DVD, which you can view as many times as you want, and show to family and friends:
DVD = $24.50

Bryan Rosner Presenting on Sunday Morning In Seattle

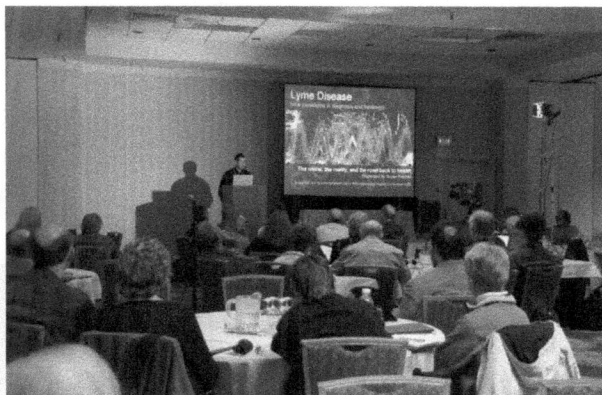

**DVD
93 Minutes
$24.50**

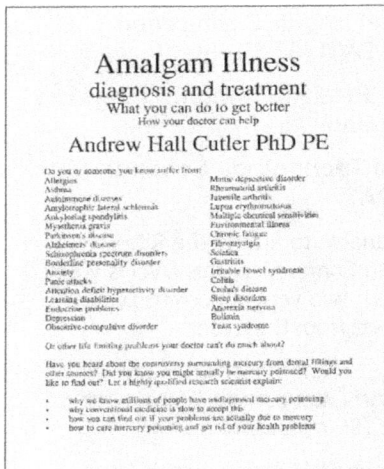

Amalgam Illness
diagnosis and treatment
What you can do to get better
How your doctor can help

Andrew Hall Cutler PhD PE

Book • $35

Amalgam Illness, Diagnosis and Treatment: What You Can Do to Get Better, How Your Doctor Can Help

By Andrew Cutler, PhD

This book was written by a chemical engineer who himself got mercury poisoning from his amalgam dental fillings. He found that there was no suitable educational material for either the patient or the physician. Knowing how much people can suffer from this condition, he wrote this book to help them get well. With a PhD in chemistry from Princeton University and extensive study in biochemistry and medicine, Andrew Cutler uses layman's terms to explain how people become mercury poisoned and what to do about it. The author's research shows that mercury poisoning can easily be cured at home with over-the-counter oral chelators – this book explains how.

In the book you will find practical guidance on how to tell if you really have chronic mercury poisoning or some other problem. Proper diagnostic procedures are provided so that sick people can decide what is wrong rather than trying random treatments. If mercury poisoning is your problem, the book tells you how to get the mercury out of your body, and how to feel good while you do that. The treatment section gives step-by-step directions to figure out exactly what mercury is doing to you and how to fix it.

"Dr. Cutler uses his background in chemistry to explain the safest approach to treat mercury poisoning. I am a physician and am personally using his protocol on myself."

- Melissa Myers, M.D.

Sections also explain how the scientific literature shows many people must be getting poisoned by their amalgam fillings, why such a regulatory blunder occurred, and how the debate between "mainstream" and "alternative" medicine makes it more difficult for you to get the medical help you need.

This down-to-earth book lets patients take care of themselves. It also lets doctors who are not familiar with chronic mercury intoxication treat it. The book is a practical guide to getting well. Sections from the book include:

- Why worry about mercury poisoning?
- What mercury does to you – symptoms, laboratory test irregularities, diagnostic checklist.
- How to treat mercury poisoning easily with oral chelators.
- Dealing with other metals including copper, arsenic, lead, cadmium.
- Dietary and supplement guidelines.
- Balancing hormones during the recovery process.
- How to feel good while you are chelating the metals out.
- How heavy metals cause infections to thrive in the body.
- Politics and mercury.

This is the world's most authoritative, accurate book on mercury poisoning.

Paperback book, 8.5 x 11", 226 pages, $35

Hair Test Interpretation: Finding Hidden Toxicities

By Andrew Cutler, PhD

Hair tests are worth doing because a surprising number of people diagnosed with incurable chronic health conditions actually turn out to have a heavy metal problem; quite often, mercury poisoning. Heavy metal problems can be corrected. Hair testing allows the underlying problem to be identified – and the chronic health condition often disappears with proper detoxification.

Hair Test Interpretation: Finding Hidden Toxicities is a practical book that explains how to interpret **Doctor's Data, Inc.** and **Great Plains Laboratory** hair tests. A step-by-step discussion is provided, with figures to illustrate the process and make it easy. The book gives examples using actual hair test results from real people.

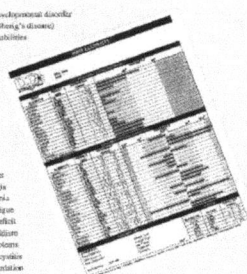

Hair Test Interpretation: Finding Hidden Toxicities

Andrew Hall Cutler, Ph. D., P. E.

Toxicity Causes Health Problems

Book • $35

One of the problems with hair testing is that both conventional and alternative health care providers do not know how to interpret these tests. Interpretation is not as simple as looking at the results and assuming that any mineral out of the reference range is a problem mineral.

Interpretation is complicated because heavy metal toxicity, especially mercury poisoning, interferes with mineral transport throughout the body. Ironically, if someone is mercury poisoned, hair test mercury is often low and other minerals may be elevated or take on unusual values. For example, mercury often causes retention of arsenic, antimony, tin, titanium, zirconium, and aluminum. An inexperienced health care provider may wrongfully assume that one of these other minerals is the culprit, when in reality mercury is the true toxicity.

"This new book of Andrew's is the definitive guide in the confusing world of heavy metal poisoning diagnosis and treatment. I'm a practicing physician, 20 years now, specializing in detoxification programs for treatment of resistant conditions. It was fairly difficult to diagnose these heavy metal conditions before I met Andrew Cutler and developed a close relationship with him while reading his books. In this book I found his usual painful attention to detail gave a solid framework for understanding the complexity of mercury toxicity as well as the less common exposures. You really couldn't ask for a better reference book on a subject most researchers and physicians are still fumbling in the dark about."
- Dr. Rick Marschall

So, as you can see, getting a hair test is only the first step. The second step is figuring out what the hair test means. Andrew Cutler, PhD, is a registered professional chemical engineer with years of experience in biochemical and healthcare research. This clear and concise book makes hair test interpretation easy, so that you know which toxicities are causing your health problems.

Paperback book, 8.5 x 11", 298 pages, $35

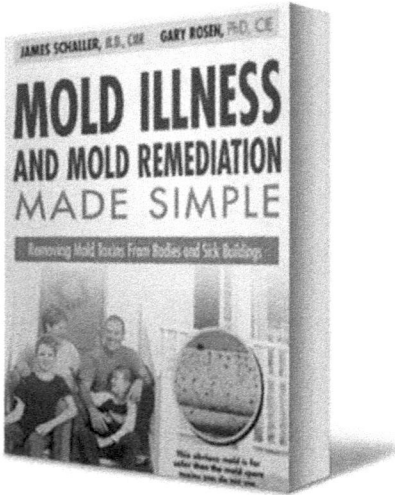

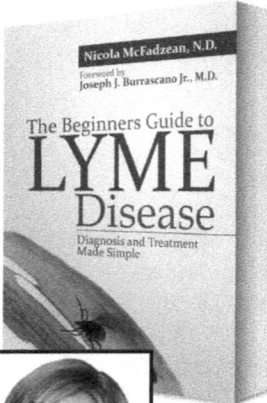

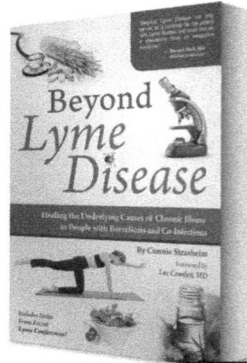

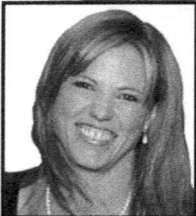

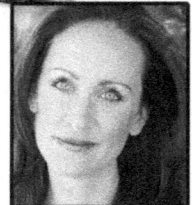

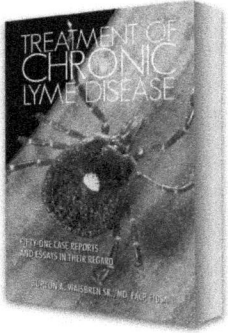

Treatment of Chronic Lyme Disease: 51 Case Reports and Essays In Their Regard

By Burton Waisbren Sr., MD, FACP, FIDSA

DON'T MISS THIS BOOK! A MUST-HAVE RESOURCE. What sets this Lyme disease book apart are the credentials of its author: he is not only a Fellow of the Infectious Diseases Society of America (IDSA), he is also one of its Founders! With 57+ years experience in medicine, Dr. Waisbren passionately argues for the validity of chronic Lyme disease and presents useful information about 51 cases of the disease which he has personally treated. His position is in stark contrast to that of the IDSA, which is a very powerful organization. **Quite possibly the most important book ever published on Lyme disease, as a result of the author's experience and credentials.**

Book • $24.95

Paperback book, 6x9", 169 pages, $24.95

Bartonella: Diagnosis and Treatment

By James Schaller, M.D.

2 Book Set • $99.95

As an addition to his growing collection of informative books, Dr. James Schaller penned this excellent 2-part volume on Bartonella, a Lyme disease co-infection. The set is an ideal complementary resource to his Babesia textbook (next page).

Bartonella infections occur throughout the entire world, in cities, suburbs, and rural locations. It is found in fleas, dust mites, ticks, lice, flies, cat and dog saliva, and insect feces.

This 2-book set provides advanced treatment strategies as well as detailed diagnostic criteria, with dozens of full-color illustrations and photographs.

Both books in this 2-part set are included with your order.

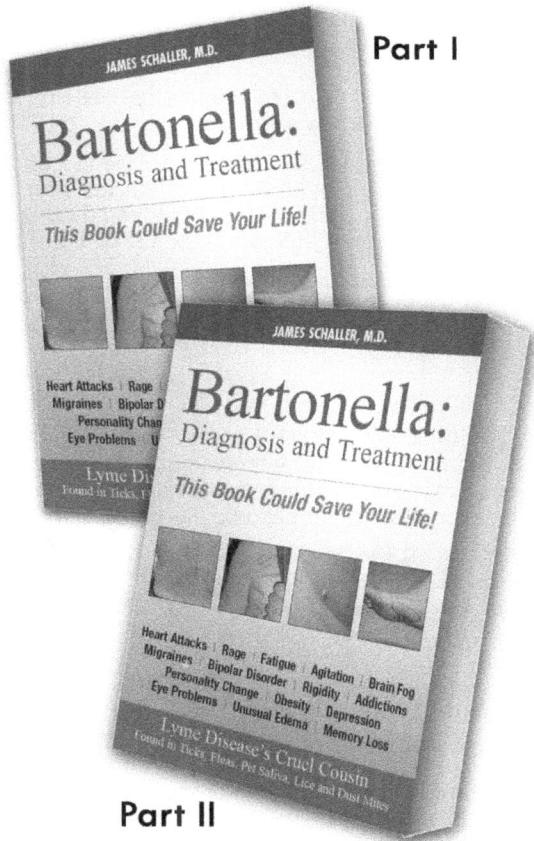

Part I

Part II

2 paperback books included, 7 x 10", 500 pages, $99.95

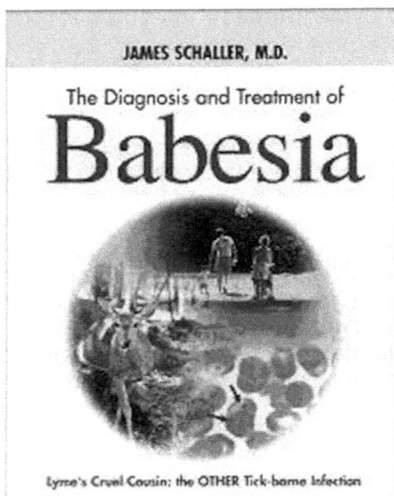

JAMES SCHALLER, M.D.

The Diagnosis and Treatment of

Babesia

Lyme's Cruel Cousin: the OTHER Tick-borne Infection

Book • $55

The Diagnosis and Treatment of Babesia: Lyme's Cruel Cousin – The Other Tick-Borne Infection

By James Schaller, M.D.

Do you or a loved one experience excess fatigue? Have you ever had unusually high fevers, chills, or sweats? You may have Babesia, a very common tick-borne infection. Babesia is often found with Lyme disease and, like all tick-borne infections, is rarely diagnosed and reported accurately.

The deer tick which carries Lyme disease and Babesia may be as small as a poppy seed and injects a painkiller, an antihistamine, and an anticoagulant to avoid detection. As a result, many people have Babesia and do not know it. Numerous forms of Babesia are carried by ticks. This book introduces patients and health care workers to the various species that infect humans and are not routinely tested for by sincere physicians.

Dr. Schaller, who practices medicine in Florida, first became interested in Babesia after one of his own children was infected with it. None of the elite pediatricians or child specialists could help. No one tested for Babesia or considered it a possible diagnosis. His child suffered from just two of these typical Babesia symptoms:

- Significant Fatigue
- Coughing
- Dizziness
- Trouble Thinking
- Fevers
- Memory Loss

- Chills
- Air Hunger
- Headache
- Sweats
- Unresponsiveness to Lyme Treatment

With 374 pages, this book is the most current and comprehensive book on Babesia in the English language. It reviews thousands of articles and presents the results of interviews with world experts on the subject. It offers you top information and broad treatment options, presented in a clear and simple manner. All treatments are explained thoroughly, including their possible side effects, drug interactions, various dosing strategies, pros/cons, and physician experiences.

"Once again Dr. Schaller has provided us with a much-needed and practical resource. This book gave me exactly what I was looking for."

- Thomas W., Patient

Finally, the book also addresses many other aspects of practical medical care often overlooked in this infection, such as treatment options for managing fatigue. Plainly stated, this book is a must-have for patients and health care providers who deal with Lyme disease and its co-infections. Dr. Schaller's many years in clinical practice give the book a practical angle that many other similar books lack. Don't miss this user-friendly resource!

Paperback book, 7 x 10", 374 pages, $55

Also available on our website as an eBook!

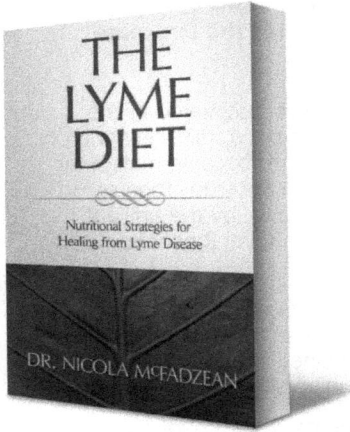

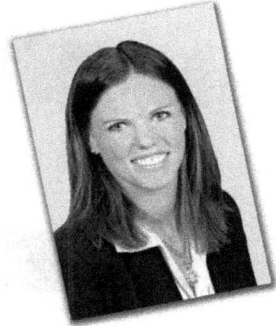

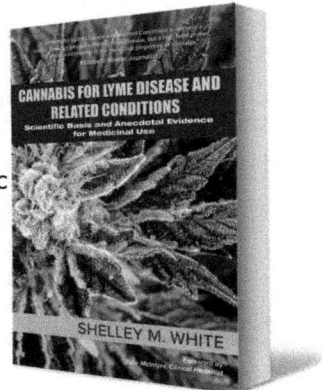

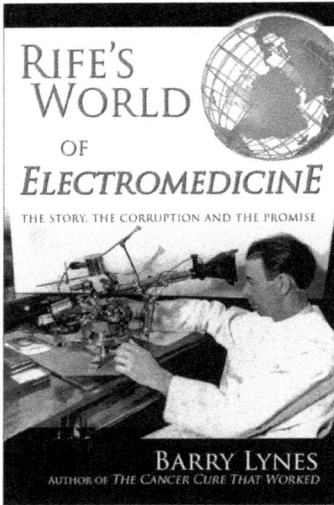

Book • $17.95

Rife's World of Electromedicine: The Story, the Corruption and the Promise

By Barry Lynes

The cause of cancer was discovered in the early 1930's. It was a virus-sized, mini-bacteria or "particle" that induced cells to become malignant and grow into tumors. The cancer microbe or particle was given the name BX by the brilliant scientist who discovered it: Royal Raymond Rife.

Laboratory verification of the cause of cancer was done hundreds of times with mice in order to be absolutely certain. Five of America's most prominent physicians helped oversee clinical trials managed by a major university's medical school.

Sixteen cancer patients were brought by ambulance twice a week to the clinical trial location in La Jolla, California. There they were treated with a revolutionary electromedicine that painlessly, non-invasively destroyed only the cancer-causing microbe or particle named BX. After just three months of this therapy, all patients were diagnosed as clinically cured. Later, the therapy was suppressed and remains so today.

In 1987, Barry Lynes wrote the classic book on Rife history (*The Cancer Cure That Worked*, see catalog page 14). *Rife's World* is the sequel.

Paperback book, 5.5 x 8.5", 90 pages, $17.95

Physicians' Desk Reference (PDR) Books (opposing page)

Most people have heard of *Physicians' Desk Reference* (PDR) books because, for over 60 years, physicians and researchers have turned to PDR for the latest word on prescription drugs.

You may not know that Thomson Healthcare, publisher of PDR, offers PDR reference books not only

THOMSON

"I relied heavily on the PDRs during the research phase of writing my books. Without them, my projects would have greatly suffered."
- Bryan Rosner

for drugs, but also for herbal and nutritional supplements. No available books come even close to the amount of information provided in these PDRs—*PDR for Herbal Medicines* weighs 5 lbs and has over 1300 pages, and *PDR for Nutritional Supplements* weighs over 3 lbs and has more than 800 pages.

We carry all three PDRs. Although PDR books are typically used by physicians, we feel that these resources are also essential for people interested in or recovering from chronic disease. For the supplements, herbs, and drugs included in the books, you will find the following information: Pharmacology, description and method of action, available trade names and brands, indications and usage, research summaries, dosage options, history of use, pharmacokinetics, and much more! Worth the money for years of faithful use.

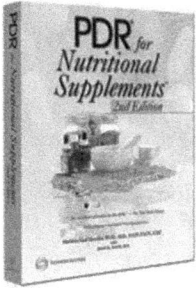

PDR for Nutritional Supplements *2ⁿᵈ Edition!*

This PDR focuses on the following types of supplements:

- Vitamins
- Minerals
- Amino acids
- Hormones
- Lipids
- Glyconutrients
- Probiotics
- Proteins
- Many more!

"In a part of the health field not known for its devotion to rigorous science, [this book] brings to the practitioner and the curious patient a wealth of hard facts."

- Roger Guillemin, M.D., Ph.D., Nobel Laureate in Physiology and Medicine

Book • $69.50

The book also suggests supplements that can help reduce prescription drug side effects, has full-color photographs of various popular commercial formulations (and contact information for the associated suppliers), and so much more! Become educated instead of guessing which supplements to take.

Hardcover book, 11 x 9.3", 800 pages, $69.50

PDR for Herbal Medicines *4ᵗʰ Edition!*

PDR for Herbal Medicines is very well organized and presents information on hundreds of common and uncommon herbs and herbal preparations. Indications and usage are examined with regard to homeopathy, Indian and Chinese medicine, and unproven (yet popular) applications.

In an area of healthcare so unstudied and vulnerable to hearsay and hype, this scientifically referenced book allows you to find out the real story behind the herbs lining the walls of your local health food store.

Use this reference before spending money on herbal products!

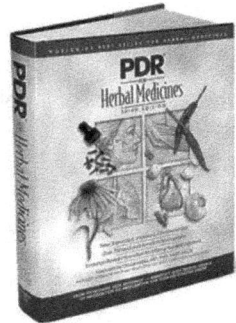

Book • $69.50

Hardcover book, 11 x 9.3", 1300 pages, $69.50

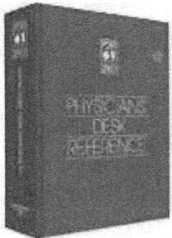

PDR for Prescription Drugs *Current Year's Edition!*

With more than 3,000 pages, this is the most comprehensive and respected book in the world on over 4,000 drugs. Drugs are indexed by both brand and generic name (in the same convenient index) and also by manufacturer and product category. This PDR provides usage information and warnings, drug interactions, plus a detailed, full-color directory with descriptions and cross references for the drugs. A new format allows dramatically improved readability and easier access to the information you need now.

Book • $99.50

Hardcover book, 12.5 x 9.5", 3533 pages, $99.50

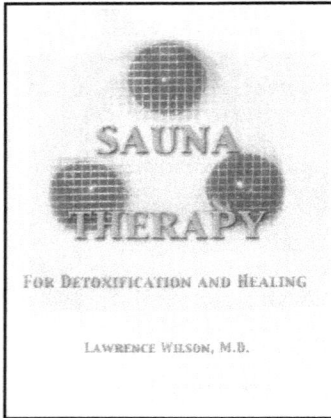

Sauna Therapy for Detoxification and Healing

By Lawrence Wilson, MD

This book provides a thorough yet articulate education on sauna therapy. It includes construction plans for a low-cost electric light sauna. The book is well referenced with an extensive bibliography.

Sauna therapy, especially with an electric light sauna, is one of the most powerful, safe and cost-effective methods of natural healing. It is especially important today due to extensive exposure to toxic metals and chemicals.

Fifteen chapters cover sauna benefits, physiological effects, protocols, cautions, healing reactions, and many other aspects of sauna therapy.

Book • $22.95

Dr. Wilson is an instructor of Biochemistry, Hair Mineral Analysis, Sauna Therapy and Jurisprudence at various colleges and universities including Yamuni Institute of the Healing Arts (Maurice, LA), University of Natural Medicine (Santa Fe, NM), Natural Healers Academy (Morristown, NJ), and Westbrook University (West Virginia). His books are used as textbooks at East-West School of Herbology and Ohio College of Natural Health. Go to www.LymeBook.com for free book excerpts!

Paperback book, 8.5 x 11", 167 pages, $22.95

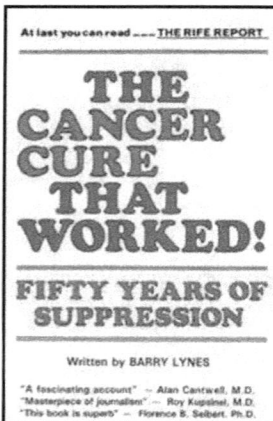

The Cancer Cure That Worked: Fifty Years of Suppression

At Last You Can Read… The Rife Report

By Barry Lynes

Investigative journalism at its best. Barry Lynes takes readers on an exciting journey into the life work of Royal Rife. We are now the official publisher of this book. Call or visit us online for wholesale terms.

Book • $19.95

Over 50,000 Copies Sold!

"A fascinating account…"
-Alan Cantwell, MD

"This book is superb."
-Florence B. Seibert, PhD

"Barry Lynes is one of the greatest health reporters in our country. With the assistance of John Crane, longtime friend and associate of Roy Rife, Barry has produced a masterpiece…" -Roy Kupsinel, M.D., editor of *Health Consciousness Journal*

Paperback book, 5 x 8", 169 pages, $19.95

Rife Video Documentary
2-DVD Set, Produced by
Zero Zero Two Productions

Must-Have DVD set for your Rife technology education!

In 1999, a stack of forgotten audio tapes was discovered. On the tapes were the voices of several people at the center of the events which are the subject of this documentary: a revolutionary treatment for cancer and a practical cure for infectious disease.

The audio tapes were over 40 years old. The voices on them had almost faded, nearly losing key details of perhaps the most important medical story of the 20th Century.

But due to the efforts of the Kinnaman Foundation, the faded tapes have been restored and the voices on them recovered. So now, even though the participants have all passed away...

...they can finally tell their story.

2-DVD Set • $39.95

"These videos are great. We show them at the Annual Rife International Health Conference."
-Richard Loyd, Ph.D.

"A mind-shifting experience for those of us indoctrinated with a conventional view of biology."
-Townsend Letter for Doctors and Patients

In the summer of 1934 at a special medical clinic in La Jolla, California, sixteen patients withering from terminal disease were given a new lease on life. It was the first controlled application of a new electronic treatment for cancer: the Beam Ray Machine.

Within ninety days all sixteen patients walked away from the clinic, signed-off by the attending doctors as cured.

What followed the incredible success of this revolutionary treatment was not a welcoming by the scientific community, but a sad tale of its ultimate suppression.

The Rise and Fall of a Scientific Genius documents the scientific ignorance, official corruption, and personal greed directed at the inventor of the Beam Ray Machine, Royal Raymond Rife, forcing him and his inventions out of the spotlight and into obscurity. **Just converted from VHS to DVD and completely updated.**

Includes bonus DVD with interviews and historical photographs! Produced in Canada.

Visit our website today to watch a FREE PREVIEW CLIP!

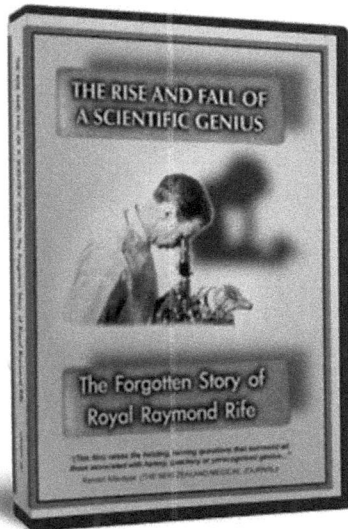

2 DVD-set, including bonus DVD, $39.95

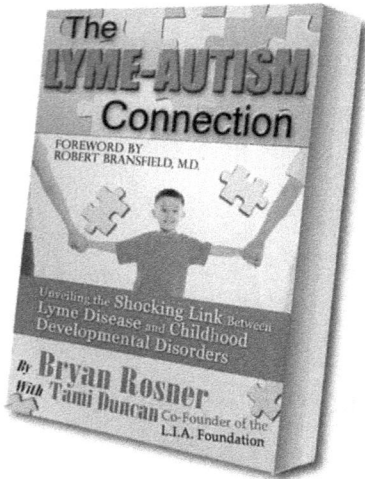

The Lyme-Autism Connection: Unveiling the Shocking Link Between Lyme Disease and Childhood Developmental Disorders

By Bryan Rosner & Tami Duncan

Did you know that Lyme disease may contribute to the onset of autism?

This book is an investigative report written by Bryan Rosner and Tami Duncan. Duncan is the co-founder of the *Lyme Induced Autism (LIA) Foundation*, and her son has an autism diagnosis.

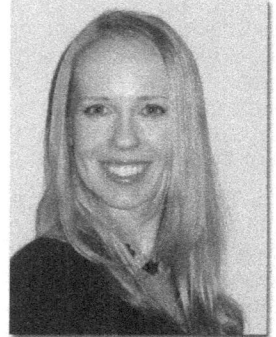

Book • $25.95

Tami Duncan, Co-Founder of the Lyme Induced Autism (LIA) Foundation

Awareness of the Lyme-autism connection is spreading rapidly, among both parents and practitioners. *Medical Hypothesis*, a scientific, peer-reviewed journal published by Elsevier, recently released an influential study entitled *The Association Between Tick-Borne Infections, Lyme Borreliosis and Autism Spectrum Disorders*. Here is an excerpt from the study:

> *"Chronic infectious diseases, including tick-borne infections such as Borrelia burgdorferi, may have direct effects, promote other infections, and create a weakened, sensitized and immunologically vulnerable state during fetal development and infancy, leading to increased vulnerability for developing autism spectrum disorders. An association between Lyme disease and other tick-borne infections and autistic symptoms has been noted by numerous clinicians and parents."*

—Medical Hypothesis Journal.
Article Authors: Robert C. Bransfield, M.D., Jeffrey S. Wulfman, M.D., William T. Harvey, M.D., Anju I. Usman, M.D.

Nationwide, 1 out of 150 children are diagnosed with Autism Spectrum Disorder (ASD), and the LIA Foundation has discovered that many of these children test positive for Lyme disease/Borrelia related complex—yet most children in this scenario never receive appropriate medical attention. This book answers many difficult questions: How can infants contract Lyme disease if autism begins before birth, precluding the opportunity for a tick bite? Is there a statistical correlation between the incidences of Lyme disease and autism worldwide? Do autistic children respond to Lyme disease treatment? What does the medical community say about this connection? Do the mothers of affected children exhibit symptoms? **Find out in this book.**

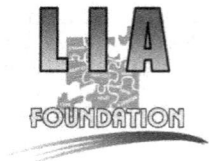

Paperback book, 6x9", 287 pages, $25.95

**Dietrich Klinghardt, M.D., Ph.D.
"Fundamental Teachings"
5-DVD Set**

Includes Disc Exclusively For Lyme Disease!

Dietrich Klinghardt, M.D., Ph.D. is a legendary healer known for discovering and refining many of the cutting-edge treatment protocols used for a variety of chronic health problems including Lyme disease, autism and mercury poisoning.

Now you can find out all about this doctor's treatment methods from the privacy of your own home! This 5-DVD set includes the following DVDs:

- **DISC 1**: The Five Levels of Healing and the Seven Factors
- **DISC 2**: Autonomic Response Testing and Demonstration
- **DISC 3**: Heavy Metal Toxicity and Neurotoxin Elimination / Electrosmog
- **DISC 4:** Lyme disease and Chronic Illness
- **DISC 5**: Psycho-Emotional Issues in Chronic Illness & Addressing Underlying Causes

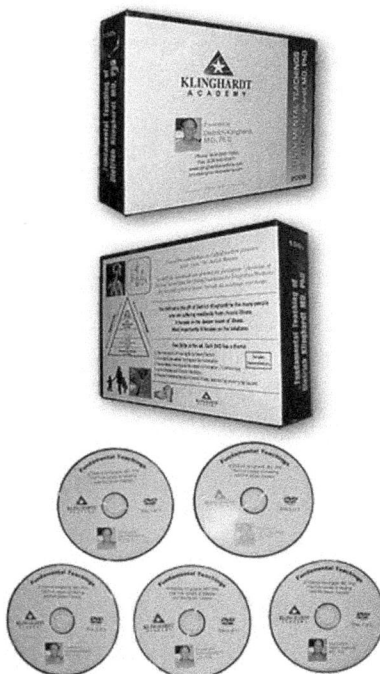

5-DVD Set • $125

Dr. Dietrich Klinghardt is one of the most important contributors to modern integrative treatment for Lyme disease and related medical conditions. This comprehensive DVD set is a must-have addition to your educational library.

5-DVD Set, $125

Our catalog has space limitations, but our website does not! Visit www.LymeBook.com to see even more exciting products.

Don't Miss These New Books & DVDs, Available Online:
- Babesia Update by James Schaller, M.D.
- Bryan Rosner's Anti-Lyme Journal/Newsletter
- Cure Unknown, by Pamela Weintraub
- The Experts of Lyme Disease, by Sue Vogan
- The Lyme Disease Solution, by Ken Singleton, M.D.
- **Lots of Free Chapters and Excerpts Online!**

Don't use the internet? No problem, just call (530) 573-0190.

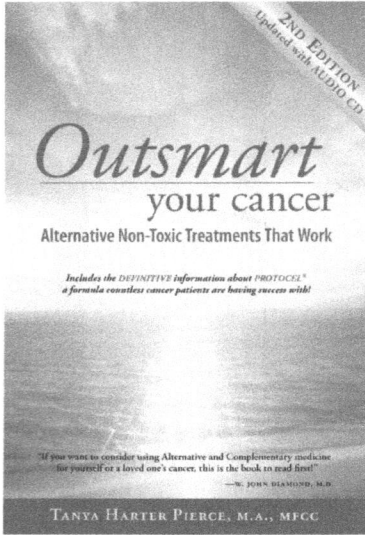

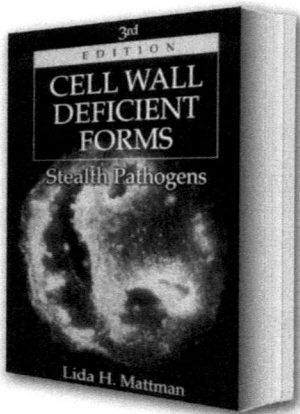

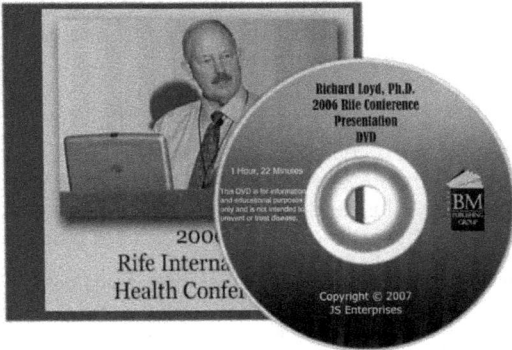

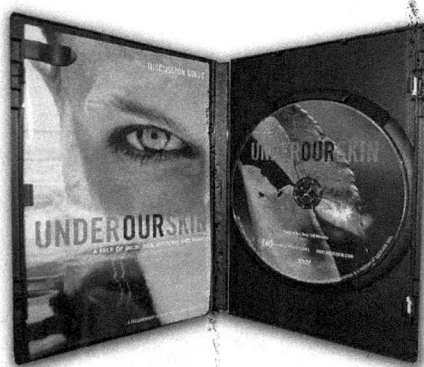

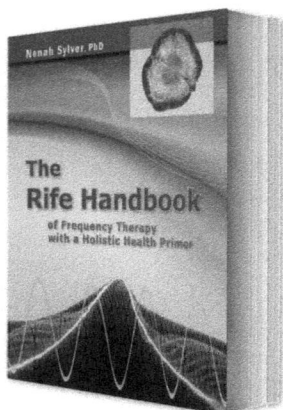

www.ingramcontent.com/pod-product-compliance
Lightning Source LLC
Chambersburg PA
CBHW080408270326
41929CB00018B/2942